COMPLEMENTARY HEALTH AND DIABETES:
A Focus on Dietary Supplements

Laura Shane-McWhorter,
PharmD, BCPS, BC-ADM, CDCES, FASCP, FADCES

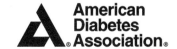

American Diabetes Association®

Director, Book Operations, Victor Van Beuren; *Managing Editor, Books,* John Clark; *Associate Director, Book Marketing,* Annette Reape; *Acquisitions Editor,* Jaclyn Konich; *Design and Composition,* Jeska Horgan-Kobelski; *Editor,* Zach VandeZande; *Cover Design:* Jenn French Designs; *Printer,* Lightning Source.

Printed in the United States of America

1 3 5 7 9 10 8 6 4 2

The suggestions and information contained in this publication are generally consistent with the Standards of Medical Care in Diabetes and other policies of the American Diabetes Association, but they do not represent the policy or position of the Association or any of its boards or committees. Reasonable steps have been taken to ensure the accuracy of the information presented. However, the American Diabetes Association cannot ensure the safety or efficacy of any product or service described in this publication. Individuals are advised to consult a physician or other appropriate health care professional before undertaking any diet or exercise program or taking any medication referred to in this publication. Professionals must use and apply their own professional judgment, experience, and training and should not rely solely on the information contained in this publication before prescribing any diet, exercise, or medication. The American Diabetes Association—its officers, directors, employees, volunteers, and members—assumes no responsibility or liability for personal or other injury, loss, or damage that may result from the suggestions or information in this publication.

American Diabetes Association titles may be purchased for business or promotional use or for special sales. To purchase more than 50 copies of this book at a discount, or for custom editions of this book with your logo, contact the American Diabetes Association at the address below or at booksales@diabetes.org.

American Diabetes Association
2451 Crystal Drive, Suite 900
Arlington, VA 22202

DOI: 10.2337/9781580407687

Library of Congress Control Number: 2021931789

Acknowledgements

I would like to thank my family, including all my children and grandchildren, as well as my friends, who have provided encouragement and counsel. I would most especially like to express my love and appreciation for my husband, Jerry McWhorter, for his unwavering support while I was writing this book.

I would also like to thank Victor van Beuren, of the American Diabetes Association, who believed this was a worthwhile endeavor.

Contents

Introduction   1

Botanical and Non-botanical Products for Glucose Lowering   19
   Aloe (*Aloe vera L.*)   20
   Banaba (*Lagerstroemia speciosa L*)   24
   Berberine (*Coptis chinensis [Huanglian or French]*)   28
   Bilberry (*Vaccinium myrtillus L.*)   34
   Bitter Melon (*Momordica charantia*)   39
   Chia (*Salvia hispanica L.*)   45
   Chromium   49
   Cinnamon (*Cinnamomum cassia*) or (*Cinnamomum zeylanicam*)   56
   Fenugreek (*Trigonella foenum-graecum Linn.*)   62
   Flaxseed (*Linum Usitassimum L.*)   68
   Ginseng (Asian or Korean [*Panax ginseng C.A. Meyer*]
     and American [*Panax quinquefolius L.*])   75
   Gymnema (*Gymnema sylvestre R. Br.*)   82
   Holy Basil (*O tenuiflorum L.*; Formerly Known as *Ocimum sanctum L.*)   87
   Honey (Sometimes Known as Manuka Honey)   91
   Ivy Gourd (*Coccinia indica*, Also Known as *Coccinia cordifolia*
     and *Coccinia grandis*)   96
   Magnesium   100
   Milk Thistle (*Silybum marianum*)   106
   Mulberry (*Morus alba Linn.*)   112
   Nopal (*Opuntia streptacantha lemaire*)   117
   Probiotics   122
   Psyllium (*Plantago ovata*)   129
   Tea (*Camellia sinensis*)   134
   Turmeric (*Curcuma longa Linn*)   141
   Vinegar (*Acetic acid*)   147
   Zinc   152

Botanical and Nonbotanical Products Used for Diabetes Comorbidities 159
    α-Lipoic Acid   160
    Benfotiamine (Also Known as Vitamin Bl, Allithiamines)   166
    Coenzyme Q10   170
    Fish Oil (Ω-3 Fatty Acids)   180
    Garcinia (*Garcinia cambogia*)   189
    Garlic (*Allium sativum*)   193
    Ginkgo (*Gingko biloba L.*)   198
    Glucomannan (*Amorphophallus konjac K. Koch*)   204
    Hibiscus (*Hibiscus sabdariffa L.*)   208
    Pine Bark Extract (*Pinus pinaster ait*)   214
    Red Yeast Rice (*Monascus purpureus went*)   219
    St. John's Wort (*Hypericum perforatum L.*)   225
    Vitamin D   229

Closing Comments and Advice for Clinicians   237
    Case Study   242

Appendix: Tables 1 and 2   245

Index   287

Introduction

Diabetes affects millions of individuals and has continued to increase at an alarming rate. The World Health Organization reports that there are over 400 million people who have diabetes.[1] Appropriate diabetes care and management involves three major tenets—healthy nutrition, physical activity, and effective pharmacotherapies. However, many persons with diabetes (PWD) gravitate towards nontraditional treatments for diabetes, such as complementary and alternative medicine (CAM) modalities. The National Institutes of Health National Center for Complementary and Integrative Health (NCCIH) has updated its terminology and now uses the term "complementary health approaches" instead of CAM to include two major modalities.[2]

These two major modalities include natural products and mind and body practices. Natural products include botanical products (such as herbs), vitamins and minerals, and probiotics. Mind and body practices include yoga, chiropractic and osteopathic manipulation, massage therapy, acupuncture, relaxation techniques, Qigong, and several other modalities of treatment. The NCCIH uses the term "complementary health approaches" (CHA) when referring to "nonmainstream practices" and "integrative health" when incorporating complementary approaches into mainstream or conventional healthcare. Nevertheless, the term "CAM" is still frequently used.

The National Health Interview Survey (NHIS) is administered every five years to a group of up to 40,000 U.S. citizens and includes questions on CHA.[3] Per the 2012 NHIS, the most commonly used CHA was non-vitamin and non-mineral natural products, which was used by 17.7% of respondents.[3] Different articles in the literature may refer to these oral products not only as natural products but also as CAM supplements, natural product supplements, herbs, botanical dietary supplements or nonbotanical dietary supplements, or simply as dietary supplements. Per the NCCIH, these terms all mean the same thing, and they are all dietary supplements. Dietary supplements are marketed as tablets, capsules, powders, softgels, gelcaps, or liquids. The Dietary Supplement Health and Education Act (DSHEA) of 1994 requires that these products should be labeled as such—as a dietary supplement.[4] Furthermore, DSHEA states these products are intended to supplement the diet and may contain one or more dietary ingredients (including vitamins, minerals, herbs or other botanicals, amino acids, and certain other substances) or their constituents.[4]

Consumer spending reflects Americans' support of the dietary supplement industry. The NHIS reported that approximately 59 million persons spent an estimated $30.2 billion USD out of pocket. The highest amount was spent on visits to CHA practitioners: $14.7 billion USD. Self-care approaches (homeopathic medicines or self-help materials related to complementary health topics, such as CDs or books) accounted for $2.7 billion USD spent. The report stated that consumers spent $12.8 billion USD on natural product supplements.[5]

However, other sources report different monetary amounts. According to the Natural Medicines website, total supplement sales in 2018 were $42.6 billion USD.[6] In 2020, the journal of the American Botanical Council (ABC) reported herb sales reached $9.6 billion USD for 2019.[7] The ABC market report listed the top 40 products sold, and many of those are used by PWD, and will be discussed in this book.

Epidemiology of Use

The allure of dietary supplements is far-reaching and appeals to many who believe they are devoid of any pharmacologic activity and thus have no side effects or other adverse consequences. It is unknown exactly how many persons with diabetes use supplements, since there are different surveys that report varying numbers. One survey found that PWD are 1.6 times more likely to use complementary strategies than individuals without diabetes.[8] Two other surveys reported that one third of individuals with diabetes use CAM.[9,10] A survey of adults with diabetes reported that 67% used some type of supplement or vitamin.[11] A different evaluation found that vitamins and herbs were used by an average of 82% of PWD.[12] This survey of 806 individuals also found that 85.6% of Hispanics, 84.1% of African Americans, 79.6% of Asians, 77.8% of Native Americans, and 66.1% of Pacific Islanders used supplements for diabetes. This survey also reported that the type of supplement used by PWD varied according to ethnicity.[12] For instance, Hispanics mainly used nopal (prickly pear cactus) or aloe vera, Asians used ginkgo biloba, and Native Americans used American ginseng or aloe vera.[12] Medication histories of 459 PWD found that 55% used supplements on a daily basis.[13] Use of complementary health approaches is not restricted to adults. A survey of parents reported that 18% were administering CHA to their children with type 1 diabetes, which included modified diet, homeopathy, and supplements such as cinnamon and aloe vera.[14] Thus, use may vary from 18% in children up to 82% in adults.

There are various reasons that PWD use supplements. Overall, 85% of adults use natural products for wellness, while over 40% use these products for treatment of a health condition.[15]

Cross-sectional evaluation of the 2012 NHIS reported that 26.2% of adults with diabetes had used CAM in the previous year.[16] In this report, reasons for CAM use were categorized as treatment only, wellness only, or a combination of treatment plus wellness. A total of 56.7% of PWD reported using CAM for both treatment and wellness. However, 28.3% reported using CAM only for wellness, and 15% reported using CAM for treatment only. The most common type of CAM treatment was herbal therapies, reported by 56.9% of those surveyed.[16] Furthermore, herbal therapies were more commonly used for wellness. The report did not specify that these patients were using CAM for diabetes, only for overall wellness. The same authors reported on CAM use by older persons with diabetes, using the same data from the 2012 NHIS.[17] They reported that 25% of older adults with diabetes used CAM in the previous year. The most commonly used treatments were herbal therapies by 62.8% of those surveyed. The report indicated that 45.7% of older persons used herbal therapies for treatment only, 67.6% for wellness only, and 66.4% for both treatment and wellness.[17]

Some reports have intimated that increased medication costs or provider visit costs may steer individuals in the direction of seeking more accessible products.[13] Since supplements are viewed as "natural," some individuals may feel that supplement use allows them to avoid side effects of allopathic medications. Alternative explanations include the powerful influence of the media and significant others, which may sway them towards supplement use or the feeling that even when used, conventional treatments fail to cure diseases.[18] An earlier NHIS report suggested that those with more severe diabetes had nearly twice the odds of using CAM. In this report, severity was based on a count of measures, such as five or more years since diagnosis, use of insulin or oral hypoglycemics, at least one functional limitation secondary to the diabetes, and three known diabetes complications. There was a 66% increase in use by those who had a 10-year or longer diagnosis of diabetes and a 74% greater likelihood of CAM use if they had a functional limitation due to their diabetes.[19] Other predictors of CAM use by PWD included female gender, having a university education, attending exercise classes and social or support groups, experiencing moderate pain, having depression or anxiety, and having "other" chronic conditions (such as arthritis or body aches).[20]

Because PWD are 1.6 times more likely to use CAM, they may be more vulnerable to problems that may arise.[8] Two immediate concerns are adverse effects and drug interactions.

Adverse Effects

A 2015 report in the *New England Journal of Medicine* noted that 23,000 visits to the ER are secondary to side effects from supplement use.[21] The report may have been exaggerated, because a large percentage of visits were due to inadvertent exposures in children or swallowing difficulties in elderly patients. However, the problematic visits still amounted to 10,000 incidents. Most of the adverse reactions (73%) were cardiac in nature (chest pain, tachycardia, palpitations) and were mostly due to energy supplements.[21] Other problematic supplements in the report were for weight loss and men's health. An important reminder for clinicians is that diabetes co-morbidities may include decreased energy, obesity, and sexual dysfunction. Thus, patients with diabetes may turn to these products and potentially experience adverse effects from using these supplements.

An example of a problematic supplement used for weight loss is *Garcinia cambogia,* used to manage obesity. A potential side effect is hepatotoxicity, which may culminate in the need for liver transplantation.[22]

Hepatotoxicity secondary to herbal and dietary supplements has been increasingly cited as a problem.[23] Per 2013-2014 data from the NIH-funded Drug-Induced Liver Injury Network (DILIN) study, 20% of all drug-induced liver injury is due to supplements. Some of the culpable ingredients include anabolic steroids inadvertently found in bodybuilding supplements, green tea for weight loss, and multi-ingredient products.[23] Another hepatotoxic ingredient in weight-loss supplements was aegeline, the major alkaloid found in the bael tree, *Aegele marmelos.*[23] A useful resource for clinicians is the LiverTox website, developed by the Liver Disease Research Branch of the National Institute of Diabetes and Digestive and Kidney Diseases (NIDDK) in conjunction with the National Library of Medicine.[24]

Drug Interactions

Drug interactions may also occur when combining supplements with conventional medications. This could cause problems if an individual with diabetes is taking supplements in addition to other prescription medications.[19] For instance, depression is a common problem in PWD and is commonly treated with selective serotonin reuptake inhibitors (SSRIs), such as fluoxetine (Prozac®) or sertraline (Zoloft®), or escitalopram (Lexapro®). An example of a drug interaction may be serotonin toxicity due to excess serotonin (called serotonin syndrome) if *Garcinia cambogia* is combined with a serotonergic antidepressant. Serotonin toxicity is characterized by diaphoresis, muscle rigidity, tremor, clonus, hypertension, and tachycardia as well as other symptoms. A case report describes a patient who had been on escitalopram for a year prior to taking *Garcinia cambogia*.[25] Serotonin syndrome occurred when the patient took *Garcinia cambogia* in combination with the escitalopram. After re-challenge with a different SSRI (sertraline), serotonin syndrome recurred.[25]

St. John's wort (SJW) is a popular supplement used for depression. Depressed PWD may believe that this is a benign nonprescription product and then perhaps take it to self-treat depression. However, SJW may interact with many prescription products that PWD may be taking, such as oral contraceptives, angiotensin receptor blockers, statins, or even some sulfonylureas.[26] In these cases, SJW may lower serum concentrations and thus diminish efficacy of these important medications.

Another example of a potential drug interaction may occur when *Ginkgo biloba* is combined with warfarin.[27] *Ginkgo biloba* is used for a variety of reasons, such as intermittent claudication, or peripheral vascular disease. An analysis of retrospective data from a large medical record database found that gingko use is associated with a 38% increased risk of bleeding when taken concurrently with warfarin.[27]

Overall issues with side effects and drug interactions may potentially occur for a variety of reasons. One issue is a lack of patient ability to effectively communicate with their health care provider. PWD are often vulnerable underserved individuals who may have health disparities and difficulty communicating with their health care provider. Persons who believe their provider has better language concordance, better interpersonal communication scores, and provides better medical explanations are more likely to disclose use of CHA to that provider.[28] However, a major reason for nondisclosure of supplement use may be that clinicians do not always ask patients whether they are taking supplements. Patients do not consistently disclose supplement use to their providers; the most common stated reason is that providers did not ask.[29] A critical time when clinicians should ask about supplement use is when a patient is scheduled for surgery. Some products may cause problems during surgery, such as bleeding, sedation, or interaction with anesthetics.[30]

Other Potential Concerns

Other potential issues include problems with product content and labeling. For instance, clinical studies may not verify the actual supplement content.[31] Product content mislabeling may also be problematic. For instance, star anise is a supplement used for respiratory infections and flu. However, there are two types of star anise products—one is Chinese in origin, and one is Japanese. The Chinese product is benign but the Japanese product is highly toxic.[32] Thus, mislabeling or lack of complete labeling may result in toxicity.

Furthermore, there may be product variability, contamination, misidentification, and issues with standardization. An example of product variability occurred in an analysis of ω-3 fatty acid supplements. More than 70% of tested products did not contain the stated label content of eicosapentanoic acid (EPA) or docosahexanoic acid (DHA). Only 21% of the tested supplements had 100% of the stated label EPA amount and only 25% had 100% of the stated DHA label amount.[33] A different analysis of ω-3 fatty acids showed not only variability in the product content but also that the product was in the beginning stages of rancidity.[34]

Yet another example in variability and contamination or adulteration is provided by kratom, a product from Southeast Asia used for pain, including neuropathic pain. Addictive plant alkaloids have been found in kratom products.[35] Other variability issues include the possibility of contamination with not only toxic plants but also molds, pesticides, or fertilizers.[36]

A different example of product variability has been noted with berberine, a supplement used for diabetes management.[37] A study of this popular supplement evaluated the potency of 15 products. The average content was found to be 75% of what was claimed on the label, but potency varied from 33 to 100%. Of the tested products, 60% failed to meet potency standards of 90 to 110% of labeled claims. This discrepancy may contribute to inconsistency in safety and/or effectiveness.[37] Another example is contaminants in products that athletes may use. Sometimes, even with due diligence and product investigation, there may be inadvertent contaminants that may result in disqualification of an athlete from a competitive event. For instance, a product that was reputed to increase muscle mass and improve strength was contaminated with clenbuterol, a β agonist with anabolic characteristics.[38]

Another factor affecting variability has been phytochemical variation, which affects plants' chemical makeup.[39] Plants may contain different chemical constituents based on geography, climate, environment, and growth stage at harvest. An example study assessed the impact of climate on chemical constituents. The researchers grew five medicinal plants in two different climates and altitudes and found significant differences in the flavonoid and phenol concentrations.[40]

In addition, constituents may differ between plant parts (roots, stems, bark, flowers, and leaves). For instance, *Ginkgo biloba* leaves are the only part that contain the appropriate concentrations of the active chemical constituents, and the desired amounts are found primarily during the fall.[39] Another example is cinnamon; there are multiple forms, and the active ingredients vary between products. NCCIH found that powdered cinnamon products were not comprised of a single species. However, they found that cinnamon sticks were more genetically pure than the powdered form.[39] Cinnamon aqueous extracts and powders from pulverized bark contain different chemical constituents and may differ in bioavailability.[41]

Another example in variability is provided by the collaboration between a research agency, the National Toxicology Program (NTP), and the dietary supplement industry in finding information that may affect public safety. The National Cancer Institute nominated *Aloe vera* to be studied by NTP because it is widely used and there is concern that some constituents are carcinogenic. Manufacturers use a charcoal filtration process to decolorize constituents in the outer leaf pulp that contains aloe latex, which includes anthraquinones (with laxative activity). In a two-year study in rats, NTP found that *non*-decolorized whole leaf Aloe vera extract exhibited carcinogenicity.[42] Interestingly, carcinogenicity was not found when decolorized products were tested. Aloin in the aloe latex component is theorized to be the carcinogenic anthraquinone. It is unknown how much aloin may be in a product consumed by humans, and manufacturers are not required to list aloin content in consumer products.

The inclusion of undeclared ingredients in supplements has been a major safety issue. A 2018 quality-improvement study conducted by the FDA's Center for Drug Evaluation and Research published a report on tainted supplement products.[43] The study found that supplements evaluated by the FDA between 2007 and 2016 contained 776 prescription drugs. Of these, 45.5% were for sexual enhancement, 40.9% were for weight loss, and 11.9% were for muscle building. More than one unapproved ingredient was found in 20.2% of products. The most common contaminants were sildenafil (Viagra®) in sexual enhancement supplements (47.0%), sibutramine (a prescription weight loss medication taken off the market due to cardiotoxicity) in weight loss supplements (84.9%), and steroids or steroid-like ingredients in muscle building supplements (89.1%).[43] To further corroborate such findings in this report, lorcaserin (Belviq®), a prescription weight loss drug, has also been found in a weight loss dietary supplement.[44] In this report, each capsule contained 6.6 mg of loracserin. As a reference point, the prescription dose is 10 mg twice daily. Lorcaserin was removed from the market in 2020. Furthermore, phosphodiesterase-5-inhibitors other than sildenafil have been found in supplements for men's sexual health.[45]

Undeclared ingredients such as anabolic steroids may contribute to side effects such as hepatotoxicity.[23] The issue of including anabolic steroids in bodybuilding supplements has been called a public health risk.[46]

Toxicity due to lead or arsenic contamination of different supplements continues to be a problem.[47] Mis-identification of products is also a safety concern. Perhaps the best example of misidentification of a product ingredient has to do with the toxicity produced by *Aristolochia serpentaria*, substituted for *Stephania tetranda* in a weight loss compounded product, and resultant nephrotoxicity.[48]

A unique "contamination" issue is that of economic adulteration, where a lower cost ingredient or filler is substituted for, or added to, a higher cost ingredient.[49]

A different issue is that of standardization. Some supplements are available as standardized forms or extracts. Ideally, standardization should guarantee consistency from batch to batch as well as active ingredient stability. However, the active chemical constituents are unknown for many products, making standardization difficult. A standardized constituent may be consistent between products, but it may be controversial as to which is the active ingredient. For instance, St. John's wort has two major marker constituents—hypericin and hyperforin. Both forms have been effective in studies. Many researchers believe that hyperforin may be primarily responsible for the antidepressant effect as well as responsible for drug interactions.[26]

Strategies are emerging to evaluate the quality of ingredients used in natural products[50]; there are government agencies that are committed to helping consumers and professionals navigate the incredible amount of information regarding supplements. The Dietary Supplement Health and Education Act of 1994 authorized the establishment of the Office of Dietary Supplements (ODS) at the National Institutes of Health (NIH).[4] The ODS is the federal agency dedicated to the scientific evaluation of supplements. It supports and conducts research to enhance the knowledge of dietary supplements to improve health and quality of life. One strategy has been to develop fact sheets on ingredients in supplements in an easy-to-read format for consumers along with a detailed version for professionals.[51]

Dietary Supplement Regulation

One of the most challenging concerns is the task of regulating dietary supplements. Clinical data that appropriately and thoroughly evaluates supplement safety and efficacy is insufficient to recommend use. When DSHEA was first established, there were approximately 4000 supplements on the market. However, the supplement industry has exploded, and it is estimated that now there are over 85,000 marketed supplements.[52] Per DSHEA, supplements are regulated as foods, not drugs, thus there may be many issues with the manufacturing oversight of available products.[4] Dietary supplements are regulated by the FDA, but not in the same way as prescription medications. A difference is that there is no approval process for supplements. Supplements must contain ingredients that were used before DSHEA was enacted or determined to be safe in order to be marketed and sold. However, prescription drugs must undergo an extensive evaluation process before being marketed. Thus, prescription medications are considered unsafe until proven safe, but supplements are considered safe until proven otherwise.

Although PWD might elect to use supplements to treat diabetes, DSHEA forbids manufacturers from stating that the products are FDA-approved for diabetes or other disease states. The labeling is confusing because DSHEA does allow claims regarding ability to maintain body "structure and function." The statement, "this product *supports* normal blood glucose," may be misconstrued to mean that the product is appropriate to treat diabetes. However, if a product makes a "structure and function" statement, then the following wording must appear on the label: "This statement has not been evaluated by FDA. This product is not intended to diagnose, treat, cure, or prevent any disease."[53] Only FDA-approved drugs may make that claim. Another example of a "structure and function" claim is "helps maintain vision acuity"; a patient may interpret that statement to mean the product has proven to prevent vision loss. Thus, it is easy to see how PWD may misconstrue "structure and function" claims. To add further food for thought, a 2015 Harris Poll of 2252 adults reported that "alternative treatments" are viewed as safe, effective, and reliable by 69%, 63%, and 50% of Americans, respectively.[54] According to this poll, 48% of uninsured people were more likely to use alternative treatments, and millennials were more likely to use alternative treatment products than those older than 70 years of age.

Many consumers are unaware that the FDA does not have the authority to review supplement product content for safety and effectiveness before they are marketed.[55] However, a manufacturer must inform the FDA in advance of marketing a new supplement ingredient that was not on the market prior to the enactment of DSHEA (October 15, 1994). Since DSHEA was first enacted, thousands of products have been marketed, but up to 2011, the FDA only received 700 premarket notifications.[56] Issues with supplement regulation are very confusing for consumers.

Many clinicians believe that supplements are completely unregulated, but manufacturers must comply with Good Manufacturing Practices.[57] Moreover, per the Consumer Protection Act, manufacturers must report serious adverse events to the FDA if they occur.[58] This was a notable legislative event. Over half of Class 1 drug recalls (those that result in serious harm or death) were from supplements.[59]

As discussed in the previous sections, there are issues with ingredient identification, contamination and adulteration, adverse event reporting, appropriate analytical methods for assuring quality of supplements, as well as safety and efficacy concerns. All of these issues are compounded by the human factor in that many individuals wish to take supplements for a variety of reasons; one of the most compelling is they are viewed as "natural." A further issue that clinicians should consider is that some PWD may even be taking multiple supplement product ingredients (called "stacking") which may lead to further problems.

Supplement Verification Programs

In caring for PWD, it is important to provide useful information about dietary supplements such as how to select an appropriate product. Different dietary supplement testing programs evaluate labeling and ingredient purity (although not efficacy). For instance, the U.S. Pharmacopeia (USP) has a Dietary Supplement Verification Program. The "USP-verified mark" on the label indicates the product ingredients are accurately labelled, that the potency is accurate, that the product is free of contaminants (such as heavy metals, pesticides, molds, or undeclared pharmaceutical ingredients), and that the product will dissolve properly.[60]

An agency that provides certification for dietary supplements is NSF® International.[61] It tests, inspects, and certifies different products, including dietary supplements. Services provided are to identify and quantify dietary ingredients that are declared on the label, ensure there are no unsafe contaminant levels, and to do a GMP facility inspection.

ConsumerLab.com is a different certification company that tests certain products for purity and accuracy of labeled ingredient content.[62] To maintain the approval seal, the supplement must pass yearly random sample testing.

The Consumers Union also provides information regarding different supplements and testing companies in its publication, *Consumer Reports*.[63]

Consumer Information

Although DSHEA has tried to promote a more secure marketplace, supplement safety, quality, and efficacy may vary or yet still be unknown. Thus, it is still important to provide other useful information for consumers. Therefore, the FDA has created different FDA websites to foster consumer safety. One such website is "Tips for the Savvy Supplement User."[64] This website provides recommendations and information to the supplement user, such as checking with their doctor about supplement use, thinking about their total diet, and raising the issue of drug interactions or adverse effects.

A website to guide older individuals is "Tips for Older Dietary Supplement Users."[65] This website focuses on potential problems older individuals may encounter. For instance, the site helps educate older individuals about undesirable effects of supplements during surgery and the dangers of some particular products that may be harmful to older individuals.

A different FDA website helps advise patients to be wary of supplement scams.[66] Some statements that warrant caution include the claim that the product is natural—since there are many natural products that may be very dangerous. Other claims that may be misleading include stating that a product may benefit a wide range of diseases ("it is good for everything"), that the disease may be cured quickly in a matter of days or weeks, and personal testimonials such as "it cured my diabetes," or that it is a "miracle cure." Another common misleading statement is that the product is FDA-approved, since supplements are not approved before marketing (only a new dietary ingredient must be approved).[66]

Clinicians may wish to refer patients to the online handout "FDA 101: Health Fraud Awareness" since one category mentioned is "diabetes fraud" with claims such as "drop your blood sugar 50 points in 30 days" and "reduce or eliminate the need for diabetes drugs or insulin."[67] The FDA has tried to make consumers aware of information regarding illegal claims such as "eliminating the need to take diabetes medications" or "being a natural diabetes cure."[68]

Clinicians may also help consumers learn how to evaluate information on the internet.[69] Some important questions to consider would be who runs the website, what is the source of information, and is the information too good to be true. Other important points to address include whether the website states what references are provided for evidence or when the website was last updated.

Despite numerous challenges regarding supplement regulation, in February 2019, the FDA announced plans to strengthen dietary supplement oversight.[70] Three priorities have been cited for this new plan: protecting consumer safety; corroborating product integrity by ensuring that supplements contain the ingredients stated on the label and that quality manufacturing is consistent; and advocating for informed decision-making through patient and provider dialogue. As examples of this strengthened oversight, the FDA announced it sent several letters to manufacturers of products making illegal claims to prevent, cure, or treat Alzheimer's disease. Another example of a new effort to protect consumers is the launch of the Dietary Supplement Ingredient Advisory List located on the FDA's website, a new tool to quickly notify the public when the FDA learns of ingredients that are unlawfully marketed in supplements.[71]

How to Navigate this Book

This book will discuss the use of commonly used supplements not only used to treat diabetes but also its co-morbidities. There are hundreds of different natural products used to treat diabetes; one published manuscript stated there are over 1,200 natural products used to treat diabetes.[72] Interestingly, metformin (the most commonly used medication to initiate type 2 diabetes treatment) is a biguanide related to a botanical product, *Galega officinalis L.*, or goat's rue.[73]

In managing the care of PWD, it is important for clinicians to respect patients' health beliefs and address questions in an unbiased manner. First, clinicians should ask about supplement use. Then, instead of merely telling patients they should not use supplements, it is important to be non-judgmental and unbiased. Thus, patients may inform clinicians what supplements they are taking. Clinicians may then establish a dialogue to discuss and advise patients in an open manner. It is imperative that clinicians remain up to date on information regarding theoretical mechanism of action, adverse effects, and drug interactions with supplements. It is the intent of this book to provide useful information to clinicians regarding supplements for PWD.

Clinicians should strive to educate their patients about studies that evaluate supplements, and thus provide evidence-based information. For instance, the study design is important—such as whether it is a randomized, double-blind, and placebo-controlled trial, whether it includes a small or large number of subjects, whether the study has well-defined events or endpoints, and whether the results have been diligently evaluated by appropriate statistical analysis.

Botanical and nonbotanical products for glucose lowering include aloe vera, banaba, berberine, bilberry, bitter melon, chia, chromium, cinnamon, fenugreek, flaxseed, ginseng, gymnema, holy basil, honey, ivy gourd, magnesium, milk thistle, mulberry, nopal, probiotics, psyllium, tea, turmeric, vinegar, and zinc. Products discussed for co-morbidities include alpha-lipoic acid, benfotiamine, coenzyme Q10, fish oil, Garcinia cambogia, garlic, Ginkgo biloba, glucomannan, hibiscus, pine bark extract, red yeast rice, St. John's wort, and vitamin D.

In the individual monographs of commonly used products for diabetes and glucose lowering, the following will be presented: traditional uses, chemical constituents, theorized mechanism of action, adverse effects and drug interactions, examples of clinical studies, an overall summary, as well as references for each section. The first reference for each monograph will be information from the Natural Medicines website.[74] This is a premiere evidence-based database that is frequently updated and has provided monographs for over 1,400 supplements. Each monograph in this book is discussed in Natural Medicines. The Natural Medicines website reference will be followed by references specific to each monograph. Table 1 lists information for supplements used for diabetes, and Table 2 lists information for comorbidities. The Natural Medicines rating for degree of efficacy is also provided for each product in Tables 1 and 2.

References

1. World Health Organization. Diabetes. Available from https://www.who.int/news-room/fact-sheets/detail/diabetes. Accessed January 27, 2020
2. National Institutes of Health. National Center for Complementary and Integrative Health. Complementary, alternative, or integrative health: what's in a name? Available from https://www.nccih.nih.gov/health/complementary-alternative-or-integrative-health-whats-in-a-name. Accessed January 27, 2020

3. Clarke TC, Black LI, Stussman BJ, Barnes PM, Nahin RL. Trends in the use of complementary health approaches among adults: United States, 2002-2012. National health statistics reports; no. 79. Hyattsville, MD: National Center for Health Statistics. 2015

4. U.S. Food and Drug Administration. Dietary Supplement Health and Education Act of 1994. Public Law No. 103–417, 108 Stat. 4325–4335; October 25 1994. 103rd Congress. Available from https://ods.od.nih.gov/About/DSHEA_Wording.aspxhttps://ods.od.nih.gov/About/DSHEA_Wording.aspx. Accessed January 27, 2020

5. Nahin RL, Barnes PM, Stussman BJ. Expenditures on complementary health approaches: United States, 2012. National health statistics reports; no 95. Hyattsville, MD: National Center for Health Statistics. 2016

6. Dietary supplement sales soar: find out which market segments lead the surge. *Natural Medicines*; September 2019. Available from https://natural-medicines.therapeuticresearch.com/news/news-items/2019/september/dietary-supplement-sales-soar-find-out-which-market-segments-lead-the-surge.aspx. Accessed January 29, 2020

7. Smith T, May G, Eckl V, Morton Reynolds C. Market report. Herbal Gram 2020;127:54-67.

8. Egede LE, Ye X, Zheng D, Silverstein MD. The prevalence and pattern of complementary and alternative medicine use in individuals with diabetes. *Diabetes Care* 2002;25:324–329

9. Ryan EA, Pick ME, Marceau C. Use of alternative medicines in diabetes mellitus. *Diabet Med* 2001;18:342–345

10. Yeh GY, Eisenberg DM, Davis RB, Phillips RS. Use of complementary and alternative medicine among persons with diabetes mellitus: results of a national survey. *Am J Pub Health* 2002;92:1648–1652

11. Garrow D, Egede LE. Association between complementary and alternative medicine use, preventive care practices, and use of conventional medical services among adults with diabetes. *Diabetes Care* 2006;29:15–19

12. Villa-Caballero L, Morello CM, Chynoweth ME, et al. Ethnic differences in complementary and alternative medicine use among patients with diabetes. *Complement Ther Med* 2010;18:241–248

13. Odegard PS, Janci MM, Foeppel MP, Beach JR, Trence DL. Prevalence and correlates of dietary supplement use in individuals with diabetes mellitus at an academic diabetes care clinic. *Diabetes Educ* 2011;37:419–425

14. Dannemann K, Hecker W, Haberland H, et al. Use of complementary and alternative medicine in children with type 1 diabetes mellitus – prevalence, patterns of use, and costs. *Pediatr Diabetes* 2008;9:228–235

15. Stussman BJ, Black LI, Barnes PM, Clarke TC, Nahin RL. Wellness-related use of common complementary health approaches among adults: United

States, 2012. National health statistics reports; no 85. Hyattsville, MD: National Center for Health Statistics. 2015

16. Rhee TG, Westberg SM, Harris IM. Complementary and alternative medicine in US adults with diabetes: reasons for use and perceived benefits. *J Diabetes* 2018;10:310–319

17. Rhee TG, Westberg SM, Harris IM. Use of complementary and alternative medicine in older adults with diabetes. *Diabetes Care* 2018;41:e95–96

18. Palinkas LA, Kabongo ML. San Diego Unified Practice Research in Family Medicine Network. The use of complementary and alternative medicine by primary care patients. A SURF*NET study. *J Fam Pract* 2000;49:1121–1130

19. Nahin RL, Byrd-Clark D, Stussman BJ, Kalyanaraman N. Disease severity is associated with the use of complementary medicine to treat or manage type 2 diabetes: data from the 2002 and 2007 National Health Interview Survey. *BMC Complement Altern Med* 2012;12:193

20. Canaway R, Manderson L. Quality of life, perceptions of health and illness, and complementary therapy use among people with type 2 diabetes and cardiovascular disease. *J Altern Complement Med* 2013;19:882–890

21. Geller AI, Shehab N, Weidle NJ, et al. Emergency department visits for adverse events related to dietary supplements. *N Engl J Med* 2015;373;1531–1540

22. Crescioli G, Lombardi N, Bettiol A, et al. Acute liver injury following Garcinia cambogia weight-loss supplementation: case series and literature review. *Intern Emerg Med* 2018;13:857–872

23. Navarro V, Khan I, Bjornsson E, Seef LB, Serrano J, Hoofnagle JH. Liver injury from herbal and dietary supplements. *Hepatology* 2017;65:363–373.

24. LiverTox. Clinical and research drug information on drug-induced liver injury. Available from https:/www.livertox.nih.gov. Accessed March 21 2019

25. Lopez AM, Kornegay J, Hendrickson RG. Serotonin toxicity associated with garcinia cambogia over-the-counter supplement. *J Med Toxicol* 2014;10:399–401.

26. Soleymani S, Bahramsoltani R, Rahimi R, Abdollahi M. Clinical risks of St John's Wort (Hypericum perforatum) co-administration. *Expert Opin Drug Metab Toxicol* 2017;13(10):1047–1062

27. Stoddard GJ, Archer M, Shane-McWhorter L, Bray BE, Redd DF, Proulx J, Zeng-Treitler Q. Ginkgo and Warfarin interaction in a large veterans administration population. *AMIA Annu Symp Proc* 2015 Nov 5;2015:1174–1183

28. Chao MT, Handley MA, Quan J, et al. Disclosure of complementary health approaches among low income and racially diverse safety net patients with diabetes. *Patient Educ Couns* 2015;98:1360–66

29. Jou J, Johnson PJ. Nondisclosure of complementary and alternative medicine use to primary care physicians: findings of the 2012 National health interview survey (research letter). *JAMA Intern Med* 2016;176:545–546

30. Abe A, Kaye AD, Gritsenko K, Urman RD, Kaye AM. Perioperative analgesia and the effects of dietary supplements. *Best Practice & Research Clinical Anaesthesiology* 2014;28:183–9

31. Wolsko PM, Solondz DK, Phillips RS, et al. Lack of herbal supplement characterization in published randomized controlled trials. *Am J Med* 2005;118:1087–1093

32. Vermaak I, Viljoen A, Lindstrom SW. Hyperspectral imaging in the quality control of herbal medicines – the case of neurotoxic Japanese star anise. *J Pharm Biomed Anal* 2013;75:207–213

33. Kleiner AC, Cladis DP, Santerre CR. A comparison of actual versus stated label amounts of EPA and DHA in commercial omega-3 dietary supplements in the United States. *J Sci Food Agric* 2015;95:1260–1267

34. Opperman M, Benade S. Analysis of the omega-3-fatty acid content of South African fish oil supplements: a follow-up study. *Cardiovasc J Afr* 2013;24:297–302

35. Lydecker AG, Sharma A, McCurdy CR, et al. Suspected adulteration of commercial kratom products with 7-hydroxymitragynine. *J Med Toxicol* 2016;12:341–349

36. Gupta RC, Srivastava A, Lall R. Toxicity potential of nutraceuticals. *Methods Mol Biol* 2018;1800:367–394

37. Funk RS, Singh RK, Winefield RD, et al. Variability in potency among commercial preparations of berberine. *J Diet Suppl* 2018;15:343–351

38. Mathews NM. Prohibited contaminants in dietary supplements. *Sports Health* 2018;10:19–30

39. Shipkowski KA, Betz JM, Birnbaum LS, et al. Naturally complex: perspectives and challenges associated with botanical dietary supplement safety assessment. *Food Chem Toxicol* 2018;118:963–971.

40. Kaur T, Bhat R, Vyas D. Effect of contrasting climates on antioxidant and bioactive constituents in five medicinal herbs in Western Himalayas. *J Mt Sci* 2016;13:484–492

41. Cheng DM, Kuhn P, Poulev A, et al. In vivo and in vitro antidiabetic effects of aqueous cinnamon extract and cinnamon polyphenol-enhanced food matrix. *Food Chem* 2012;135:2994–3002

42. National Institute of Environmental Health. Aloe vera fact sheet. Available from https://www.niehs.nih.gov/health/materials/aloe_vera_508.pdf. Accessed January 27, 2020

43. Tucker J, Fischer T, Upjohn L, Mazzera D, Kumar M. Unapproved pharmaceutical ingredients included in dietary supplements associated with US Food and Drug Administration warnings. *JAMA Netw Open* 2018;1(6):e183337

44. Hachem R, Malet-Martino M, Gilard V. First identification and quantification of lorcaserin in an herbal slimming dietary supplement. *J Pharm Biomed Anal* 2014;98:94–99

45. Venhuis BJ, de Kaste D. Towards a decade of detecting new analogues of sildenafil, tadalafil and vardenafil in food supplements: a history, analytical aspects and health risks. *J Pharm Biomed Anal* 2012;69:196–208

46. Abbate V, Kicman AT, Evans-Brown M, et al. Anabolic steroids detected in bodybuilding dietary supplements – a significant risk to public health. *Drug Test Anal* 2015;7:609–618

47. Mikulskia MA, Wichmanb MD, Simmons DL, et al. Toxic metals in ayurvedic preparations from a public health lead poisoning cluster investigation. *Int J Occup Environ Health* 2017;23:187–192

48. Grollman AP, Marcus DM. Global hazards of herbal remedies: lessons from Aristolochia. *EMBO Rep* 2016;17:619–625

49. Cohen PA. The FDA and adulteration of supplements: dereliction of duty. *JAMA Netw Open* 2018;1(6):e183329. doi:10.1001/jamanetworkopen.2018.3329

50. Betz JM, Brown PN, Roman MC. Accuracy, precision, and reliability of chemical measurements in natural products research. *Fitoterapia* 2011;82:44–52

51. NIH Office of Dietary Supplements. Dietary supplement fact sheets. Available from https://ods.od.nih.gov and https://ods.od.nih.gov/factsheets/list-all/. Accessed January 27, 2020

52. Dwyer JT, Coates PM, Smith MJ. Dietary supplements: regulatory challenges and research resources. *Nutrients* 2018;10:41; doi:10.3390/nu10010041

53. U.S. Food and Drug Administration: Regulations on statements made for dietary supplements concerning the effect of the product on the structure or function of the body. Fed Register 2000;65:1000–1050

54. Harris Poll. Health and Healing in America: Majorities See Alternative Therapies as Safe and Effective. Harris Poll® #36, May 10, 2016. Available from https://www.prnewswire.com/news-releases/health-and-healing-in-america-majorities-see-alternative-therapies-as-safe-and-effective-300265772.html. Accessed January 27, 2020

55. U.S. FDA Food Facts - Dietary Supplements. Available from https://www.fda.gov/downloads/Food/DietarySupplements/UCM240978.pdf. Accessed January 27, 2020

56. U.S. Food and Drug Administration. Draft guidance for industry: dietary supplements new dietary ingredient notifications and related issues. Available from https://www.fda.gov/food/dietary-supplements/new-dietary-ingredients-ndi-notification-process. Accessed January 27, 2020

57. U.S. Food and Drug Administration. Current good manufacturing practice in manufacturing, packaging, labeling, or holding operations for dietary supplements: final rule. *Fed Reg* 2007;72(121): 34752-8/ Available from https://www.fda.gov/food/guidanceregulation/cgmp/ucm079496.htm. Accessed April 6, 2019.

58. U.S. Food and Drug Administration. Dietary Supplement and Non-Prescription Drug Consumer Protection Act. (Public Law No. 109-462, 109th Congress. Available from https://www.congress.gov/109/crpt/srpt324/CRPT-109srpt324.pdf. Accessed January 27, 2020.

59. Harel Z, Harel S. Wald R, Mamdani M, Bell CM. The frequency and characteristics of dietary supplement recalls in the United States. *JAMA Intern Med* 2013;173:926–928.

60. U.S. Pharmacopeia Convention. USP Verification Services. Available from http://www.usp.org/verification-services/dietary-supplements-verification-program. Accessed January 27,2020

61. NSF International: NSF certified dietary supplements. Available from http://www.nsf.org/services/by-industry/nutritional-products/supplement-safety. Accessed January 27, 2020.

62. ConsumerLab.com. About Consumer.Lab.com. Available fromhttps://www.consumerlab.com/aboutcl.asp). Accessed January 27, 2020

63. Consumer Reports. How to Choose Supplements Wisely. Available from https://www.consumerreports.org/supplements/how-to-choose-supplements-wisely/. Accessed January 27, 2020

64. US FDA. Tips for Dietary Supplement Users. Making Informed Decisions and Evaluating Information. Available from https://www.fda.gov/food/dietarysupplements/usingdietarysupplements/ucm110567.htm. Accessed January 27, 2020.

65. US FDA. Tips for Older Dietary Supplement Users. Available from https://www.fda.gov/Food/DietarySupplements/UsingDietarySupplements/ucm110493.htm. Accessed January 27, 2020

66. US FDA. Some imported dietary supplements and non-prescription drug products may harm you. Available from https://www.fda.gov/ForConsumers/ConsumerUpdates/ucm466588.htm. Accessed January 27, 2020

67. FDA Consumer Health Information. FDA 101: health fraud awareness. Available from https://www.fda.gov/files/about%20fda/published/FDA-101--Health-Fraud-Awareness----PDF.pdf. Accessed January 27, 2020.

68. US FDA. Beware of illegally marketed diabetes treatments. Available from https://www.fda.gov/ForConsumers/ConsumerUpdates/ucm361487.htm. Accessed January 27, 2020

69. NIH Office of Dietary Supplements. How to evaluate health information on the internet – questions and answers. Available from https://ods.od.nih.gov/Health_Information/How_To_Evaluate_Health_Information_on_the_Internet_Questions_and_Answers.aspx. Accessed January 27, 2020

70. US FDA. Statement from FDA commissioner Scott Gottlieb, M.D., on the agency's new efforts to strengthen regulation of dietary supplements by modernizing and reforming FDA's oversight. Available from https://www.fda.gov/news-events/press-announcements/statement-fda-commissioner-scott-gottlieb-md-agencys-new-efforts-strengthen-regulation-dietary. Accessed January 27, 2020.

71. US FDA. Dietary supplement ingredient advisory list. Available from https://www.fda.gov/food/dietary-supplement-products-ingredients/dietary-supplement-ingredient-advisory-list. Accessed January 27, 2020

72. Chang CL, Lin Y, Bartlome AP, et al. Herbal therapies for type 2 diabetes mellitus: chemistry, biology, and potential application of selected plants and compounds. *Evid Based Complement Alternat Med* 2013;2013:378657.

73. Bailey CJ, Day C: Metformin: its botanical background. *Pract Diab Int* 2004;21:115–117.

74. Natural Medicines (Natural Medicines Database search engine). Available from https://naturalmedicines.therapeuticresearch.com. Accessed April 8, 2019.

Botanical and Nonbotanical Products for Glucose Lowering

Aloe	20		Honey	91
Banaba	24		Ivy Gourd	96
Berberine	28		Magnesium	100
Bilberry	34		Milk Thistle	106
Bitter Melon	39		Mulberry	112
Chia	45		Nopal	117
Chromium	49		Probiotics	122
Cinnamon	56		Psyllium	129
Fenugreek	62		Tea	134
Flaxseed	68		Turmeric	141
Ginseng	75		Vinegar	147
Gymnema	82		Zinc	152
Holy Basil	87			

ALOE (*Aloe vera L.*)

Aloe is a cactus-like succulent and is a member of the Liliaceae family. It grows well in warm climates, including several areas of the United States. There are two major components—aloe latex and aloe gel. Dried aloe leaf juice is part of the aloe latex, and in the past it was used as a laxative due to the anthraquinone constituent. Aloe gel has been used topically to treat dermatological conditions and wounds. Aloe gel has also been used in oral formulations to treat diabetes, hyperlipidemia, and obesity.[1]

Chemical Constituents and Mechanism of Action

Aloe contains various ingredients, including acemannan, aloeresin A, and different phenolic and saponin constituents.[1,2] The definitive mechanism of glucose lowering action in humans is unknown. However, animal studies have shown an increase in pancreatic insulin production, increased hepatic gluconeogenesis, and decreased insulin resistance by activation of adenosine monophosphate (AMP) active muscle protein kinase. Aloeresin may have possible α-glucosidase inhibition. Fiber content may delay or prevent glucose absorption, and acemannan may promote probiotic effects.[1-3]

Adverse Effects and Drug Interactions

Side effects have included gastrointestinal irritation such as abdominal pain and diarrhea.[1] Diarrhea may be caused by products that may contain ingredients from the pericyclic cells obtained just beneath the leaf skin—the aloe latex—which contains anthraquinones with laxative activity. Some of the anthraquinone ingredients are theorized to be carcinogenic.[1] Acute hepatitis and thyroid dysfunction has been noted in a few case reports.[4-6] Aloe may not be safe in pregnant women due to the possibility of inducing abortion; furthermore, some of the ingredients may pass into breast milk.[1]

Hypokalemia has been reported, possibly secondary to aloe latex. Hypokalemia has been cited as a possible cause of elevated digoxin concentrations, which may result in digoxin toxicity.[1] An unusual case report included excessive blood loss in a surgical case where the anesthetic agent, sevoflurane, was used. The cause may be impaired platelet aggregation and subsequent bleeding.[7] Additive hypoglycemia may theoretically occur if combined with secretagogues, although this was not reported in a study where aloe was combined with a sulfonylurea.[8]

Clinical Studies

Although an initial report of aloe used in a very small sample of patients with type 2 diabetes reported benefit, further studies have been done with better study design. In a single-blind, placebo-controlled study, 40 patients with newly-diagnosed type 2 diabetes received one tablespoon of aloe gel twice daily or placebo for 6 weeks.[9] Fasting glucose declined from 250 mg/dL (13.9 mmol/L) at baseline to 142 mg/dL (7.9 mmol/L) after 6 weeks in the aloe group ($P = 0.01$). Triglycerides decreased significantly (220 mg/dL to 123 mg/dL [2.5 mmol/L to 1.4 mmol/L]; $P = 0.01$) but total cholesterol remained unchanged.

In another 6-week single-blind controlled trial, 40 patients with type 2 diabetes added one tablespoon of aloe gel or placebo twice daily to a sulfonylurea (glibenclamide).[8] Fasting glucose declined significantly in the aloe group from 288 mg/dL to 148 mg/dL (16 mmol/L to 8.2 mmol/L); $P = 0.01$ vs. control. Total cholesterol remained unchanged (230 mg/dL [5.95 mmol/L] to 226 mg/dL [5.8 mmol/L]). However, triglycerides declined significantly from 265 mg/dL to 128 mg/dL (3 mmol/L to 1.5 mmol/L); $P = 0.01$ vs. control.

A 2-month randomized controlled study compared aloe gel in 30 persons with type 2 diabetes on oral medications (sulfonylureas and metformin) with placebo in another 30 persons with type 2 diabetes.[10] A1C declined by 0.7% from 7.3% to 6.6% in the aloe group compared with a 0.5% increase from 7.3% to 7.8% in the placebo group ($P = 0.036$). Fasting glucose decreased from 173 to 168 mg/dL (9.6 to 9.3 mmol/L) in the aloe group and increased from 185 to 191 mg/dL (10.3 to 10.6 mmol/L) in the placebo group ($P = 0.036$). LDL declined significantly in the aloe group ($P = 0.004$). Although triglycerides decreased, the results were not significant.

A 2016 meta-analysis of nine studies in 283 subjects of various aloe formulations found significant decreases in A1C (1.05%; $P = 0.004$) in five of the studies and fasting glucose (47 mg/dL [2.6 mmol/L]; $P < 0.0001$) in the nine studies.[11] Limitations with these studies included not specifying which plant part was studied, small sample size, and heterogeneous study design. One issue was that studies in persons with prediabetes were included in the analysis.

Prediabetes is emerging as a consideration for aloe use. A study compared two doses of aloe vera (two 300-mg or two 500-mg capsules/day) to placebo for 8 weeks in 72 individuals with prediabetes.[12] Fasting glucose decreased significantly by 4 and 7 mg/dL (0.22 and 0.39 mmol/L), respectively, with both doses ($P = 0.001$ and $P < 0.001$, respectively). A1C decreased by 0.2% and 0.4% with the lower and higher doses ($P = 0.042$ and $P = 0.011$, respectively). LDL cholesterol also decreased in the higher dose group ($P = 0.01$).

A 2016 systematic review and meta-analysis of randomized controlled trials evaluated aloe vera in prediabetes and type 2 diabetes.[13] The analysis included eight randomized controlled trials—three in prediabetes (with 235 subjects) and five (also with 235 subjects) in type 2 diabetes. In the prediabetes trials, fasting glucose declined slightly but significantly (4 mg/dL [0.22 mmol/L] decrease; $P < 0.0001$). However, A1C did not decrease in prediabetes. In the diabetes trials fasting glucose and A1C declined significantly by 21 mg/dL (1.17 mmol/L; $P = 0.05$) and 1.77% ($P = 0.01$), respectively.[13]

A different 2016 systematic review and meta-analysis evaluated aloe treatment in five trials in 415 individuals with prediabetes or early diabetes (and not yet on treatment).[14] Although all the studies stated that randomization was done, only two studies reported how this was done. The five trials, lasting from 6–12 weeks, found that fasting glucose decreased significantly by 30 mg/dL (1.67 mmol/L); $P = 0.02$. Two studies evaluated A1C and found a significant decrease of 0.41% ($P < 0.00001$).[14] Four of the studies found a significant decrease in total cholesterol and triglycerides. Three studies reported a significant decrease in LDL and significant increase in HDL.

Summary

Doses of aloe are variable, ranging from 100–1,000 mg or 15–150 mL per day.[1] Aloe gel contains acemannan, a polysaccharide that is high in fiber and may slow or prevent glucose absorption. Other research indicates that aloe vera may have extensive action in inhibiting α-glucosidase activity, decreasing insulin resistance and inflammation and stimulating production of beneficial gut microbes. However, aloe latex contains cathartics, and there is concern that there may be inadvertent inclusion of these components in aloe supplements. Moreover, aloe whole leaf extract may contain carcinogenic ingredients.[1] Aloe is found as capsules, tablets, or liquids. It is highly used by Hispanics (the Spanish word for aloe is *sábila*) in shakes and smoothies. A case report of prolonged bleeding when used with the anesthetic agent sevoflurane warrants discontinuation 2 weeks before surgery. Cases of acute hepatitis and thyroid dysfunction have been reported. There is insufficient evidence for use of aloe as an oral product in diabetes or prediabetes. Short-term use has decreased fasting glucose, triglycerides, LDL, and A1C. However, long-term supplementation is not recommended, especially due to the potential contamination with cathartic or carcinogenic ingredients, and problems with fluid and electrolyte disturbances.

References

1. Natural Medicines (Natural Medicines Database search engine). Available from https://naturalmedicines.therapeuticresearch.com. Accessed April 8, 2019

2. Pothuraju R, Sharma RK, Onteru AK, Singh S, Hussain SA. Hypoglycemic and hypolipidemic effects of aloe vera extract preparations. *Phytother Res* 2016;30:200–207

3. Chang CL, Lin Y, Bartolome AP, Chen YC, Chiu SC, Yang WC. Herbal therapies for type 2 diabetes mellitus: chemistry, biology, and potential

application of selected plants and compounds. *Evid Based Complement Alternat Med* 2013;2013:378657

4. Bottenburg MM, Wall GC, Harvey RL, et al. Oral aloe vera-induced hepatitis. *Ann Pharmacother* 2007;41:1740–1743
5. Rabe C, Musch A, Schirmacher P, et al. Acute hepatitis induced by an aloe vera preparation: a case report. *World J Gastroenterol* 2005;11:303–304
6. Pigatto PD, Guzzi G. Aloe linked to thyroid dysfunction. *Arch Med Res* 2005;36:608
7. Lee A, Chui PT, Aun CS, Gin T, Lau AS. Possible interaction between sevoflurane and aloe vera. *Ann Pharmacother* 2004;38:1651–1654
8. Bunyapraphatsara N, Yongchaiyudha S, Rungpitarangsi Chokechaijaroenporn O. Antidiabetic activity of Aloe vera L. juice. II. Clinical trial in diabetes mellitus patients in combination with glibenclamide. Phytomedicine 1996;3:245–248
9. Yongchaiyudha S, Rungpitarangsi V, Bunyapraphatsara N, Chokechaijaroenporn O. Antidiabetic activity of Aloe vera L. juice. I. Clinical trial in new cases of diabetes mellitus. Phytomedicine 1996;3:241–243
10. Husseini HF, Kianbakht S, Hajiaghaee R, Dabaghian FH. Anti-hyperglycemic and antihypercholesterolemic effects of Aloe vera leaf gel in hyperlipidemic type 2 diabetic patients: a randomized double-blind placebo-controlled clinical trial. Planta Med 2012;78:311–316
11. Dick WR, Fletcher EA, Shah SA. Reduction of fasting blood glucose and hemoglobin A1c using oral aloe vera: a meta-analysis. J Altern Complement Med 2016;22:450–457
12. Alinejad-Mofrad S, Foadoddini M, Saadatjoo SA, Shayesteh M. Improvement of glucose and lipid profile status with Aloe vera in pre-diabetic subjects: a randomized controlled trial. J Metab Disord 2015;14:1–7
13. Suksomboon N, Poolsup N, Punthanitisarn S. Effect of Aloe vera on glycemic control in prediabetes and type 2 diabetes: a systematic review and meta-analysis. J Clin Pharm Ther 2016; 41:180–188.
14. Zhang Y, Liu W, Liu D, Zhao T, Tian H. Efficacy of aloe vera supplementation on prediabetes and early non-treated diabetic patients: a systematic review and meta-analysis of randomized controlled trials. Nutrients 2016;8, pii:E388; doi 10.3390/nu8070388

BANABA (*Lagerstroemia speciosa L*)

Banaba is a type of crepe myrtle that grows in the Philippines, India, Malaysia, and Australia.[1,2] Banaba is also known as queen's crape myrtle, queen's flower, and pride of India.[1] The tree has flowers that are a bright pink to purple.[1] It is used as a folk medicine in the Philippines and a tea made from the leaves is used to treat diabetes.[2] Banaba has become increasingly popular in the United States. It is used for diabetes, prediabetes, hyperlipidemia, and weight loss.[1]

Chemical Constituents and Mechanism of Action

Active ingredients include corsolic acid and ellagitannins. Ellagitannins include lagerstroemin, flosin B and reginin A, and mechanistically may be glucose transport enhancers.[3] Ellagitannins are plant polyphenols, which reportedly bind to several polypeptides such as the regulatory subunit of protein kinase A. Ellagitannins are theorized to stimulate glucose uptake and have insulin-like activity. The latter activity is thought to be secondary to activation of insulin receptor tyrosine kinase or the inhibition of tyrosine phosphatase. Essentially, insulin-like actions are accompanied by the increased tyrosine-phosphorylation of the β-subunit of insulin receptors.[4]

Adverse Effects and Drug Interactions

Reported adverse effects have occurred with combination products of banaba and cinnamon inner bark extract—it is unknown whether it was the banaba, cinnamon, or the combination that was responsible.[5,6] The adverse effects included stomach upset, dizziness, weakness, diaphoresis, palpitations, and tremor. Another more serious adverse effect has been lactic acidosis in a person with impaired renal function who was also taking a non-steroidal anti-inflammatory (NSAID) agent (which in and of itself may be nephrotoxic).[7]

Banaba may lower blood pressure,[5,6] and in combination with antihypertensives, hypotension may occur. Theoretically, banaba may cause excessive lowering of blood glucose if combined with drugs that can cause hypoglycemia, such as sulfonylureas, or with complementary therapies that have hypoglycemic activity (gymnema sylvestre, American ginseng, etc.).[1] However, banaba has been studied in combination with oral diabetes medications and hypoglycemia has not been reported.[6]

Banaba inhibits the organic anion-transporting polypeptide (OATP),[8] which is responsible for the absorption of some drugs that may be used in diabetes, such as statins, sulfonylureas (glyburide), some β blockers, some angiotensin receptor blockers, and fluoroquinolones. Thus, banaba may decrease the absorption of these drugs.

A 15-day randomized control trial was done in 10 subjects with type 2 diabetes and fasting glucose levels between 140 (7.8 mmol/L) and 250 mg/dL (13.9 mmol/L).[2] Diabetes medications were stopped for 45 days prior to the study. The authors used a 1% corsolic acid extract called Glucosol™. Three different doses of banaba (16, 32, or 48 mg) in either a soft gel or hard gel formulation were used. Five subjects in each group received the three different doses for 15 days, with a 10-day washout between doses. Basal glucose was measured by a fasting blood sample seven days before starting treatment. During the study, three samples were drawn and an average of the three readings was compared to the basal value. The 32- and 48-mg soft gel formulations showed 11% and 30% decrease, respectively, from basal values after 15 days of treatment ($P \le 0.01$ and $P \le 0.002$, respectively). Only the 48-mg hard gel formulation showed a significant decrease of 20% ($P \le 0.001$) but the effect was still less than the soft gel formulation.

Studies published in the Japanese language have shown 13–17% decreases in glucose.[9,10] In a double-blind crossover study, 31 subjects with impaired glucose tolerance were administered 10 mg of corsolic acid or placebo five minutes prior to a 75-g glucose tolerance test.[11] Glucose was measured at 30, 60, 90, 120, and 180 minutes. Banaba decreased glucose at 60 and 120 minutes, but the decrease was statistically significant at 90 minutes ($P < 0.05$).[11]

In recent studies, banaba has been combined with other ingredients in persons with diabetes. A representative study was an open-label study of 50 persons on metformin and other diabetes medications, who did not have the American Diabetes Association target A1C of less than 7%.[5] A combination of Lagerstroemia speciosa and Cinnamomum burmanii (100 mg daily) in addition to their diabetes medications was administered for 12 weeks. One-hour postprandial glucose decreased by 26 mg/dL (1.44 mmol/L) from a baseline of 275 mg/dL (15.3 mmol/L); ($P = 0.021$) and A1C decreased 0.65% from a baseline of 9.7% to 9.02% ($P = 0.001$). There was no significant decrease in fasting glucose. Blood pressure also decreased.

Other studies have evaluated banaba in combination with cinnamon for prediabetes, with resultant improved insulin sensitivity.[6] In combination with several other supplements such as red yeast rice, coenzyme Q10, and others, lipids have also decreased.[12,13]

Summary

Banaba is a tropical plant that shows potential benefit in treating type 2 diabetes. It is increasingly being included as an ingredient in multi-ingredient products for diabetes, prediabetes, hyperlipidemia, and even weight loss.[1] The active ingredients are thought to stimulate cell glucose uptake by insulin-like activity. Because adverse effects have been reported in multi-ingredient products, it is difficult to ascertain whether these effects are due to banaba or the other ingredients. The reported adverse effects have included stomach upset, diaphoresis, dizziness, palpitations, and tremor. Additive blood glucose and blood pressure lowering may occur with diabetes and antihypertensive medications, respectively. Doses of these medications or complementary therapies with these effects may have to be adjusted to prevent excessive lowering of blood glucose or blood pressure. In combination with an NSAID, nephrotoxicity and lactic acidosis were reported. In the one study where different doses of banaba were used as single agents the authors only reported percent lowering of blood glucose and did not report actual values.[2] Frequently, banaba is combined with other plant or supplement ingredients for diabetes, to lower lipids, or for weight loss.[1,5,6,12,13] These added complementary therapies have included cinnamon derivatives as well as berberine, turmeric, alpha lipoic acid, chromium, folic acid, artichoke, red yeast rice, and coenzyme Q10.[5,6,12,13] There is no long-term information available. The dose is 48 mg/day of the 1% corsolic acid extract, using the soft gel formulation,[3] or 100 mg of the banaba-cinnamon combination.[5]

References

1. Natural Medicines (Natural Medicines Database search engine). Available from https://naturalmedicines.therapeuticresearch.com. Accessed April 8, 2019
2. Judy WV, Hari SP, Stogsdill WW, et al. Antidiabetic activity of a standardized extract (GlucosolTM) from Lagerstroemia speciosa leaves in type II diabetics: a dose-dependence study. *J Ethnopharmacol* 2003;87:115–117
3. Hayashi T, Maruyama H, Kasai R, et al. Ellagitannins from Lagerstroemia speciosa as activators of glucose transport in fat cells. *Planta Med* 2002;68:173–175
4. Hattori K, Sukenobu N, Sasaki T, et al. Activation of insulin receptors by lagerstroemin. *J Pharmacol Sci* 2003;93:69–73
5. Tjokroprawiro A, Murtiwi S, Tjandrawinata RR. DLBS3233, a combined bioactive fraction of Cinnamomum burmanii and Lagerstroemia speciosa, in type-2 diabetes mellitus patients inadequately controlled by metformin and other oral antidiabetic agents. *J Complement Integr Med* 2016;13(4):413–420
6. Manaf A, Tjandrawinata RR, Malinda D. Insulin sensitizer in prediabetes: a clinical study with DLBS3233, a combined bioactive fraction of Cinnamomum burmanii and Lagerstroemia speciosa. *Drug Des Devel Ther* 2016;10:1279–1289
7. Zheng JQ, Zheng CM, Lu KC: Corsolic acid-induced acute kidney injury and lactic acidosis in a patient with impaired kidney function. *Am J Kidney Dis* 2010;56:419–420

8. Fuchikami H, Satoh H, Tsujimoto M, Ohdo S, Ohtani H, Sawada Y. Effects of herbal extracts on the function of human organic anion-transporting polypeptide OATP-B. *Drug Metab Dispos* 2006;34:577–582
9. Ikeda Y, Chen JT, Matsuda T: Effectiveness and safety of banabamin tablet containing extract from banaba in patients with mild type 2 diabetes (In Japanese). *Jpn Pharmacol Ther* 1999;27:829–835
10. Ikeda Y, Noguchi M, Kishi S, et al: Blood glucose controlling effects and safety of single and long-term administration on the extract of banaba leaves (in Japanese). *J Nutr Food* 2002;5:41–53
11. Fukushima M, Matsuyama F, Ueda N, et al. Effect of corsolic acid on post-challenge plasma glucose levels. *Diab Res Clin Pract* 2006;73:174–177
12. Cicero AFG, Colletti A, Fogacci F, et al. Effects of a combined nutraceutical on lipid pattern, glucose metabolism and inflammatory parameters in moderately hypercholesterolemic subjects: a double-blind, crossover, randomized clinical trial. *High Blood Press Cardiovasc Prev* 2017;24:13–18
13. Cicero AFG, Fogacci F, Morbini M, et al. Nutraceutical effects on glucose and lipid metabolism in patients with impaired fasting glucose: a pilot, double-blind, placebo-controlled, randomized clinical trial on a combined product. *High Blood Press Cardiovasc Prev* 2017;24:283–288

BERBERINE (*Coptis chinensis [Huanglian or French]*)

Berberine is a yellow, bitter-tasting isoquinoline alkaloid extracted from the roots and rhizomes of many different plants, such as the Chinese herb Coptis chinensis (Huanglian or French), tree turmeric, and European barberry, among others. It is a component of goldenseal (Hydrastis canadensis), a well-known botanical supplement. Berberine was found to lower glucose when used to treat bacterial diarrhea in persons with diabetes.[1] Besides lowering glucose, it also has been shown to lower lipids, blood pressure, and weight.[1-12] Berberine has also been used to treat metabolic syndrome and non-alcoholic fatty liver disease (NAFLD).[1]

Chemical Constituents and Mechanism of Action

Berberine is an isoquinoline plant alkaloid. The mechanism of glucose lowering is multimodal. It may increase or enhance glucose-stimulated insulin secretion and increase insulin receptor expression, facilitate GLUT4 translocation, exert α-glucosidase inhibitor activity, enhance adenosine monophosphate activated protein kinase (AMPK), exhibit PPAR γ activity, and stimulate gut microbiota.[1-5] Animal research has suggested berberine may increase secretion of glucagon-like peptide-1 (GLP-1).[2] Berberine lowers lipids through a variety of mechanisms, including decreased cholesterol absorption and increased bile acid synthesis.[1] Berberine also promotes LDL uptake and decreases proprotein convertase subtilisin/kesin type 2 (PCSK9) secretion.[4] Berberine may lower blood pressure via alpha-2 agonist activity (similar to clonidine) or through blocking alpha-adrenergic activity.[1] Additionally, berberine also inhibits aldose reductase, which may be beneficial in decreasing risk of microvascular complications, such as nephropathy.[12]

Adverse Effects and Drug Interactions

The main side effects are abdominal upset, constipation, diarrhea, headache, and muscle pain.[1,2,6] Some persons have used it intravenously since it is a vasodilator, but cardiac adverse effects have been reported.[1] Pregnant women should not use it, due to possible uterine contractions, and it should be avoided in lactating women because it may be transferred in breast milk. It should also not be used in infants, because it may result in fatal kernicterus.[1]

Caution is warranted when used with other agents because berberine may inhibit certain Cytochrome P450 enzymes (CYP3A4, 2C9, 2D6) and thus increase levels of drugs metabolized by these enzymes (for example: cyclosporine, certain statins, some calcium channel blockers and other antihypertensives, psychiatric medications, and warfarin). Taking berberine with diabetes medications, antihypertensives, or central nervous system (CNS) depressants may result in hypoglycemia, hypotension, or sedation, respectively.[1]

Berberine was compared with placebo in a 3-month randomized controlled trial in 116 persons with newly diagnosed type 2 diabetes mellitus (T2DM) and hyperlipidemia.[10] Subjects were randomized to 0.5 g twice daily of berberine or placebo. A1C significantly decreased, as did fasting and postprandial glucose in the berberine group compared with placebo ($P < 0.0001$ for each parameter). A1C decreased from 7.5% to 6.6% in the berberine group and 7.6% to 7.3% in the placebo group. Fasting glucose declined from 126 to 101 mg/dL (7 mmol/L to 5.6 mmol/L) in the berberine group versus 122 to 115 mg/dL (6.8 to 6.4 mmol/L) in the placebo group. Postprandial glucose decreased from 216 to 160 mg/dL (12 to 8.9 mmol/L) on berberine versus 220 to 198 mg/dL (12.2 to 11 mmol/L) on placebo. There were also significant decreases favoring berberine in LDL cholesterol ($P < 0.0001$), weight ($P = 0.034$), and systolic blood pressure ($P = 0.038$).

A different randomized study evaluated 97 persons with T2DM for 2 months.[9] Of these, 50 were randomized to berberine (1 g daily), 26 to metformin (1.5 g daily), and 21 to rosiglitazone (4 mg daily). Fasting glucose and A1C decreased significantly from baseline in all three groups. A1C decreased from 8.3% to 6.8% in the berberine group, 9.4% to 7.2% in the metformin group, and 8.3% to 6.8% in the rosiglitazone group ($P < 0.001$ for berberine and metformin; $P < 0.01$ for rosiglitazone). Triglycerides decreased significantly only in the berberine group ($P < 0.01$).

Another randomized controlled trial evaluated two groups with T2DM—one group was newly diagnosed and the other was poorly controlled.[11] The newly-diagnosed group of 36 subjects took berberine or metformin for three months. In both groups, there was a statistically significant decline from baseline in A1C, fasting glucose, and postprandial glucose ($P < 0.01$ compared with baseline). A1C decreased from 9.5% to 7.5% in the berberine group and from 9.2% to 7.7% in the metformin group. Fasting glucose decreased from 191 to 123 mg/dL in the berberine group (10.6 to 6.85 mmol/L), and from 179 to 129 mg/dL (9.96 to 7.2 mmol/L) in the metformin group. For postprandial glucose, the decrease was 357 to 199 mg/dL (19.8 to 11.1 mmol/L) on berberine and 370 to 232 mg/dL (20.5 to 12.9 mmol/L) on metformin. The authors did not provide a statistical analysis of the comparison between berberine and metformin, but the numbers were very similar. Patients in the poorly controlled group (48 subjects) continued their medications (oral agents or insulin) with added berberine (1.5 g/day) for three months. A1C decreased from 8.1% to 7.3%; fasting glucose decreased from 173 to 137 mg/dL (9.6 to 7.6 mmol/L), and postprandial glucose decreased from 266 to 175 mg/dL (14.8 to 9.7 mmol/L). The decreases were all statistically significant ($P < 0.001$ for all three parameters).

Various meta-analyses have been published evaluating berberine for diabetes only, and others that include evaluations for hypertension or hyperlipidemia. A

2012 meta-analysis by Dong, et. al. of 14 randomized controlled trials in 1068 persons evaluated berberine for diabetes.[6] The analysis compared berberine in combination with lifestyle modification to lifestyle modification alone, or a comparison of berberine combined with oral hypoglycemics (metformin, glipizide, or rosiglitazone) versus hypoglycemics alone, or berberine alone versus the hypoglycemics.[6] Berberine in combination with lifestyle versus lifestyle alone resulted in an overall decrease in A1C of 0.72% ($P < 0.00001$). Fasting glucose decreased by 16 mg/dL (0.87 mmol/L) and postprandial glucose by 31 mg/dL (1.72 mmol/L). The P value for both was < 0.00001. The combined berberine plus oral hypoglycemics evaluation resulted in a decreased A1C of 0.53% ($P = 0.01$). For this group, fasting glucose decreased 11 mg/dL (0.59 mmol/L; $P < 0.00001$) and postprandial glucose decreased 19 mg/dL (1.05 mmol/L; $P = 0.0003$). For berberine compared to oral hypoglycemics, there was no significant difference in A1C ($P = 0.28$) or fasting glucose ($P = 0.21$)[6] The authors noted problematic issues in the studies included, such as poor methodology quality, small sample sizes, and possible bias.

A 2019 systematic review and meta-analysis of 28 studies by Liang, et. al. evaluated berberine for diabetes in 2,313 individuals.[7] The included studies exhibited a complex array of different comparisons between berberine as monotherapy or in combination with other treatments such as lifestyle modification or diabetes medications. For instance, six trials compared berberine plus lifestyle versus lifestyle monotherapy or lifestyle with placebo. Thirteen compared berberine plus one oral diabetes agent with a control of the same oral diabetes agent as monotherapy. Two studies compared berberine plus two oral diabetes agents versus the same oral agents as monotherapy. Fourteen compared berberine plus one oral diabetes agent versus berberine monotherapy. Four trials compared a combination of berberine plus oral diabetes medications with berberine monotherapy. Study duration ranged from 14 days to two years. Overall, fasting glucose in 28 studies decreased 9.7 mg/dL (0.54 mmol/L; $P < 0.001$). Postprandial glucose measured in 20 studies decreased 17 mg/dL (0.94 mmol/L; $P < 0.001$). A1C measured in 19 studies decreased 0.5% (0.54 mmol/L; $P = 0.007$).[7] The analysis was fraught with issues due to the heterogeneity of studies, methodology quality, varying doses, and varying diabetes medications used, as well as missing details of randomization and blinding.

A 2015 meta-analysis of 27 studies in 2569 persons also evaluated effects on diabetes (17 trials), lipids (six trials), and blood pressure (four trials).[8] The analysis found that the combination of berberine with oral agents (for diabetes, hyperlipidemia, or hypertension) had greater efficacy than the individual oral agents as monotherapy for those disease states. The combination of berberine with lifestyle versus lifestyle or berberine versus placebo found a similar A1C lowering to the 2012 meta-analysis by Dong et al. (0.71%; $P < 0.00001$).[6] The combined berberine plus oral hypoglycemics versus hypoglycemics alone also yielded a similar decrease in A1C to the 2012 meta-analysis by Dong et al. (0.58%; $P = 0.002$).[6] In this combination group, fasting glucose decreased 12 mg/dL (0.67 mmol/L; $P < 0.00001$) and postprandial glucose decreased 17.6 mg/dL (0.98 mmol/L; $P = 0.0006$). As In the 2012 meta-analysis by Dong et al., there were no significant differences between berberine and oral hypoglycemics for A1C lowering ($P = 0.41$), but oral hypoglycemics had a slightly lower fasting glucose than berberine of 3.6 mg/dL (0.2 mmol/L; $P = 0.05$). For berberine plus lifestyle compared to placebo plus lifestyle, total cholesterol decreased 26 mg/dL (0.66 mmol/L; $P = 0.0002$), LDL cholesterol decreased 25 mg/dL (0.65 mmol/L; $P < 0.00001$), triglycerides decreased 34.5 mg/dL (0.39 mmol/L; $P = 0.0001$), and HDL increased 2.7 mg/dL (0.07 mmol/L; $P < 0.00001$). Combined with lipid-lowering medications, berberine was more effective than the lipid-lowering agents as monotherapy in lowering total cholesterol ($P = 0.003$) LDL cholesterol ($P < 0.00001$), and increasing HDL cholesterol ($P < 0.00001$). However, triglyceride lowering was not significant ($P = 0.07$). For systolic blood pressure, the decrease was significant for berberine compared to control (6 mm Hg; $P = 0.0003$) as was diastolic blood pressure (3 mm Hg; $P = 0.03$).[8] Results for both systolic and diastolic blood pressure lowering were similar when berberine was combined with antihypertensives.

A 2018 systematic review and meta-analysis of berberine for dyslipidemia analyzed 16 trials and 2147 subjects (approximately half on berberine and half on placebo) treated for 1–24 months.[13] Total cholesterol decreased by 18.2 mg/dL (0.47 mmol/L); LDL cholesterol decreased by 14.7 mg/dL (0.38 mmol/L), triglycerides decreased by 24.8 mg/dL (0.28 mmol/L), and HDL increased by 3.1 mg/dL (0.08 mmol/L). Total cholesterol and LDL lowering were both significant ($P < 0.00001$ for each) as was triglyceride lowering ($P = 0.002$). The HDL increase was also significant ($P = 0.001$).[13] A 2017 systematic review of 12 randomized controlled trials of berberine (alone and combined with other supplements) for hyperlipidemia found that LDL decreased by 20–50 mg/dL (0.52 to 1.3 mmol/L) and triglyceride reductions ranged from 25–55 mg/dL (0.28 to 0.62 mmol/L).[14]

Summary

Berberine may work in a variety of ways to lower glucose by modulating insulin secretion or working on different enzyme systems and even stimulating gut microbiota. For lipid-lowering effects, berberine may work on upregulating LDL receptors and modifying PCSK9 activity. Berberine may inhibit cholesterol absorption and increase bile acid synthesis.[1] The main side effects are abdominal upset and constipation, and a major caution is that it should not be used by pregnant women or in lactating women or infants.[1] Caution is warranted when used with other agents because berberine may inhibit certain Cytochrome P450 enzymes (CYP3A4, 2C9, 2D6) and thus increase levels of drugs metabolized by these enzymes (for example cyclosporine, certain statins, some calcium channel blockers, warfarin, certain antihypertensives, and psychiatric medications).[1] It also may excessively lower glucose If combined with secretagogues.

Berberine is a highly studied supplement, and has been evaluated in several different trials. As stated in the background section, one issue that warrants caution is that there may be variability in the potency of different commercial products. Some trials study diabetes only, whereas others evaluate patients with diabetes, hyperlipidemia, and hypertension. All of these clinical disorders have responded to berberine treatment, particularly when combined with conventional medications to treat these conditions. Meta analyses evaluating berberine have also shown efficacy, but are fraught with problematic study design and heterogeneity.

Berberine is being studied in combination with milk thistle, a different glucose lowering supplement, and may have greater A1C lowering than berberine monotherapy.[15] Berberine is a promising supplement since it not only works for lowering glucose but also has lipid and blood pressure lowering effects. It is found in combination with other supplements, such as red yeast rice, to treat hyperlipidemia.[14] Doses used in studies have ranged from 500 mg two to three times daily. However, it is important to recognize that target goals for diabetes and its co-morbidities as well as impact on mortality have not been shown.

References

1. Natural Medicines (Natural Medicines Database search engine). Available from https://naturalmedicines.therapeuticresearch.com. Accessed April 8, 2019
2. Chang W, Chen L, Hatch GM. Berberine as a therapy for type 2 diabetes and its complications: from mechanism of action to clinical studies. *Biochem Cell Biol* 2015;93:479–486.
3. Rios JL, Francini F, Schinella GR: Natural products for the treatment of type 2 diabetes mellitus. *Planta Med* 2015;81:975–994
4. Pirillo A, Catapano AL. Berberine, a plant alkaloid with lipid and glucose-lowering properties: from in vitro evidence to evidence to clinical studies. *Atherosclerosis* 2015;243:449-461
5. Li Z, Geng YN, Jiang JD, Kong WJ. Antioxidant and anti-inflammatory activities of berberine in the treatment of diabetes mellitus. *Evid Based Complement Alternat Med* 2014;2014:289264
6. Dong H, Wang N, Zhao L, Lu F. Berberine in the treatment of type 2 diabetes mellitus: a systematic review and meta-analysis. *Evid Based Complement Alternat Med* 2012;2012:591654. doi:10.1155/2012/591654
7. Liang Y, Xu X, Yin M, et al. Effects of berberine on blood glucose in patients with type 2 diabetes mellitus: a systematic literature review and a meta-analysis. *Endocrine J* 2019;66:51–63

8. Lan J, Zhao Y, Dong F, et al. Meta-analysis of the effect and safety of berberine in the treatment of type 2 diabetes mellitus, hyperlipemia, and hypertension. *J Ethnopharmacol* 2015;161:69–81

9. Zhang H, Wei J, Xue R, et al. Berberine lowers blood glucose in type 2 diabetes mellitus patients through increasing insulin receptor expression. *Metabolism: Clinical and Experimental* 2010;59:285–292.

10. Zhang Y, Li X, Zou D, et al. Treatment of type 2 diabetes and dyslipidemia with the natural plant alkaloid berberine. *J Clin Endocrinol Metab* 2008;93:2559–2565

11. Yin J, Xing H, Ye J. Efficacy of berberine in patients with type 2 diabetes mellitus. *Metabolism* 2008;57:712–17

12. Yin J, Ye J, Jia W. Effects and mechanisms of berberine in diabetes treatment. *Acta Pharmaceutica Sinica B* 2012;2:327–334

13. Jianqing J, Jingen L, Qian L, Hao X. Efficacy and safety of berberine for dyslipidemias: a systematic review and meta-analysis of randomized clinical trials. *Phytomedicine* 2018;50:25–34

14. Koppen LM, Whitaker A, Rosene A, Beckett RD. Efficacy of berberine alone and in combination for the treatment of hyperlipidemia: a systematic review. *J Evid Based Complementary Altern Med* 2017;22:956–968

15. Di Pierro F, Putignano P, Villanova N, et al. Preliminary study about the possible glycemic clinical advantage in using a fixed combination of Berberis aristata and Silybum marianum standardized extracts versus only Berberis aristata in patients with type 2 diabetes. *Clin Pharmacol* 2013;5;167–174

BILBERRY (*Vaccinium myrtillus L.*)

Bilberry is a shrub found in North America, Northern Europe, and now parts of Asia. It belongs to a large genus (*Vaccinium*) of plants that include the American blueberry (*Vaccinium corymbosum*), whortleberry (*Vaccinium arctostaphylos*), cranberry (*Vaccinium macrocarpum*), and huckleberry (*Vaccinium ovatum*).[1-4] It flowers from April to June, and the fruit is harvested from July to September. The word "bilberry" comes from a Danish word, "bollebar," which means dark berry.[1] The fruit and the leaves are the relevant parts. Bilberry has been used to improve nocturnal visual acuity and other ophthalmic disorders, including retinopathy. Bilberry is also used for circulatory disorders such as venous insufficiency and varicose veins, as well as for diabetes, prediabetes, metabolic syndrome, hypertension, and inflammatory disorders such as arthritis.[1-4]

Chemical Constituents and Mechanism of Action

Anthocyanoside flavonoids (anthocyanins) are the most pertinent chemical constituents in bilberry fruit that have antioxidant activity.[1-4] In vitro, anthocyanins stimulate insulin secretion in rodent pancreatic β-cells. The polyphenols in leaves include resveratrol, and other leaf constituents are flavonoids including quercetin and chromium. The varying compounds in bilberry have many different effects including anti-inflammatory and antiplatelet properties. For hypertension and retinopathy, bilberry may produce vasorelaxation and increased ocular blood flow.[1] The polyphenols may have α-glucosidase inhibitory activity.[1-4] The phenols may also inhibit glucose uptake. The leaf also contains another substance, neomirtilline, that may decrease blood glucose.[5] Although there are many purported effects, diabetes research has not been robust, and trials with good study design are missing.

Adverse Effects and Drug Interactions

Because bilberry has been consumed as a food, it is thought to be safe. The most reported adverse effects have been benign, such as mild digestive distress. However, bilberry is theorized to cause hypotension, hypoglycemia, and bleeding.[1]

There are no known drug interactions, but it may inhibit platelet aggregation and thus may interact with drugs such as warfarin, aspirin, or P2Y12 inhibitors (such as clopidogrel) and supplements that also possess antiplatelet activity, such as ginkgo or fenugreek, resulting in bleeding. Since it may affect blood glucose, a theoretical additive hypoglycemic effect may occur with secretagogues or supplements with hypoglycemic activity, such as berberine, gymnema sylvestre, or fenugreek.[1]

In spite of early enthusiasm and speculation during World War II about the beneficial effect of bilberry preserves in improving night vision in Royal Air Force pilots, this effect has not been demonstrated in controlled trials. One randomized double-blind placebo-controlled study was done in 15 men recruited from a naval air station.[6] The subjects were given 160 mg bilberry extract containing 25% anthocyanosides or placebo three times a day for 21 days. There were no differences between the groups in night visual acuity or night contrast sensitivity.

In another randomized double-blind placebo-controlled trial, 16 men with normal vision were given three different doses of anthocyanosides (12, 24, or 36 mg) or placebo once daily, with a 2-week washout between doses.[7] There were no differences in night vision between the anthocyanoside groups and placebo.

A different randomized double-blind placebo-controlled study evaluated three different night-vision tests in 18 healthy male volunteers.[8] The subjects received 12 or 24 mg anthocyanosides or placebo twice daily for 4 days, with a 2-week washout between doses. Once again, there was no difference between the treatment and placebo groups.

In a double-blind, placebo-controlled trial published in Italian, bilberry extract (160 mg twice daily; 115 mg anthocyanosides daily) was administered to 14 patients with retinopathy related to diabetes and/or hypertension.[9] The 11 patients on bilberry and 12 patients on placebo were treated for one month. The bilberry group showed significant improvement in ophthalmoscopy parameters.

Animal data has shown that bilberry administration has resulted in consistent plasma glucose decreases.[5] Studies of bilberry administration in persons with diabetes are emerging. A randomized double-blind crossover study comparing bilberry to placebo was done in eight males with type 2 diabetes or impaired glucose tolerance (IGT).[10] Subjects were not on any diabetes medications and used lifestyle only for management of hyperglycemia. Following an overnight fast, the participants were randomized to placebo or a single capsule of 0.47 g of a standardized bilberry extract containing 36% (per weight) anthocyanins (Mirtoselect®) followed by a 75-g oral glucose tolerance test. The commercial product is equivalent to 50 g of fresh bilberries. Following a 2-week washout, the participants then were crossed over to the other treatment. Although plasma glucose was measured at various time points, incremental plasma glucose was significantly lower compared to placebo only at the later time points of 120, 150, and 180 minutes ($P = 0.04$, 0.02, and 0.004, respectively) after ingesting the bilberry extract. Compared to placebo, bilberry decreased the incremental area under the curve for glucose (AUCi) by 18% ($P = 0.003$). The extract also significantly decreased the overall venous plasma insulin AUCi by 18% ($P = 0.028$). Since there was a delay in significant AUCi lowering response, the authors theorized the active ingredient might take some time to reach the gastrointestinal tract to produce its effect.

A different 12-week study evaluated ingestion of three different nutrient groups, including bilberries, fish, and whole-grain products on glucose and lipids in 106 participants with impaired glucose tolerance (IGT).[11] Participants were randomized into three intervention groups. One group consumed a combination of whole grain and low postprandial insulin response grain products (25% of their daily caloric intake), 100–150 g of fatty fish (such as salmon, redfish, mackerel, anchovy, and rainbow trout), three times/week, and three daily portions of bilberry (equivalent to 300 g of fresh bilberries). A second group ingested only a whole grain–enriched diet (the same whole grains as in group one) and were asked not to change their fish and berry intake. The third group replaced their usually consumed breads with refined wheat breads and were asked not to eat bilberries; fish was allowed no more than once weekly. A 3-hour 75-g OGTT and other metabolic parameters were measured at baseline and again at 12 weeks. In the first group where three healthy nutrients were consumed, there was a significant decrease at 2 hours in the OGTT. This value decreased from 121 mg/dL (6.7 mmol/L) at baseline to 108 mg/dL (6 mmol/L) at 12 weeks ($P = 0.027$). The glucose AUC also decreased from baseline to 12 weeks ($P = 0.027$). There was no significant decrease in the 2-hour OGTT value in the second or third group.[11] The same researchers also studied the impact on HDL in a secondary analysis of this trial and found a statistically significant increase in the triple nutrient group.[12] In these two studies, it is unknown whether the nutrient combination or individual components were primarily responsible for benefit.

Summary

Although bilberry is widely used, it is important that clinicians and patients know there is little published evidence for its use in diabetes or for visual improvement. It is consumed as a food and found fresh, frozen, and dried as well as in jams and liquids. It is also sold as supplements.[1] The benefit in diabetes may be related to α-glucosidase inhibition, and the chromium in the leaves may provide some glucose lowering activity.[1-4] Bilberry extract, 160 mg twice daily, was useful in retinopathy in a small study of 14 individuals, and this may be especially important for individuals with diabetes.[9] Per a study in 50 persons with mild senile cataracts, bilberry may help prevent cataract progression; this is of importance to persons with diabetes, since they are more prone to cataracts.[13] Bilberry has been combined with pine bark extract (pycnogenol), an antioxidant that dilates the microcirculation, to lower intraocular pressure and improve ocular blood flow.[14] This combination product (Mirtogenol®) has even been combined with prescription anti-glaucoma products to lower intraocular pressure. Even though it may be a benign agent, there is insufficient evidence to promote bilberry use. In food form, it is probably not a concern, but adulteration of bilberry extracts has been found and is a potential caution.[15] There is no known dose for diabetes, but the dose used for a study evaluating the impact of bilberry on postprandial glucose was a single capsule of 0.47 g of a standardized bilberry extract containing 36% (per weight) anthocyanins. This contains the equivalent of 50 g of fresh bilberries.[10] However, the study in impaired glucose tolerance of the three different nutrient groups used 300 g daily of bilberries.[11,12] Bilberry extract, 160 mg twice daily, has been used for retinopathy;[9] 80–160 mg of aqueous extract three times daily (standardized to 25% anthocyanosides) has also been used.[1]

References

1. Natural Medicines (Natural Medicines Database search engine). Available from https://naturalmedicines.therapeuticresearch.com. Accessed April 8, 2019

2. NCCIH. Bilberry. Available from https://nccih.nih.gov/health/bilberry. Accessed April 20, 2019

3. Chu W-k, Cheung SCM, Lau RAW, Benzie IFF. Bilberry (Vaccinium myrtillus L.). in: Benzie IFF, Wachtel-Galor S, eds. Herbal Medicine: Biomolecular and Clinical Aspects. 2nd edition. Boca Raton (FL): CRC Press, 2011

4. Anonymous: Vaccinium myrtillus (Bilberry). *Altern Med Rev* 2001;6:500–504

5. Cignarella A, Nastasi M, Cavalli E, Puglisi L. Novel lipid-lowering properties of Vaccinium myrtillus L. leaves, a traditional antidiabetic treatment, in several models of rat dyslipidaemia: a comparison with ciprofibrate. *Thrombosis Res* 1996;84:311–322

6. Muth ER, Laurent JM, Jasper P. The effect of bilberry nutritional supplementation on night visual acuity and contrast sensitivity. *Altern Med Rev* 2000;5:164–173

7. Levy Y, Glovinsky Y. The effect of anthocyanosides on night vision. *Eye* 1998;12:967–969

8. Zadok D, Levy Y, Glovinsky Y. The effect of anthocyanosides in a multiple oral dose on night vision. *Eye* 1999;13:734–736

9. Perossini M, Guidi G, Chiellini S, Siravo D. Diabetic and hypertensive retinopathy therapy with Vaccinium myrtillus anthocyanosides (Tegens): Double-blind, placebo-controlled clinical trial [in Italian]. *Ann Ottalmol Clin Ocul* 1987;113:1173–1177

10. Hoggard N, Cruickshank M, Moar K-M, et al. A single supplement of a standardized bilberry (Vaccinium myrtillus L.) extract (36% wet weight anthocyanins) modifies glycemic response in individuals with type 2 diabetes controlled by diet and lifestyle. *J Nutr Sci* 2013;2:e22.doi:10.1017/jns.2013.16 eCollection 2013

11. Lankinen M, Schwab U, Kolehmainen M, et al. Whole grain products, fish and bilberries alter glucose and lipid metabolism in a randomized, controlled trial; The Sysdimet Study. *PLoS One* 2011;6:e22646. doi:10.1371/journal.pone.0022646

12. Lankinen M, Kolehmainen M, Jaaskelainen T, et al. Effects of whole grain, fish, and bilberries on serum metabolic profile and lipid transfer protein activities: a randomized trial (Sysdimet). *PLoS One* 2014;9:e90352. doi:10.1371/journal.pone.0090352

13. Bravetti G.O, Fraboni E, Maccolini E. Preventive medical treatment of senile cataract with vitamin E and Vaccinium myrtillus anthocyanosides: clinical evaluation. *Ann Ottalmol Clin Ocul* 1989;115:109–16

14. Steigerwalt RD, Gianni B, Paolo M, Bombardelli E, Burki C, Schonlau F. Effects of Mirtogenol on ocular blood flow and intraocular hypertension in asymptomatic subjects. *Mol Vis* 2008;14:1288–1292

15. Gardana C, Ciappellano S, Mariononi L, Fachechi C, Simonetti P. Bilberry adulteration: identification and chemical profiling of anthocyanins by different analytical methods. *J Agric Food Chem* 2014;62:10998–11004

BITTER MELON (*Momordica charantia*)

Bitter melon is a plant product also known as bitter gourd, bitter apple, bitter cucumber, karolla, and karela. It is a member of the *Cucurbitaceae* family and is related to the melon family, such as honeydew, cantaloupe, Persian melon, muskmelon, and casaba.[1] Although the fruit and seeds are used for diabetes and prediabetes, bitter melon is cultivated in various parts of the world—including India, Asia, Africa, and South America—for consumption as a vegetable. Bitter melon grows as a vine with green leaves and yellow flowers. The fruit is green with a bumpy exterior, resembling a cucumber, and the interior is yellow-orange. The fruit and seeds are thought to be useful for diabetes.[1-4]

Bitter melon has also been used for psoriasis and gastrointestinal disorders. Women have used bitter melon as an emmenagogue (to help induce menstruation) and as an abortifacient. It has also been used to treat cancer and HIV.[1-4]

Chemical Constituents and Mechanism of Action

Bitter melon has chemical constituents that may have hypoglycemic activity, including the glycosides momordin and charantin, as well as momordicin, Polypeptide P (an insulin-like peptide), and vicine.[1-4] The mechanism of glucose lowering includes tissue glucose uptake, glycogen synthesis, enhanced glucose oxidation of the G6PDH pathway (an issue possibly important in persons of Mediterranean ancestry), AMPK activation, and α-glucosidase inhibition.[1-7] Other mechanisms may involve PPAR receptor γ activation and GLUT 4 translocation.[5,8]

Adverse Effects and Drug Interactions

The major side effect of bitter melon is gastrointestinal discomfort.[1] However, some very serious, isolated events have occurred, including hypoglycemic coma from a tea containing bitter melon.[1-3] Another syndrome called favism, or hemolytic anemia, has occurred; it is characterized by headache, fever, abdominal pain, and coma. Individuals of Mediterranean or Middle-Eastern ancestry, who may have a G6PDH deficiency, may be prone to hemolytic anemia.[1,2] Background articles have noted that two protein constituents, α-momorcharin and β-momorcharin, in bitter melon are known abortifacients.[1-3] Severe hypoglycemia and seizures in two children who were given bitter melon tea have been reported.[2,3]

When bitter melon is combined with sulfonylureas, hypoglycemia may occur, and this has been reported when it was combined with chlorpropamide.[9] Hypoglycemia may also occur if bitter melon is combined with supplements that lower glucose, such as berberine or gymnema sylvestre.[1]

Bitter melon may inhibit p-glycoprotein efflux and thus increase serum drug concentrations of medications that are substrates of this pathway.[10] Bitter melon may thus increase serum levels and enhance pharmacologic effects of the dipeptidyl peptidase 4 (DPP4) inhibitor, linagliptin; calcium channel blockers including diltiazem or verapamil; direct oral anticoagulants (DOACs) such as apixiban or rivaroxaban; certain chemotherapeutic agents such as vincristine, etoposide, or vinblastine; certain protease inhibitors (indinavir and ritonavir); and several other medications.

Clinical Studies

Human studies of bitter melon are often of short duration with sub-optimal study design and do not consistently provide adequate details regarding blinding and randomization. Studies have mostly been done in individuals with type 2 diabetes. One small study was done in subjects with type 1 and type 2 diabetes using injectable polypeptide-P (an insulin-like polypeptide isolated from bitter melon).[11] Five subjects with type 1 diabetes were given the active compound and compared to six subjects also with type 1 diabetes in a control group. Six subjects with type 2 diabetes were given the active compound and compared to two subjects (also with type 2 diabetes) in a control group. Fasting glucose was measured, followed by administration of injectable bitter melon. Then glucose was measured at 4, 6, 8, and 12 hours post injection. In the type 1 diabetes group, the first glucose measurement decreased from 304 mg/dL (16.9 mmol/L) to 169 mg/dL (9.4 mmol/L) after 4 hours ($P < 0.05$), and the lower glucose measurement was maintained at 6 and 8 hours after injection. Glucose did not significantly decrease in those with type 2 diabetes.[11]

The first randomized 3-month double-blind placebo-controlled study was conducted in 40 adults with newly diagnosed diabetes or persons with type 2 diabetes (all on diabetes medications) with suboptimal glycemic control.[12] The bitter melon dose was two 500-mg capsules of bitter melon three times daily with meals. The mean treatment A1C difference between the bitter melon and placebo group was 0.22% ($P = 0.483$). Although fasting glucose and cholesterol were measured, there were no other significant improvements.[12]

A 4-week randomized double-blind active-control trial compared three different doses of bitter melon (500 mg, 1,000 mg, or 2,000 mg daily of dried powder of the fruit pulp) with metformin (1,000 mg daily) in 129 persons with newly diagnosed type 2 diabetes.[13] The fructosamine in the metformin group decreased significantly from 308.3 µmol/L at baseline to 291.5 µmol/L (−16.8 µmol/L; 95% CI −31.2 to −2.4) after 4 weeks. The fructosamine in the highest dose bitter melon group (2,000 mg/day) decreased from 326.8 µmol/L to 316.6 µmol/L (−10.2 µmol/L; 95% CI −19.1 to −1.3). Thus, metformin and the highest dose of bitter melon decreased fructosamine significantly, although metformin produced a greater decrease. The difference in fructosamine between treatments was not significant. Fasting glucose decreased significantly in the metformin group, but not in the bitter melon groups. Contrary to earlier evaluations, bitter melon did not decrease 2-hour glucose levels after an oral glucose tolerance test (OGTT) challenge.[13]

A 2012 Cochrane Review evaluated four randomized trials ranging from 4 weeks–3 months in 479 subjects.[14] Trials compared bitter melon with placebo and with glyburide and metformin, and there were no significant changes in glycemic parameters. The authors stated that evaluated trials were of low methodological quality and concluded overall that there was insufficient evidence to support use of bitter melon.

Since the 2012 Cochrane Review, other studies have been published. One small pilot study in patients with type 2 diabetes was a 16-week parallel randomized double-blind placebo-controlled trial where 19 persons were assigned to 6.26 mg/day of dried fruit pulp of bitter melon and 19 to placebo.[15] In the bitter melon group, A1C declined significantly by 0.5% from 7.47% at baseline to 6.97% at endpoint ($P = 0.001$) and the decline in the placebo group was 0.2%, from 7.32% at baseline to 7.12% at endpoint ($P = 0.153$). The difference between bitter melon and placebo was significant ($P = 0.044$). This study reported that fasting glucose decrease was not significant ($P = 0.156$ for bitter melon vs. placebo) but there was a significant decline in serum advanced glycation end products ($P = 0.028$) for bitter melon vs. placebo. One notable finding in this study was that there was no change in liver function enzymes or measures of renal function.[15]

Another study was a 10-week randomized parallel group trial in 95 persons recently diagnosed with type 2 diabetes.[8] Three groups were randomized to 2 or 4 g/day of bitter melon dried powder of the fruit pulp (Group I and II, respectively), and the third group (Group III) was randomized to glibenclamide (glyburide, a sulfonylurea) for 10 weeks. The article noted two different doses of glibenclamide (in one instance 2.5 mg/day was mentioned and in another instance 5 mg/day was stated). Group I had a decrease in A1C from 8.25% at baseline to 7.4% at endpoint ($P \leq 0.05$); Group II decreased from 8.3% to 7.15% ($P \leq 0.02$) and the sulfonylurea group decreased from 8.45% to 6.9% ($P < 0.005$). There was no statistically-significant difference between the three groups. Fasting glucose decreased significantly from baseline by 13 mg/dL (0.72 mmol/L) and 15 mg/dL (0.83 mmol/L) in the two bitter melon groups, and by 26.5 mg/dL (1.47 mmol/L) in the sulfonylurea group. However, the difference between groups was significant only between the lower dose of bitter melon and the sulfonylurea ($P \leq 0.05$). This study also measured plasma sialic acid (PSA) concentrations, a marker of potential cardiovascular disease. Notably, PSA declined in both bitter melon groups, although significantly only in the higher dose group. In the sulfonylurea group, the PSA increase was not significant.[8]

A 2014 systematic review and meta-analysis evaluated impact of bitter melon on glycemic parameters in four trials ranging from 4–12 weeks in 208 subjects.[4] The authors stated they identified several studies for the analysis and also noted there were several different dosage forms and varying doses, which may have contributed to heterogeneity of evidence. Ultimately, the authors stated that only two studies reported usable data for a meta-analysis of A1C, and this showed a weighted mean difference decrease of 0.13% that was not significant. The authors also stated that only two studies reported usable data for fasting glucose, which reported a weighted mean difference decrease of 2.2 mg/dL (0.12 mmol/L) that was not significant.[4]

A 2019 systematic review and meta-analysis by Peter et al., evaluated 10 randomized controlled trials lasting 4–16 weeks, including one trial in persons with prediabetes.[16] The majority of evaluated studies used monoherbal bitter melon preparations of whole fruit, pulp, or seeds in 1,045 individuals with diabetes. In the overall evaluation, meta-analysis of five trials compared bitter melon to placebo in 243 persons and A1C decreased 0.26% ($P = 0.03$).[16] In the prediabetes study of 52 persons the decrease in fasting glucose was statistically significant (5.6 mg/dL [0.31 mmol/L], $P = 0.031$). In five trials comparing bitter melon to placebo, fasting glucose decreased 0.04 mg/dL (0.72 mmol/L; $P = 0.02$) in 231 subjects. In three trials comparing bitter melon to placebo, postprandial glucose decreased 0.08 mg/dL (1.43 mmol/L); ($P = 0.0002$) in 153 subjects. Three studies compared monoherbal bitter melon preparations to oral diabetes medications in 323 persons and, not surprisingly, found that diabetes medications were more effective than bitter melon in decreasing fasting glucose by 0.042 mg/dL (0.76 mmol/L; $P < 0.00001$).[16] However, it may be argued that these numbers may be too small to be clinically relevant.

Summary

Bitter melon is a plant product that has been highly used. In various studies, there are responders as well as nonresponders to various glycemic parameters. Most evidence supporting bitter melon has come from mostly small studies with weak study design. Meta analyses do not provide much guidance since there are only a few trials that can be included due to the heterogeneity of formulations as well as study design. Overall, study results may show some benefit, but evidence is not sufficiently robust to recommend use, and there are no long-term trials. Caution should be advised because bitter melon may cause hypoglycemia—especially when combined with conventional diabetes medications.[9] Due to p-glycoprotein inhibition, bitter melon may increase concentrations of several medications that individuals with diabetes may take, such as linagliptin, some calcium channel blockers, or direct oral anticoagulants.[10] It should be used with caution by women of childbearing age, since it may inadvertently cause miscarriage due to abortifacient constituents. There is no information regarding use in lactating women, so it should also be avoided in this population. Children should not use bitter melon, since serious adverse effects have been reported, including hypoglycemic coma. Individuals of Mediterranean or Middle-Eastern descent with known G6PDH deficiency or those who have allergies to the melon family should also avoid use. Studies evaluating the role of bitter melon supplements continue to be done, and it is unknown which dosage forms are the most appropriate. Different forms have been used, including juice, powder, vegetable pulp suspensions, extracts, and even injectable forms. Doses have varied, but powdered bitter melon fruit 2–4 g daily and extracts have been used. Overall evidence does not justify its use, but it is important to acknowledge that many persons throughout the world consume it as a vegetable as part of their diet.

References

1. Natural Medicines (Natural Medicines Database search engine). Available from https://naturalmedicines.therapeuticresearch.com. Accessed April 8, 2019
2. Basch E, Gabardi S, Ulbricht C. Bitter melon (Momordica charantia): a review of efficacy and safety. *Am J Health-Syst Pharm* 2003;60:356–359
3. Raman A, Lau C. Anti-diabetic properties and phytochemistry of Momordica charantia L. (Cucurbitacease). *Phytomedicine* 1996;2:349–362
4. Yin RV, Lee NC, Hirpara H, Phung OJ. The effect of bitter melon (Momordica charantia) in patients with diabetes mellitus: a systematic review and meta-analysis. *Nutr Diabetes* 2014;4:e145
5. Alam MA, Uddin R, Subhan N, et al. Beneficial role of bitter melon supplementation in obesity and related complications in metabolic syndrome. *J Lipids* 2015;2015:496169. doi: 10.1155/2015/496169
6. Tan MJ, Ye JM, Turner N, et al. Antidiabetic activities of triterpenoids isolated from bitter melon associated with activation of the AMPK pathway. *Chem Biol* 2008;15:263–273
7. Nhiem NX, Kiem PV, Minh CV, et al. Alpha-Glucosidase inhibition properties of cucurbitane-type triterpene glycosides from the fruits of Momordica charantia. *Chem Pharm Bull (Tokyo)*. 2010;58:720–724
8. Rahman IU, Khan RU, Rahman KU, Bashsir M. Lower hypoglycemic but higher antiatherogenic effects of bitter melon than glibenclamide in type 2 diabetic patients. *Nutr J* 2015;14:13. doi: 10.1186/1475-2891-14-13
9. Aslam M, Stockley IH: Interaction between curry ingredient (karela) and drug (chlorpropamide) (Letter). *Lancet* 1979;1:607
10. Konishi T, Satsu H, Hatsugai Y, et al. Inhibitory effect of a bitter melon extract on the P-glycoprotein activity in intestinal Caco-2 cells. *Br J Pharmacol* 2004;143:379–387
11. Khanna P, Jain SC, Panagariya A, Dixit VP. Hypoglycemic activity of polypeptide-p from a plant source. *J Nat Prod* 1981;44:648–55

12. Dans AM, Villarruz MVC, Jimeno CA, et al. The effect of Momordica charantia capsule preparation on glycemic control in type 2 diabetes mellitus needs further studies. *J Clin Epidemiol* 2007;60:554–559
13. Fuangchan A, Sonthisombat P, Seubnukarn T, et al. Hypoglycemic effect of bitter melon compared with metformin in newly diagnosed type 2 diabetes patients. *J Ethnopharmacol* 2011;134:422–428
14. Ooi CP, Yassin Z, Hamid TA. Momordica charantia for type 2 diabetes mellitus. Cochrane Database Syst Rev 2012;8:CD007845
15. Trakoon-osot W, Sotanaphun, U, Phanachet P, et al. Pilot study: hypoglycemic and antiglycation activities of bitter melon (Momordica charantia L.) in type 2 diabetic patients. *J Pharm Res* 2013;6:859–864
16. Peter EL, Kasali FM, Deyno S, et al. Momordica charantia L. lowers elevated glycaemia in type 2 diabetes mellitus patients: systematic review and meta-analysis. *J Ethnopharmacol* 2019;231:311–324

CHIA (*Salvia Hispanica L.*)

Chia seeds have been used as a food for thousands of years. It belongs to the family *Lamiaceae,* and is also known as Spanish sage, Mexican chia, and black chia. The word "chia" comes from an Aztec word meaning "oily." It is grown commercially in Mexico, Central, and South America. The plant comes from the mint family, grows to about 1 meter in height, and produces white or purple flowers during the summer.[1-3]

Chia seeds have also been used in folk medicine and cosmetics. The seeds are used in supplements as medicinal agents for disease states such as diabetes, hypertension, obesity, metabolic syndrome, and cardiovascular disease. Topically it has been used for pruritus.[1]

Chemical Constituents and Mechanism of Action

Chia contains a plant source of ω-3 fatty acids—alpha-linolenic acid—but also contains fiber, protein, calcium, phosphorous, magnesium, iron, and antioxidants. The antioxidants include chlorogenic acid, caffeic acid, quercetin, kaempferol, and myricetin.[2] Therapeutic benefit may include decreased levels of post-meal glucose; other beneficial effects may be due to the high fiber content.[1-2,4-6] A specific product called Salba has been cultivated to provide a high fiber and concentrated alpha linolenic acid content.[4] Decreased blood pressure may possibly be due to some chemical constituents with angiotensin converting enzyme inhibition activity.[2]

Adverse Effects and Drug Interactions

The main adverse effects are possible minor gastrointestinal upset[7] and possible allergic reactions.[8]

A theoretical side effect of chia is a potential increase in triglycerides,[1] but a study using Salba did not show increased triglycerides in the patients who used it.[4] Another potential side effect is that high alpha-linolenic acid intake may increase the risk for advanced prostate cancer, although this finding has been controversial.[9]

Evaluation of laboratory parameters of lipids, renal function, and coagulation factors has not shown any adverse effects.[4] There are no reports of drug interactions.[1]

Clinical Studies

A controversy surrounds what type of chia seed to use in supplements, since both black and white seeds have been used. Some individuals recommend the black chia seeds instead of white as they are less expensive. One study used the white chia seeds in the form of a specific manufactured product called Salba. The single-blind crossover study was done in 20 individuals with type 2 diabetes.[4] Patients were randomized to receive a daily dose of 37 g a day of chia or wheat bran (the control). After 12 weeks, the patients were crossed over to the other group after a washout period of 4–6 weeks. The A1C decrease was statistically significant from a baseline of 6.9% to 6.7% ($P < 0.05$) in the chia group but did not change in the control group (6.7% at baseline and 12 weeks). The difference between chia and control was not statistically significant. The systolic blood pressure (SBP) decrease was statistically significant in the chia group from 129 at baseline to 123 mm Hg at endpoint ($P < 0.001$), but increased in the control group (122–129 mm Hg). Compared to the control, the decrease in SBP in the chia group was statistically significant ($P < 0.05$). Diastolic blood pressure (DBP) also decreased in the chia group, but the change was not statistically significant (81 to 78 mm Hg). The DBP increased but was not statistically significant in the control group (76 to 79 mm Hg). There were no statistically significant changes in lipids in either group. Other markers of cardiovascular disease also improved in the chia group, including C-reactive protein and the von Willebrand factor.[4]

In a different 6-month double-blind randomized controlled trial, 77 overweight and obese subjects with type 2 diabetes were given 30 g/1000 kcal/day of Salba chia or 36 g/1000 kcal/day of oat bran.[7] The primary endpoint was weight change, but impact on glucose was also assessed. Weight loss was greater in the chia group than the control group (1.9 vs. 0.3 kg; $P < 0.02$). Both the chia and oat bran groups had a decrease in A1C, although the decrease was greater in the latter (0.1 vs. 0.3%; $P = 0.231$). Fasting glucose did not change in the chia group but remained at 133.2 mg/dL (7.4 mmol/L) after 6 months. Fasting glucose decreased slightly in the oat bran group (135 mg/dL [7.5 mmol/L] to 131.4 mg/dL [7.3 mmol/L]). The difference was not statistically significant ($P = 0.351$). Adiponectin increased and was statistically significant in the chia group compared to control ($P = 0.022$).[7]

In a randomized controlled crossover trial, the impact of chia whole and ground seeds on postprandial glucose was evaluated in 13 healthy volunteers.[6] Blood samples were collected at 15, 30, 45, 60, 90, and 120 minutes for three different breads—one was a white bread alone, and the other two breads contained whole or ground chia seeds. A statistically significant difference was found between the two chia seed breads and the control ($P = 0.04$) but not between the two different chia seed breads ($P = 0.98$). Thus, the study confirmed that there was no difference in the benefit of whole or ground chia seeds.[6]

Chia has also been shown to decrease blood pressure in hypertensive subjects.[10] In a 12-week trial, 26 hypertensive subjects were randomized to one of three groups. One group of nine comprised untreated hypertensive subjects randomized to chia; a second group of 10 comprised treated hypertensives assigned to chia; the last group of seven treated hypertensives were assigned to placebo. The treatment groups received 35 g of chia flour, added to beverages typically consumed, including fruit juices, water, yogurt, and vitamins. The SBP decrease of the two pooled chia groups was statistically significant and decreased from 146.2 mm Hg at baseline to 136.3 mm Hg after 12 weeks ($P < 0.01$), while the decrease in the placebo group was not statistically significant (144 to 141.2 from baseline to 12 weeks). The DBP in the pooled chia group decreased from 94.2 mm Hg at baseline to 85.5 mm Hg after 12 weeks ($P < 0.001$). The decrease in the placebo group was not statistically significant (90.1 mm decreased to 87.8 mm Hg after 12 weeks). Per ambulatory blood pressure monitoring, mean blood pressure decreased significantly in the pooled chia group (98.1 mm Hg at baseline to 92.8 mm Hg at 12 weeks; $P < 0.05$).[10]

Summary

Chia has been described as a superfood, and is recognized as a novel food in the European Union. It contains alpha-linolenic acid, a ω-3 fatty acid that is a precursor to eicosapentanoic acid and docosahexanoic acid, as well as other minerals and antioxidants.[3] It decreases postprandial glucose as well as blood pressure and may benefit certain metabolic parameters. Persons who may be allergic to certain plants should be cautious regarding possible allergies. Men with pre-existing prostate cancer should avoid chia seed consumption, though the research in support of this warning is controversial. The dose that has been used in studies is 37 g daily of chia, in a specific product called Salba. Although it has been widely consumed as a food, studies evaluating its use in diabetes are now emerging; the impact on A1C and fasting glucose in studies has been modest. However, its role may be to lower postprandial glucose. Chia and other high fiber products, such as flaxseed, have recently become popular. In a small study of 15 healthy individuals, comparison of chia and flaxseed to a control group found that both products lower postprandial glucose.[11] However, the chia group reduced peak glucose and decreased the appetite score to a greater extent than the flax. A trial in persons with metabolic syndrome who followed a dietary pattern consisting of chia seeds, nopal, oats, and soy protein reported a decrease in body weight and triglycerides.[12] Although chia is safe as a food, its role in diabetes requires further study.

References

1. Natural Medicines (Natural Medicines Database search engine). Available from https://naturalmedicines.therapeuticresearch.com. Accessed April 8, 2019
2. Ullah R, Nadeem N, Khalique A, et al. Nutritional and therapeutic perspectives of Chia (Salvia hispanica L.): a review. *J Food Sci Technol* 2016;53:1750–1758

3. Parker J, Schellenberger AN, Roe AL, Oketch-Rabah H, Calderon AI. Therapeutic perspectives on chia seed and its oil: a review. *Planta Med* 2018;84:606–612

4. Vuksan V, Whitham D, Sievenpiper JL, et al. Supplementation of conventional therapy with the novel grain Salba (Salvia hispanica L.) improves major and emerging cardiovascular risk factors in type 2 diabetes: results of a randomized controlled trial. *Diabetes Care* 2007;30:2804–2810

5. Vuksan V, Jenkins AL, Dias AG, et al. Reduction in postprandial glucose excursion and prolongation of satiety: possible explanation of the long-term effects of whole grain Salba (Salvia hispanica L.). *Eur J Clin Nutr* 2010;64:436–438

6. Ho H, Lee AS, Jovanovski E, et al. Effect of whole and ground Salba seeds (Salvia Hispanica L.) on postprandial glycemia in healthy volunteers: a randomized controlled, dose-response trial. *Eur J Clin Nutr* 2013;67:786–788

7. Vuksan V, Jenkins AL, Brissette C, et al. Salba-chia (Salvia hispanica L.) in the treatment of overweight and obese patients with type 2 diabetes: a double-blind randomized controlled trial. *Nutr Metab Cardiovasc Dis* 2017;27:138–146

8. García Jiménez S, Pastor Vargas C, de las Heras M, et al. Allergen characterization of chia seeds (Salvia hispanica), a new allergenic food. *J Investig Allergol Clin Immunol* 2015;25:55–56

9. Brouwer IA, Katan MB, Zock PL. Dietary alpha-linolenic acid is associated with reduced risk of fatal coronary heart disease, but increased prostate cancer risk: a meta-analysis. *J Nutr* 2004;134:919–922

10. Toscano LT, da Silva CS, Toscano LT, et al. Chia flour supplementation reduces blood pressure in hypertensive patients. *Plant Foods Hum Nutr* 2014;69:392–398

11. Vuksan V, Choleva L, Jovanovski E, et al. Comparison of flax (Linum usitatissimum) and Salba-chia (Salvia hispanica L.) seeds on postprandial glycemia and satiety in healthy individuals: a randomized, controlled, crossover study. *Eur J Clin Nutr* 2017;71:234–238

12. Guevara-Cruz M, Tovar AR, Aguilar-Salinas CA, et al. A dietary pattern including nopal, chia seed, soy protein, and oat reduces serum triglycerides and glucose intolerance in patients with metabolic syndrome. *J Nutr* 2012;142:64–69

CHROMIUM

Chromium is a trace element found in trivalent or hexavalent forms. The hexavalent form is a carcinogen associated with industrial exposure and is not found in foods. Trivalent forms include chromium picolinate, nicotinate, and chloride. The nontoxic trivalent form is found in whole grains, high-bran cereals, egg yolks, brewer's yeast, meat, nuts, cheese, broccoli and other fresh vegetables, and even in some wines.[1,2] In past years, Brewer's yeast was thought to contain an unrecognized dietary ingredient known as glucose tolerance factor, or GTF, which is chromium.[2]

Chromium deficiency may occur when a person is on total parenteral nutrition, is pregnant, or has a poor diet, high glucose intake, or poor glucose control.[1-4]

Besides glucose control, chromium has been used for a variety of purposes, including weight loss, treating impaired glucose tolerance, improving lipids, and its ergogenic properties.[1,4] Since increased chromium excretion may occur with steroid use, chromium supplementation has been used to reverse corticosteroid-induced diabetes.[5]

The Food and Nutrition Board of the Institute of Medicine has determined there is not sufficient evidence to set an estimated average requirement for chromium.[6] The adequate intake is 35 μg/day for young men and 25 μg/day for young women, ages 19 to 50 years old. The adequate intake is 30 μg/day and 20 μg/day, respectively, for men and women older than 50 years of age.[4,6] There is no accurate assay for body chromium stores. Thus, it is difficult to determine if an individual has chromium deficiency and whether supplementation may correct it. Increased chromium levels with supplementation is not the factor that improves hyperglycemia. The concept of chromium responders versus nonresponders has been suggested.[7] Responders are more likely to have higher baseline fasting glucose and A1C and are more likely be more insulin resistant than nonresponders

Chemical Constituents and Mechanism of Action

Trivalent chromium is used therapeutically. The exact mechanism by which chromium affects glucose metabolism is unknown. The trivalent form is believed to play a role in enhancing cellular effects of insulin.[2] Chromium may affect insulin action through enhanced activity of tyrosine kinase (the enzyme required for phosphorylation) at the insulin receptor. In effect, chromium may increase insulin receptor numbers, insulin binding, and/or insulin activation. The proposed overall effect of chromium may be to increase insulin receptor or β-cell sensitivity.[2,4]

Other effects include enhanced GLUT-4 transport and increased AMPK activity resulting in suppression of the sterol regulatory element binding protein (SREBP-1), which contributes to synthesis and uptake of cholesterol, triglycerides, and fatty acids. Chromium may inhibit 3-hydroxy-3-methyl-glutaryl-CoA reductase (HMG-Co-A-reductase). Chromium also may inhibit acetyl-CoA carboxylase resulting in decreased malonyl CoA. It may also help degrade free fatty acids.[8]

Adverse Effects and Drug Interactions

Reported side effects of chromium are rare; mostly gastrointestinal upset (nausea, diarrhea, gas, constipation, and headache) has been reported.[1,8] Excessive consumption has resulted in renal toxicity, including severe interstitial nephritis as well as severe systemic illness, including hemolysis, thrombocytopenia, hepatic dysfunction, and renal failure.[9-11] Other adverse effects have included dermatologic reactions[12] and mood disturbances.[1] However, studies have demonstrated the safety of large doses of chromium picolinate,[13] and long-term administration and adverse effects have not occurred.[2,6]

There are unique effects of other drugs on chromium. Steroids may deplete chromium, and histamine blockers (famotidine) and proton pump inhibitors (omeprazole) may block chromium absorption. Certain drugs and vitamins, such as anti-inflammatory drugs (ibuprofen) and vitamin C, respectively, may increase chromium absorption.[1,4] Coadministration with zinc may decrease absorption of both nutrients. Chromium may decrease serum levels of levothyroxine.[1] Chromium also complexes with iron for binding to ferritin and thus may result in iron deficiency. Additive hypoglycemia with insulin or insulin secretagogues is a theoretical possibility.[1,4]

Beneficial interactions may also occur. β blockers may increase triglycerides and decrease HDL, the beneficial component of cholesterol. Since chromium may decrease triglycerides and increase HDL, chromium supplementation may offset β blocker-induced adverse effects on certain lipids.[14]

When combined with vitamins C or E, there may be increased insulin sensitivity and enhanced adiponectin expression.[1] Furthermore, if co-administered with biotin, there may be synergistic activity to help decrease hepatic glucose output and gluconeogenesis.[15] Biotin also suppresses phosphoenolpyruvate, the rate-limiting enzyme in gluconeogenesis.[1]

Clinical Studies

An often-cited study is one conducted by Anderson and colleagues in China.[13] The trial was a randomized double-blind placebo-controlled trial in 180 Chinese patients. Patients were randomized to placebo or to either 500 μg twice daily or 100 μg twice daily of chromium picolinate for 4 months. Fasting blood glucose and A1C levels decreased significantly in the group taking 1,000 μg/day of chromium picolinate compared with the 200-μg/day group and placebo group.[13] Fasting glucose decreased significantly in the 1,000-μg/day group at 2 and 4 months (baseline numbers were not given; results were reported in graph form). The authors reported that at 4 months, fasting glucose was 158 mg/dL (8.8 mmol/L) in the placebo group, 155 mg/dL (8.6 mmol/L) in the 200-µg/day group, and 128 mg/dL (7.1 mmol/L) in the 1,000-µg/day group ($P < 0.05$ for the 1,000-µg group vs. the other two groups). From graph interpretation, baseline A1C was 9.4% in the two chromium groups and 9.2% in the placebo group. After 4 months, A1C in the placebo, 200-µg/day, and 1,000-µg/day groups was 8.5%, 7.5%, and 6.6%, respectively. Thus, A1C decreased by 2.8% in the highest dose group and by 1.9% in the other chromium group ($P < 0.05$, reduction for both chromium groups vs. placebo). Overall, effects were dose-dependent and were seen at 2 and 4 months.[13] The main critique of this study is that it took place in China, where poor nutritional status was more likely, and the subjects may have had different dietary chromium intake than average Western populations.

Numerous trials have been conducted, and several systematic reviews and meta-analyses have been done. A 2002 meta-analysis of 15 randomized controlled trials in 618 subjects evaluated the effects of chromium supplementation.[16] In the analysis, 193 subjects had type 2 diabetes and 425 were healthy or had impaired glucose tolerance (IGT). An evaluation of 14 trials showed that fasting glucose declined by 0.027 mmol/L (0.5 mg/dL) (95% confidence interval of –0.09 to 0.15 mmol/L; or –1.6 to 2.7 mg/dL) but was not statistically significant. For A1C, the decrease in persons with IGT was also not statistically significant and declined by 0.3%. In persons with diabetes, only one trial showed a dose-dependent statistically-significant decrease in A1C; thus, the authors stated that data were inconclusive and recommended more studies be done to evaluate the role of chromium supplementation in diabetes.[16]

Other analyses have also shown there is insufficient evidence to make definitive conclusions. A systematic review of 38 studies in 1198 subjects found varying effects where four different chromium formulations were administered.[17] Studies ranged from 3 weeks–8 months and involved primarily subjects with type 2 diabetes, although there were some individuals with IGT and T1DM. A1C was calculated in 14 studies; in subjects with T2DM, A1C decreased significantly by 0.6% (95% CI –0.9% to –0.2%). Fasting glucose decreased significantly with one formulation by 1 mmol/L (18 mg/dL), with 95% CI of –1.4 to –0.5 mmol/L (–25 to –9 mg/dL). Other formulations produced differing results. The author noted significant heterogeneity in doses used and stated that many studies lacked adequate power and acknowledged that poor study design was a significant limitation, and thus concluded that further study was required.[17]

A 2014 systematic review and meta-analysis by Suksomboon et. al. evaluated subjects with both type 1 and type 2 diabetes.[8] The researchers evaluated 25 randomized controlled trials that analyzed the efficacy and safety of chromium. Twenty-two trials evaluated chromium monosupplementation, two trials included a combination with biotin, and one combined chromium with vitamins C and E.

The trials evaluated the treatment groups versus placebo. There were 1,284 patients in the 22 trials using monosupplementation. Trials lasted four to 24 weeks. In the 14 trials that assessed A1C, the decrease was 0.55% ($P = 0.001$) and in the 24 studies that evaluated fasting glucose, the decrease was 20.7 mg/dL (1.15 mmol/L; $P = 0.001$) versus placebo. Chromium monosupplemenation lowered triglycerides by 26.6 mg/dL (0.30 mmol/L; $P = 0.002$) and high density lipoprotein increased 4.6 mg/dL (0.12 mmol/L; $P = 0.01$). Decreases in total and low density lipoprotein cholesterol were not statistically significant.[8]

Researchers reported use of improved methodology to evaluate data in a 2014 meta-analysis of 16 studies.[18] The analysis included 809 subjects (440 with diabetes, and 369 without). This analysis failed to show benefit of chromium supplementation.

An analysis of 14 randomized controlled trials in 875 participants lasting eight to 24 weeks reviewed various formulations of chromium.[19] The formulations included chromium chloride, chromium picolinate, brewer's yeast, and chromium yeast. Twelve trials reported A1C, but the overall decrease varied for each formulation and was not significant. For fasting glucose, only the brewer's yeast formulation produced a statistically significant decrease (19.23 mg/dL [1.07 mmol/L; 95% CI of −35.3 to −3.16]).[19]

A 2018 pooled analysis by Huang, et. al., of 28 randomized placebo-controlled studies with 1295 participants having type 2 diabetes reported positive results.[20] Trials lasted six to 24 weeks. Sixteen trials reported A1C, and the weighted mean difference (WMD) decrease in A1C was 0.54%, which was statistically significant ($P = 0.0002$). Fasting glucose results were available for 21 trials; WMD decrease was 17.8 mg/dL (0.99 mmol/L) and was statistically significant ($P = 0.008$). Triglyceride WMD decrease was 11.71 mg/dL (0.132 mmol/L; $P = 0.0006$) and HDL WMD increase was 1.73 mg/dL (0.044 mmol/L; $P = 0.006$). This analysis also evaluated impact on blood pressure and found a decrease that was not statistically significant.[20]

A rigorous analysis by Costello et. al., of 20 randomized controlled trials involving subjects with type 2 diabetes noted many important messages that may meaningfully be applied to research involving supplements.[21] The 20 trials evaluated supplementation of seven different chromium formulations for 3 weeks to 6 months using doses of 1.28 μg/day to 1,000 μg/day. The authors defined certain clinical outcomes as being clinically meaningful—a fasting glucose ≤ 129.6 mg/dL (≤7.2 mmol/L), A1C ≤ 7%, or a ≥ 0.5% decrease in A1C. Most studies used chromium picolinate. Eleven trials used the rigorous intent to treat (ITT) study design, and nine used the weaker per protocol design. Overall, this evaluation determined that there was no benefit of chromium supplementation. The A1C decreased only in studies where diabetes medications were used concomitantly with supplements, and in some studies, even the placebo group showed a decrease. The authors of this analysis thus noted that it is unknown what may have been responsible for the decrease—whether improved medication adherence or lifestyle adherence may have played a role. The evaluation also reported that mean fasting glucose decreased only slightly and rarely reached target values. Target A1C goals were achieved in 21% (3 of 14) of the studies, fasting glucose goals in 25% (5 of 20), and both in 7% (1 of 14) of studies. Only 36% of studies (5 of 14) achieved a ≥ 0.5% decrease in A1C. The authors did not perform a meta-analysis and noted that it is not appropriate to perform such an analysis of trials that have such great variability in treatment formulations, treatment duration, and populations. They evaluated results of previous published meta-analyses, and commented that these analyses did not use the Preferred Reporting Items for Systematic Reviews and Meta-Analyses (PRISMA) criteria or a checklist to improve rigor when conducting systematic reviews or meta analyses. The authors of this rigorous analysis concluded that overall there was no documented benefit of chromium supplementation and, at best, chromium supplementation perhaps provides only a small benefit.[21]

The rigorous evaluation by Costello, et. al., did not include the 2018 analysis by Huang et. al. in subjects with type 2 diabetes.[20] The 2018 analysis did have some issues with heterogeneity—there were six different types of formulations and a wide range in doses (1.28–3,000 μg/day). The authors of this analysis stated that the evaluation compared chromium only to placebo, but one study did include sulfonylureas as part of both the treatment and control group. There was wide age variability—mean age ranged from 36–83 years. In addition, the authors stated that only five of the studies reported adequate random sequence generation. On a positive note, however, the authors stated that they used random-effect meta-regression analysis to assess the impact of dose and duration, and indicated there was no impact. Overall, the authors of this pooled 2018 analysis concluded that chromium may be considered adjunctively with pharmacologic management in type 2 diabetes.[20]

Summary

Chromium is a trace element that is deficient in certain circumstances, possibly including diabetes.[1] Chromium may work as an insulin sensitizer and enhance β-cell function. However, studies of chromium in impaired glucose tolerance, type 1, and type 2 diabetes have shown variable effects. Short-term, dose-related responses have been shown, and doses up to 1,000 μg/day for several months have not shown adverse effects, but more study is needed.[13] Positive effects of chromium have been reported in persons with type 1 or type 2 diabetes, gestational diabetes, or impaired glucose tolerance.[2] Studies have shown variable benefits for hyperlipidemia. Results from chromium research are not conclusive, particularly in light of the lack of information regarding the most appropriate biomarkers for chromium or the most appropriate formulation. Doses for diabetes have ranged from

200 µg/day–1,000 µg/day of chromium picolinate, although other doses have also been used.[1] The most recent nutrition consensus guidelines state there is insufficient evidence to recommend chromium supplementation in the absence of a deficiency.[22] However, its popularity continues.

References

1. Natural Medicines (Natural Medicines Database search engine). Available from https://naturalmedicines.therapeuticresearch.com. Accessed April 8, 2019

2. Cefalu WT, Hu FB. Role of chromium in human health and in diabetes. *Diabetes Care* 2004;27:2741–2751

3. Anderson R, Polansky M, Bryden N, Canary J. Supplemental chromium effects on glucose, insulin, glucagon, and urinary chromium losses in subjects consuming controlled low-chromium diets. *Am J Clin Nutr* 1991;54:909–916

4. NIH Office of Dietary Supplements. Chromium. Dietary Supplement Fact Sheet. Available from https://ods.od.nih.gov/factsheets/Chromium-HealthProfessional/. Accessed May 4, 2019

5. Ravina A, Slezak L, Mirsky N, Bryden NA, Anderson RA. Reversal of corticosteroid-induced diabetes mellitus with supplemental chromium. *Diabet Med* 1999;16:164–167

6. Institute of Medicine, Food and Nutrition Board. Dietary reference intakes for vitamin A, vitamin K, arsenic, boron, chromium, copper, iodine, iron, manganese, molybdenum, nickel, silicon, vanadium, and zinc. Washington, D.C., National Academy Press, Washington, DC, 2001. Available from www.nap.edu/books/0309072794/html. Accessed May 4, 2019

7. Cefalu WT, Rood J, Pinsonat P, et al. Characterization of the metabolic and physiologic response to chromium supplementation in subjects with type 2 diabetes mellitus. *Metabolism* 2010;59:755–762

8. Suksomboon N, Poolsup N, Yuwanakorn A. Systematic review and meta-analysis of the efficacy and safety of chromium supplementation in diabetes. *J Clin Pharm Ther* 2014;39:292–306

9. Wasser WG, Feldman NS, D'Agati VD. Chronic renal failure after ingestion of over the counter chromium picolinate (letter). *Ann Intern Med* 1997;126:410

10. Cerulli J, Grabe DW, Gauthier I, Malone M, McGoldrick MD. Chromium picolinate toxicity. *Ann Pharmacotherapy* 1998;32:428–431

11. Martin WR, Fuller RE. Suspected chromium picolinate-induced rhabdomyolysis. *Pharmacotherapy* 1998;18:8602.

12. Young PC, Turiansky GW, Bonner MW, Benson PM: Acute generalized exanthematous pustulosis induced by chromium picolinate. *J Am Acad Dermatol* 1999;41:820–823

13. Anderson RA, Cheng N, Bryden NA, et al. Elevated intakes of supplemental chromium improves glucose and insulin variables in individuals with type 2 diabetes. *Diabetes* 1997; 46:1786–1791

14. Roeback JR, Hla KM, Chambless LE, Fletcher RH. Effects of chromium supplementation on serum high-density lipoprotein cholesterol levels in men taking beta blockers. *Ann Intern Med* 1991;115:917–924

15. Albarracin CA, Fuqua BC, Evans JL, Goldfine ID. Chromium picolinate and biotin combination improves glucose metabolism in treated, uncontrolled overweight to obese patients with type 2 diabetes. *Diabetes Metab Res Rev* 2008;24:41–51

16. Althuis MD, Jordan NE, Ludington EA, Wittes JT: Glucose and insulin responses to dietary chromium supplements: a meta-analysis. *Am J Clin Nutr* 2002;76:148–155

17. Balk EM, Tatsioni A, Lichtenstein AH, Lau J, Pittas AJ. Effect of chromium supplementation on glucose metabolism and lipids: a systematic review of randomized controlled trials. *Diabetes Care* 2007;30:2154–2163

18. Bailey CH. Improved meta-analytic methods show no effect of chromium supplements on fasting glucose. *Biol Trace Elem Res* 2014;157:1–8

19. Yin RV, Phung OJ. Effect of chromium supplementation on glycated hemoglobin and fasting plasma glucose in patients with diabetes mellitus. *Nutr J* 2015;14:14. doi: 10.1186/1475-2891-14-14

20. Huang H, Chen G, Dong Y, Zhu Y, Chen H. Chromium supplementation for adjuvant treatment of type 2 diabetes mellitus: results from a pooled analysis. *Mol Nutr Food Res* 2018;62:1700438

21. Costello RB, Dwyer JT, Bailey RL. Chromium supplements for glycemic control in type 2 diabetes: limited evidence of effectiveness. *Nutr Rev* 2016;74:455–468

22. Evert AB, Dennison M, Gardner CD, et al. Nutrition therapy for adults with diabetes or prediabetes: a consensus report. *Diabetes Care* 2019;42:731–754

CINNAMON (*Cinnamomum cassia*) or (*Cinnamomum zeylanicam*)

Cinnamon is a well-known spice that comes primarily from one of two sources— the trunk bark or quills of *Cinnamomum cassia* (or *Cinnamomum aromaticum*) or the inner bark from the shoots of *Cinnamomum verum (Cinnamomum zeylanicum)*. Although *Cinnamomum zeylanicum* is referred to as "true cinnamon," the cassia species has been the most studied in humans.[1-3] Other cinnamon species, such as *Cinnamomum loureiroi* (Saigon cinnamon) or *Cinnamomum burmanii* are also available.[1] Cinnamon has been used in both type 1 diabetes and type 2 diabetes, prediabetes, arthritis, and for gastrointestinal (GI) complaints such as dyspepsia and flatulence. Various cinnamon species have been used in combination with other botanical ingredients to treat diabetes. Cinnamon is frequently used as a flavoring agent to different foods, and is prepared as a beverage, such as tea.[1-4]

Chemical Constituents and Mechanism of Action

The active ingredient is thought to be cinnamaldehyde, a polyphenolic polymer that may enhance the effect of insulin.[1-5] Other ingredients include eugenol and coumarins. The cassia species may contain more coumarins than the zeylanicum species.[3] There are various forms used—aqueous or organic solvent extracts as well as pulverized bark powders. Each form may have unique bioavailability and potency properties.[4]

Cinnamon is thought to work for diabetes by a variety of mechanisms. It may increase insulin receptor phosphorylation and signaling, promote cell and tissue glucose uptake, promote glycogen synthesis, and reduce postprandial glucose levels; it also inhibits alpha-glucosidases, activates peroxisome proliferator-activated receptors, promotes GLUT4 translocation, activates AMPK, and increases GLP-1 levels.[1-7] Animal data has shown that cinnamon may decrease lipids by inhibiting hepatic-3-hydroxy-methylglutaryl CoA reductase activity.[8] Although the mechanism of potential blood pressure lowering is not definitive, cinnamon may lower blood pressure through peripheral vasodilation.[9]

Adverse Effects and Drug Interactions

Adverse effects include irritation or contact dermatitis if used topically. Allergic reactions may also occur. Hepatotoxicity is possible, due to coumarin content, although the amount of coumarins is probably not sufficient to result in problems.[1]

There are no reported drug interactions. In theory, cinnamon may lower blood glucose if combined with secretagogues such as sulfonylureas or insulin. Additive hepatotoxicity may occur with hepatotoxic drugs such as acetaminophen or methotrexate or hepatotoxic supplements such as kava, comfrey, or chaparral.[1]

Cinnamon is a much-studied supplement, and there is considerable variability in the quality of studies. Numerous clinical studies and meta-analyses have evaluated cinnamon for diabetes treatment, but some analyses have also included the impact on lipids and blood pressure. One example of an early study was a 4-month randomized double-blind, placebo-controlled trial done in Germany. The investigators evaluated an aqueous cinnamon extract in 79 individuals with type 2 diabetes who were on oral diabetes medications or diet therapy.[10] Subjects were randomized to a placebo or a capsule containing 1 g cinnamon three times a day. In the cinnamon group, mean baseline fasting glucose decreased from 167 mg/dL (9.3 mmol/L) to 147 mg/dL (8.2 mmol/L) after 4 months ($P < 0.001$). The placebo group had a mean decrease from 156 mg/dL (8.7 mmol/L) to 150 mg/dL (8.3 mmol/L) that was not significant. The mean percentage difference was 10.3% in the treatment group and 3.37% in the placebo group ($P = 0.046$). The A1C did not decrease significantly. Mean A1C declined from a baseline of 6.86% to 6.83% in the cinnamon group and from 6.71% to 6.68% in the placebo group. There were no differences in lipids. Mean baseline LDL cholesterol was 134.6 mg/dL (3.48 mmol/L), and 136.1 mg/dL (3.52 mmol/L) at end point in the cinnamon group. The mean baseline and end point LDL cholesterol did not change in the placebo group and was 139.2 mg/dL (3.6 mmol/L).[10]

A 90-day randomized controlled study was done in 109 individuals with type 2 diabetes and suboptimal control. The study reported that using 1 g daily of cinnamon resulted in a significant A1C decrease of 0.83% from baseline ($P < 0.001$), while the control ("usual care") group had a 0.37% A1C reduction ($P = 0.16$) that was not significant.[11]

A larger 3-month trial was done in 150 subjects with newly diagnosed type 2 diabetes.[12] The two daily doses used were 3 g or 6 g of cinnamon compared to placebo. In the lower-dose cinnamon group, fasting glucose decreased from 227 to 116 mg/dL ($P < 0.001$), and in the higher-dose cinnamon group, fasting glucose decreased from 217 to 113 mg/dL ($P < 0.001$). The A1C in the lower-dose group decreased from 8.5% to 7.3% ($P < 0.005$) and from 8.1% to 7.25% in the higher-dose group ($P < 0.05$). Another notable change was decreases in blood pressure: systolic blood pressure (SBP) decreased from 127 to 122 mm Hg at 3 months in the higher-dose group ($P < 0.001$) and from 131 to 121 mm Hg in the lower-dose group ($P < 0.05$). Diastolic blood pressure (DBP) decreased from 83 to 80 mm Hg at 3 months in the higher-dose group ($P < 0.001$) and from 85 to 83 mm Hg in the lower-dose group ($P < 0.005$).

A 2019 systematic review and dose-response meta-analysis of randomized controlled trials addressed the impact of cinnamon on blood pressure.[9] The analysis included nine trials in 641 subjects (318 on cinnamon and 323 on control). The studies ranged from 8–16 weeks. Daily doses of 0.5–10 g of cinnamon were used in the studies. Most trials were done in subjects with type 2 diabetes, but one study was done in persons with metabolic syndrome, one in persons with hyperglycemia, and one in women with rheumatoid arthritis. For SBP, the weighted mean decrease (WMD) was 6.23 mm Hg ($P = 0.0006$), and for DBP, the WMD was 3.93 mm Hg ($P = 0.001$). The authors noted that greater lowering of SBP was shown in studies lasting longer than 12 weeks, in individuals under 50 years of age, and using daily cinnamon doses less than or equal to 2 g. The authors noted substantial heterogeneity due to varying populations and doses used.

A 3-month randomized double-blind study in 66 Chinese subjects with type 2 diabetes compared two different doses of cinnamon (120 and 360 mg daily) to placebo.[13] In all three groups, patients were taking gliclazide, a sulfonylurea. The fasting glucose decreased significantly from 162 to 144 mg/dL (9 to 8 mmol/L) in the low-dose group. The average decrease was 18.2 mg/dL (1.01 mmol/L; $P = 0.002$). In the high-dose group, fasting glucose decreased significantly from 202 to 173 mg/dL (11.2 to 9.6 mmol/L), with an average reduction of 29.2 mg/dL (1.62 mmol/L; $P = 0.00008$). The A1C decreased from 8.9% to 8.23% in the low-dose group (average reduction of 0.67%; $P = 0.003$). In the high-dose group, A1C decreased from 8.92% to 8% with an average reduction of 0.92% ($P = 0.0004$).

One of the early meta-analyses evaluated five randomized controlled trials in 282 subjects over a median period of 12 weeks.[8] Daily doses ranged from 1–6 g of cinnamon. In subjects with type 2 diabetes, the analysis reported a WMD decrease in fasting glucose of 17.15 mg/dL (0.95 mmol/L; 95% CI of −47.6 to 13.3) and a decrease in A1C of 0.01% (95% CI −0.20 to 0.22); neither result was significant. In one trial involving subjects with type 1 diabetes, the A1C decrease was 0.3% (95% CI −0.01 to 0.7), which was not significant, and the analysis did not report fasting glucose for that study. Although lipids decreased, the differences were not statistically significant. The authors reported that although overall results were not significant, potential benefits might be found in individual studies.

The Cochrane Database evaluated 10 randomized controlled studies of 577 participants with both type 1 and type 2 diabetes, using a mean cinnamon dose of 2 g daily for 4–16 weeks.[14] The mean decrease in fasting glucose for eight trials in 338 subjects was 1.44 mg/dL (0.08 mmol/L) but was not significant ($P = 0.55$). The mean decrease in A1C for six trials in 405 subjects was 0.06% ($P = 0.63$), which was not significant. Thus, the Cochrane Review reported that evidence to support use is insufficient.

A 2013 systematic review and meta-analysis of 10 randomized controlled clinical trials evaluated impact of cinnamon in 543 subjects.[15] The evaluation reported that cinnamon in doses from 120 mg–6 g daily for 4–18 weeks significantly lowered fasting glucose by 24.6 mg/dL (1.36 mmol/L; 95% CI −40.5 to −8.7), although there was a decrease of 0.16% in A1C (95% CI −0.39 to 0.06), which was not significant. Changes in lipids were statistically significant. Total cholesterol decreased by 15.6 mg/dL (0.403 mmol/L; 5% CI –29.8 to –1.44); LDL cholesterol decreased 9.4 mg/dL (0.244 mmol/L; 95% CI –17.2 to –1.63); triglycerides decreased by 29.6 mg/dL (0.334 mmol/L; 95% CI –48.8 to –10.9); and HDL increased by 1.66 mg/dL (0.043 mmol/L; 95% CI 1.09 to 2.24).

A rigorous narrative analysis of 11 randomized trials with 694 subjects reported important issues with study design in trials that evaluate cinnamon for diabetes.[4] This analysis raised some important issues, such as varying trial duration of 4–16 weeks, varying species, and varying doses. Seven studies used cassia cinnamon, one used zeylanicum cinnamon, and three did not specify the species. Doses varied from 120–1,600 mg/day. Furthermore, in 10 of the studies, subjects continued their diabetes medications, so the authors stated it is difficult to determine whether the cinnamon or perhaps increased adherence to diabetes medications or lifestyle were responsible for the benefit. The authors did not conduct a meta-analysis of the studies due to study heterogeneity. The authors concluded that decreases in A1C and fasting glucose versus comparators were modest.

Summary

In studies of varying quality, cinnamon has been reported to decrease fasting glucose, total cholesterol, LDL, and triglycerides, and increase HDL cholesterol. A meta-analysis reported that cinnamon may lower SBP by 5.39 mm Hg and DBP by 2.6 mm Hg.[9] The A1C lowering has not consistently been statistically significant. An issue with the trials is that even if results are significant, there may be substantial heterogeneity, making individual results for patients difficult to predict. There are no large long-term randomized controlled trials. Long-term safety has been questioned due to possible coumarin content in some species and subsequent hepatotoxicity. Doses used have ranged from 120 mg–6 g per day, usually in divided doses, for up to 18 weeks.[1] Many dosage forms have been used, with varying potency and bioavailability. It is unknown whether the most appropriate form is the whole powdered spice (possibly a combination of different types of cinnamon) or an aqueous extract of a polyphenolic polymer.[5,16] Overall, cinnamon used as a food is safe. Some studies in this monograph have reported benefit for diabetes[10-13,15] and blood pressure lowering[9] while others have not.[4,8,14] Studies continue to be published that garner interest. A 2020 randomized double-blind placebo-controlled trial compared cinnamon to placebo in 54 individuals with prediabetes.[16] Twenty-seven individuals took cinnamon 500 mg three times daily, and 27 took placebo for 12 weeks. The primary endpoint was fasting plasma glucose; the value remained the same in the cinnamon group but increased 4.5 mg/dL (0.25 mmol/L) in the placebo group, resulting in a between-group mean difference of approximately 5 mg/dL (0.28 mmol/L; $P < 0.01$). The area under the curve and 2-hour OGTT plasma glucose were lower in the cinnamon group ($P < 0.001$ and $P < 0.05$, respectively).[16] Even though this study showed significant results, this was only a short-term study that does not prove that cinnamon may prevent persons with prediabetes from developing diabetes. Overall, there are varying and conflicting results, but there continues to be great interest in cinnamon use for diabetes and its comorbidities.

References

1. Natural Medicines (Natural Medicines Database search engine). Available from https://naturalmedicines.therapeuticresearch.com. Accessed May 9, 2019

2. Governa P, Baini G, Borgonetti, et al. Phytotherapy in the management of diabetes: a review. *Molecules* 2018;23:pii: E105. doi: 10.3390/molecules23010105

3. Medagama AB. The glycaemic outcomes of Cinnamon, a review of the experimental evidence and clinical trials. *Nutr J* 2015;14:108

4. Costello RB, Dwyer JT, Saldanha, et al. Do cinnamon supplements have a role in glycemic control in type 2 diabetes – a narrative review? *J Acad Nutr Diet* 2016;116:1794–1802

5. Anderson RA, Broadhurst CL, Polansky MM, et al. Isolation and characterization of polyphenol type-A polymers from cinnamon with insulin-like biological activity. *J Agric Food Chem* 2004;52:65–70

6. Rafehi H, Ververis K, Karagiannis TC. Controversies surrounding the clinical potential of cinnamon for the management of diabetes. *Diabetes Obes Metab* 2012;14:493-499

7. Hlebowicz J, Darwiche G, Bjorgell O, Almer LO. Effect of cinnamon on postprandial blood glucose, gastric emptying, and satiety in healthy subjects. *Am J Clin Nutr* 2007;85:1552–1556

8. Baker WL, Gutierrez-Williams G, White CM, Kluger J, Coleman CI. Effect of cinnamon on glucose control and lipid parameters. *Diabetes Care* 2008;31:41–43

9. Mousavi SM, Karimi E, Hajishafiee M, et al. Anti-hypertensive effects of cinnamon supplementation in adults: a systematic review and dose-response meta-analysis of randomized controlled trials. *Crit Rev Food Sci Nutr* 2019; Oct 16:1–11. doi: 10.1080/10408398.2019.1678012

10. Mang B, Wolters M, Schmitt B, et al.: Effects of a cinnamon extract on plasma glucose, HbA1c, and serum lipids in diabetes mellitus type 2. *Eur J Clin Invest* 2006;36:340–344

11. Crawford P. Effectiveness of cinnamon for lowering hemoglobin A1C in patients with type 2 diabetes: a randomized, controlled trial. *J Am Board Fam Med* 2009;22:507–512

12. Sharma P, Sharma S, Agrawal RP, Agrawal V, Singhal S. A randomized double-blind placebo control trial of cinnamon supplementation on gly-

cemic control and lipid profile in type 2 diabetes mellitus. *Aust J Herbal Med* 2012;24:4–9

13. Lu T, Sheng H, Wu J, et al. Cinnamon extract improves fasting blood glucose and glycosylated hemoglobin level in Chinese patients with type 2 diabetes. *Nutr Res* 2012;32:408–412

14. Leach MJ, Kumar S. Cinnamon for diabetes mellitus. Cochrane Database Syst Rev 2012;9:CD007170

15. Allen RW, Schwartzman E, Baker WL, Coleman CI, Phung OJ. Cinnamon use in type 2 diabetes: an updated systematic review and meta-analysis. *Ann Fam Med* 2013;11:452–459

16. Romeo GR, Lee J, Mulla CM, et al. Influence of cinnamon on glycemic control in subjects with prediabetes: a randomized controlled trial. *J Endocrin Soc* 2020; doi: 10.1210/jendso/bvaa094

FENUGREEK (*Trigonella foenum-graecum Linn.*)

Fenugreek is a member of the *Leguminosae*, or *Fabaceae*, family and grows well in different parts of the world, including western Asia, parts of the Middle East, and Mediterranean regions.[1-2] The green leaves and seeds are edible, and the seeds are used medicinally.[1-3]

Not only has fenugreek been used to treat diabetes, it has also been used as a cooking spice and flavoring agent in foods and tobacco, since it tastes and smells like maple syrup. It has also been used to mask the taste of medicines.[1-3] Other uses include treatment of constipation and hyperlipidemia; antiobesity, antioxidant, anticancer, and hormonal effects (to increase testosterone levels); and use post-pregnancy to promote lactation.

Chemical Constituents and Mechanism of Action

Fenugreek contains many different chemical components, including steroidal saponins (such as diosgenin), alkaloids, flavonoids, coumarins, phenolic acid derivatives, amino acids, and other constituents.[2] The seeds contain alkaloids, including trigonelline, 4-hydroxyisoleucine, and fenugreekine, which are alkaloids with hypoglycemic activity.[1-3] A constituent of the seeds, 4-hydroxyisoleucine, may help stimulate insulin secretion.[4] Diosgenin is another constituent that may stimulate insulin secretion.[5] The seeds are also a good source of fiber and protein.[3] Sotolon is another seed constituent, used for flavoring artificial maple syrup.[1] The mechanism is multimodal: fenugreek may stimulate pancreatic βcells and help promote insulin secretion.[3] It may decrease postprandial glucose through various actions.[6] Fenugreek may also increase the number of insulin receptors in red blood cells and improve glucose utilization in peripheral tissues, thus demonstrating potential antidiabetes effects in both the pancreas and other sites.[7] Saponins in fenugreek may increase biliary cholesterol secretion, which eventually decreases serum lipids.[1]

Adverse Effects and Drug Interactions

The main side effects include diarrhea and gas, or flatulence, which subside after a few days of use.[1-3] A caution for women of childbearing age is that fenugreek consumption may cause uterine contractions and thus cause problems with pregnancy.[3]

Hypersensitivity reactions have included rhinorrhea, wheezing, and asthma exacerbations. Teratogenicity has been reported not only in animals, but also now in humans, and includes cleft palate, spina bifida, hydrocephalus, and anencephaly.[8] Cross-allergic hypersensitivity reactions may occur in persons with chickpea or peanut allergies since these are also member of the *Leguminosae* family.[1,3,8]. All of these side effects may occur in the infants of nursing mothers who use fenu-greek, since the fenugreek may be secreted in the milk.

Fenugreek contains some coumarin constituents and thus may increase the effects of anticoagulant drugs such as warfarin, P2Y12 inhibitors such as clopido-grel, or herbs with blood-thinning activity (such as ginkgo biloba, garlic, or gin-ger).[1] A case report of an interaction between warfarin and a product containing the digestive agent boldo in combination with fenugreek resulted in an increase in international normalized ratio (INR).[9] Fenugreek may also enhance the activity of diabetes medications. Thus, when used in combination with insulin or oral diabe-tes agents, the patient may experience hypoglycemia. In animal research, fenu-greek may decrease AUC of theophylline concentrations by 28%.[1]

Clinical Studies

Most studies of fenugreek involve type 2 diabetes. However, in one study, 10 patients on insulin (with type 1 diabetes) were included in a 10-day evalua-tion.[10] The patients were assigned to either placebo or twice-daily 50-g fenugreek defatted seed powder (commonly used in unleavened bread). Fasting glucose decreased from an average of 272 mg/dL (15.1 mmol/L) at baseline to 196 mg/dL (10.9 mmol/L; $P < 0.01$). Total cholesterol decreased ($P < 0.001$), as did LDL and triglycerides ($P < 0.01$ for both).

Fenugreek, at a dose of 6.3 g daily, has been studied in combination with sul-fonylureas in 69 persons with type 2 diabetes.[11] The A1C decreased from a baseline of 8.02% to 6.56% after 12 weeks of use ($P < 0.05$). Fasting glucose decreased from 155.3 to 122.2 mg/dL (8.63 mmol/L to 6.79 mmol/L), a 33-mg/dL [1.83 mmol/L] decrease after 12 weeks ($P < 0.05$). Postprandial glucose decreased from 240 to 170 mg/dL (13.34 to 9.46 mmol/L), a 70-mg/dL (3.9 mmol/L) decrease ($P < 0.01$), respectively.

A larger study involved a 6-month trial of fenugreek in 60 patients with inad-equately controlled type 2 diabetes.[12] Fenugreek seed powder, 25 g daily, was given in two equal doses at lunch and dinner. A control group consisted of 10 subjects without diabetes who were treated only with diet and without fenugreek. In sub-jects treated with fenugreek, the average fasting glucose decreased from 151 mg/dL (8.4 mmol/l) to 112 mg/dL (6.2 mmol/l) after 6 months. Glucose values 1 and 2 hours after meals also declined. Mean baseline 1-hour glucose measured by oral glucose tolerance test (OGTT) was 245 mg/dL (13.6 mmol/l) at the start of the study and decreased to 196 mg/dL (10.9 mmol/L) after 6 months ($P < 0.001$). Mean 2-hour glucose decreased from 257 mg/dL (14.3 mmol/L) to 171 mg/dL (9.5 mmol/L; $P < 0.001$). Average A1C decreased from 9.6% to 8.4% after 8 weeks ($P < 0.001$).

In a different study, 25 newly-diagnosed type 2 diabetes patients were given a hydroalcoholic fenugreek extract or placebo plus usual care of diet and exercise for

2 months.[13] The group assigned to fenugreek was given 1 g/day of the seed extract. The fenugreek group did not differ from the placebo group in fasting or postprandial glucose, although they had improved area under the curve blood glucose and insulin levels ($P < 0.001$) and an improved lipid profile for triglycerides and HDL.

A 2014 meta-analysis evaluated 10 clinical controlled trials in 278 individuals with study duration ranging from 10–84 days.[14] The study design of individual trials was heterogeneous, and various dosage forms were used. Some trials used fenugreek included in chapati bread (unleavened bread) while others used fenugreek capsules. Doses ranged from 1–100 g daily, and trials were parallel design or crossover trials. Fenugreek was compared to placebo in six studies, unspecified in one, and three compared to chapati bread without fenugreek. All 10 studies evaluated fasting glucose and there was a decrease of 17.3 mg/dL (0.96 mmol/L; $P = 0.001$). Two-hour postprandial glucose was evaluated in seven trials and showed a decrease of 39.4 mg/dL (2.19 mmol/L, $P < 0.001$). In the three trials that evaluated A1C, there was a decrease of 0.85% ($P = 0.009$). The authors stated that most trials used poor methodology and recommended future studies use higher methodology quality, with appropriate randomization, and with standardized fenugreek preparations.

A 2016 meta-analysis evaluated 12 studies (10 articles) of 1,173 subjects.[15] Varying dosage forms were used. Results were pooled to assess fasting and postprandial glucose as well as A1C. In nine studies of 877 subjects (eight with type 2 diabetes, and one with prediabetes), fasting glucose was evaluated and decreased by 15 mg/dL (0.84 mmol/L; $P = 0.002$) Eight studies of 789 subjects evaluated postprandial glucose, and the mean decrease was 23.4 mg/dL (1.3 mmol/L; $P < 0.0001$). Seven studies evaluated A1C in 752 subjects, and the mean decrease was 1.16% ($P < 0.00001$). The authors reported there was also a significant decrease in total cholesterol and triglycerides, but LDL and HDL cholesterol did not change significantly. The authors also concluded that better methodology design of future studies, with larger sample sizes, is warranted.

A randomized control study in 114 individuals with newly-diagnosed type 2 diabetes focused on lipids.[16] Half the subjects were assigned to 25 g twice daily of fenugreek seed powder solution for one month, and the other group did not receive fenugreek. The decrease in baseline and endpoint total and LDL cholesterol as well as triglycerides in the fenugreek group were statistically significant ($P \leq 0.001$), but not in the control group. The increase in HDL cholesterol was also statistically significant in the fenugreek group from baseline to endpoint ($P \leq 0.001$). The endpoint values in the fenugreek group were also statistically significant compared to control. At endpoint for fenugreek versus control, respectively, the values were 189 mg/dL(4.9 mmol/L) vs. 208 mg/dL(5.4 mmol/L) ($P \leq 0.001$) for total cholesterol; 106 mg/dL(2.7 mmol/L) vs. 144 mg/dL

(3.7 mmol/L) ($P \leq 0.001$) for LDL cholesterol; 196 mg/dL (2.2 mmol/L) vs. 244 mg/dL (2.75 mmol/L) for triglycerides ($P \leq 0.05$); and 48 mg/dL (1.24 mmol/L) vs. 36 mg/dL (0.93 mmol/L) ($P \leq 0.001$) for HDL cholesterol. A major study limitation is that the subjects' baseline characteristics were unclear—the authors stated in the abstract that treated subjects were on fenugreek and the control group was on metformin. However, in another part of the manuscript, under the "Treatment and Control Groups," the authors state that subjects in the treatment group were on fenugreek and the control group did not receive fenugreek nor any diabetes medications. Nevertheless, there were statistically significant differences between the groups at the end.

Summary

Studies of fenugreek are mostly in type 2 diabetes and are short-term, involve very few patients, and do not adequately report details about the study design and conduct. Most importantly, overall methodology is poor. In the U.S., fenugreek has GRAS (generally recognized as safe) status.[1] The most relevant chemical constituents include trigonelline and 4-hydroxyisoleucine. Fenugreek may have beneficial effects in pancreatic and other tissues and may affect glucose and carbohydrate absorption; it may even affect insulin secretion. Side effects are mostly uncomfortable gastrointestinal effects that may resolve in a few days. Pregnant women should not take fenugreek, since they may experience uterine contractions and teratogenic effects such as fetal malformations and impaired fetal neurodevelopment.[1,3,8] Women who use fenugreek as a galactogogue should be counseled that their infant may experience the side effects of this botanical, since fenugreek appears in milk. Caution is warranted in those who have a peanut allergy or are allergic to chickpeas, soybeans, or green peas or who have asthma. Individuals who take antiplatelet agents, anti-inflammatory drugs, or herbs that have blood-thinning effects should not use fenugreek. The dose used is variable, and various forms have been used. Seed powder in doses ranging from five to 100 g/day in divided doses with meals, as well as hydroalcoholic seed extracts have been used.[13] Newer formulations now include standardized seed extracts.[1] An example of a standardized extract enriched in furostanolic saponins is Fenfuro®.[17] This extract has demonstrated a significant decrease in fasting and postprandial glucose compared to placebo, but did not significantly decrease A1C. However, there are several standardized extracts being marketed.[1] Patients should be counseled about possible hypoglycemia if combined with secretagogues and the possibility of bleeding or bruising if combined with prescription medications or supplements with antiplatelet or anticoagulant effects.

References

1. Natural Medicines (Natural Medicines Database search engine). Available from https://naturalmedicines.therapeuticresearch.. Accessed May 9, 2019

2. Nagulapalli Venkata KC, Swaroop A, Bagchi D, Bishayee A. A small plant with big benefits: Fenugreek (Trigonella foenum-graecum Linn.) for disease prevention and health promotion. *Mol Nutr Food Res* 2017; 61(6). doi: 10.1002/mnfr.201600950

3. Haber SL, Keonavong J. Fenugreek use in patients with diabetes mellitus. *Am J Health-Syst Pharm* 2013;70:1196,1198,1200,1202–1203

4. Flammang AM, Cifone MA, Erexson GL, Stankowski LF Jr. Genotoxicity testing of a fenugreek extract. *Food Chem Toxicol* 2004;42:1769–1775

5. Kalailingam P, Kannaian B, Tamilmani E, Kaliaperumal R. Efficacy of natural diosgenin on cardiovascular risk, insulin secretion, and beta cells in streptozotocin (STZ)-induced diabetic rats. *Phytomedicine* 2014;21:1154-1161

6. Madar Z, Abel R, Samish S, Arad J. Glucose lowering effect of fenugreek in non-insulin dependent diabetics. Eur J Clin Nutr 1988;42:51–54

7. Raghuram TC, Sharma R, Sivakumar D, Sahay BK: Effect of fenugreek seeds on intravenous glucose disposition in non-insulin dependent diabetic patients. *Phytotherapy Res* 1994;8:83–86

8. Ouzir M, El Bairi K, Amzazi S. Toxicological properties of fenugreek (Trigonella foenum graecum). *Food Chem Toxicol* 2016;96:145–154

9. Lambert J, Cormier J: Potential interaction between warfarin and boldo-fenugreek. *Pharmacotherapy* 2001;21:509–512

10. Sharma RD, Raghuram TC, Sudhakar Rao N: Effect of fenugreek seeds on blood glucose and serum lipids in type 1 diabetes. *Eur J Clin Nutr* 1990;44:301–306

11. Lu FR, Shen L, Qin Y, Gao L, Li H, Dai Y. Clinical observation on trigonella foenum-graecum L. total saponins in combination with sulfonylureas in the treatment of type 2 diabetes mellitus. *Chin J Integr Med* 2008;14:56–60

12. Sharma RD, Sarkar A, Hazra DK, et al.: Use of fenugreek seed powder in the management of non-insulin-dependent diabetes mellitus. *Nutr Res* 1996;16:1331–1339

13. Gupta A, Gupta R, Lal B. Effect of Trigonella foenum-graecum (fenugreek) seeds on glycaemic control and insulin resistance in type 2 diabetes mellitus: a double-blind placebo-controlled study. *J Assoc Physicians India* 2001;49:1057–1061

14. Neelakantan N, Narayanan M, de Souza RJ, van Dam RM. Effect of fenugreek (Trigonella foenum-graecum L.) intake on glycemia: a meta-analysis of clinical trials. *Nutr J* 2014;13:7

15. Gong J, Fang K, Dong H, et al. Effect of fenugreek on hyperglycaemia and hyperlipidemia in diabetes and prediabetes: a meta-analysis. *J Ethnopharmacol* 2016;194:260–268

16. Geberemeskel GA, Debebe YG, Nguse NA. Antidiabetic effect of fenugreek seed powder solution (Trigonella foenum-graecum L.) on hyperlipidemia in diabetic patients. *J Diabetes Res* 2019;Article ID 8507453, Available from https://doi.org/10.1155/2019/8507453. Accessed July 12, 2020

17. Verma N, Usman K, Patel N, et al. A multicenter clinical study to determine the efficacy of a novel fenugreek seed (Trigonella foenum-graecum) extract (FenfuroTM in patients with type 2 diabetes. *Food Nutr Res* 2016;60:32382

FLAXSEED (*Linum usitassimum L.*)

Flaxseed is a fiber and food product that grows in Europe and Asia.[1] It has blue flowers that then produce small flat gold or brown seeds.[2] Flaxseed has been cultivated to make linen for thousands of years, and the oil (known as linseed oil) is used in paint and varnish.[2] It is a popular grain consumed by many individuals with and without diabetes, primarily for cardiovascular disease protection and for common maladies, such as constipation.[1,2] In diabetes and prediabetes, flaxseed is used for glucose lowering as well as hyperlipidemia, metabolic syndrome, NAFLD, inflammation, and hypertension.[1-10] Flaxseed is also used for obesity and for menopausal hot flashes.[1]

Chemical Constituents and Mechanism of Action

Flaxseed is found in various forms such as whole seed, ground seed, or flaxseed oil.[2] It is rich in soluble fiber and contains alpha linolenic acid (a plant ω-3 fatty acid), linoleic acid, and lignans (a phytoestrogen). A major plant lignan in flaxseed is secoisolariciresinol diglucoside (SDG).[1-3] Another flaxseed lignan is matairesinol.[1] Although flaxseed consumption increases plasma and red blood cell ω-3 fatty acids, the alpha-l inolenic acid in flaxseed does not have the same physiological effects as marine ω-3 fatty acids (fish oil).[11] The lignans in flaxseed are phytoestrogens with a mixed profile of estrogenic and anti-estrogenic effects.[1]

The mechanism of action is varied, and the fiber it contains helps decrease glucose absorption and delay postprandial glucose absorption, but also decreases lipids and blood pressure.[1] The SDG may lower cholesterol directly by modulating enzymes involved in lipid metabolism, 7 α–hydroxylase and acyl CoA cholesterol transferase.[2] Flaxseed may also have antioxidant activity by inhibiting peroxidation of polyunsaturated fatty acids, which may decrease LDL oxidation.[5] Besides decreasing oxidative stress, lignans may also inhibit platelet activating factor and decrease inflammation.[2] Antihypertensive action may be due to alteration of circulating oxylipins.[8]

Adverse Effects and Drug Interactions

The most common adverse effect is gastrointestinal discomfort, including fullness. Allergic and anaphylactic reactions are also possible. Unripe or raw flaxseed may contain the toxic cyanide glycosides, including linamarin, linustatin, and neolinustatin.[1] Due to possible estrogenic effects, flaxseed use is not advised during pregnancy. As with chia, due to alpha-linolenic acid properties, flaxseed may be associated with increased prostate cancer risk.[9]

Flaxseed may impair absorption of some drugs, such as acetaminophen. Additive effects may occur when flaxseed is combined with certain medications—

hypoglycemia with diabetes medications, hypotension with antihypertensives, and diarrhea with laxatives. Flaxseed may have antiplatelet properties; bleeding may occur when taken with antiplatelets. Lignans in flaxseed may interfere with estrogens binding to receptors, resulting in anti-estrogenic effects. Antibiotics may impair the conversion of lignans to other metabolites in the colon.[1]

Clinical Studies

In an evaluation of flaxseed on diabetes outcomes, 73 persons with type 2 diabetes took a flaxseed derivative (360 mg/day of the lignan, SDG) or placebo for 12 weeks.[3] After an 8-week washout, subjects were then crossed over to the other group. Fasting glucose decreased from 146 mg/dL to 141 mg/dL (8.12 mmol/L to 7.83 mmol/L) in the flaxseed group and increased slightly in the placebo group ($P = 0.829$ for flaxseed versus placebo) after 12 weeks, although results were not significant. The main benefit was a very modest but statistically significant decrease in A1C from 7.17 to 7.06%. The placebo group had a slightly increased A1C. Compared to placebo, the results were significant ($P = 0.001$). In this study, there were no significant decreases in blood pressure or lipids; thus, the lignan extract was very slightly beneficial in this study.

An open-label study evaluated 10 g/day of flaxseed powder in 18 persons with type 2 diabetes compared to 11 persons on placebo for 1 month.[4] A1C decreased 0.59% from 8.75% to 8.16% in the flaxseed group ($P < 0.001$ versus baseline) and increased 0.1% from 7.6 to 7.7% in the placebo group. Fasting glucose decreased 28.9 mg/dL (1.6 mmol/L) from 160.5 mg/dL to 131.6 mg/dL (8.9 mmol/L to 7.3 mmol/L) in the flaxseed group ($P < 0.05$ vs. baseline), but decreased slightly by 1 mg/dL (0.055 mmol/L) in the placebo group. Triglycerides decreased significantly by 29.5 mg/dL (0.33 mmol/L; $P < 0.001$ vs. baseline) and increased in the placebo group by 6.7 mg/dL (0.08 mmol/L), but the increase was not statistically significant. LDL cholesterol decreased significantly by 19.1 mg/dL (0.49 mmol/L) in the flaxseed group ($P < 0.005$ vs. baseline) and, though it decreased by 16.5 mg/dL (0.43 mmol/L) in the placebo group, the results were not significant. HDL cholesterol increased in the flaxseed group, but was not statistically significant.

In a randomized crossover study, 41 overweight or obese individuals with prediabetes were randomized to two different doses of ground flaxseed (13 or 26 g daily) or no treatment (0 g) for three different treatment periods.[5] Data was analyzed for 25 subjects. After 12 weeks on one treatment, subjects had a 2-week washout and were then crossed over to the next treatment group. Multiple analysis of variance showed a statistically significant difference for glucose ($P = 0.036$), insulin ($P = 0.013$), and homeostatic model of assessment (HOMA-IR; $P = 0.008$). Fasting glucose decreased slightly (2 mg/dL [0.11 mmol/L]), but significantly in patients on the 13-g flaxseed dose ($P = 0.036$) compared to no treatment, per paired t test. Insulin levels also decreased significantly in the 13-g group compared to the 26-g group ($P = 0.021$) and the no-treatment group ($P = 0.013$). Change in HOMA-IR was also significant for the 13-g group versus the 26-g and no-treatment groups ($P = 0.012$ and $P = 0.008$, respectively). There were no significant changes in fructosamine or inflammatory markers. Thus, lower dose flaxseed improved glucose and insulin sensitivity.

A meta-analysis of 25 randomized controlled trials in 1,879 subjects, evaluated the impact of flaxseed on glucose control.[12] Study duration ranged from 2–48 weeks, with most trials lasting 12 weeks. Pooled results for glucose reduction in 1,610 subjects in 24 studies showed a small, statistically significant decrease in glucose of 2.94 mg/dL (0.163 mmol/L; $P = 0.02$). In a subgroup analysis of studies using whole flaxseed, the decrease was 5.94 mg/dL (0.33 mmol/L; $P = 0.006$). However, in the subgroup analysis, flaxseed oil and lignin extract did not significantly reduce glucose. Overall, the results were most notable for whole flaxseed, but not the lignan extract or oil. Results were more favorable in those with baseline blood glucose $\geq$ 100 mg/dL (5.9 mmol/L). In these subjects, the glucose decreased by 5.6 mg/dL (0.31 mmol/L; $P = 0.01$). In 547 participants in 11 studies, A1C decreased by 0.045% ($P = 0.47$) but was not statistically significant. However, in individuals that had a baseline glucose higher than 100 mg/dL, A1C decreased significantly by 0.16% ($P = 0.03$). When used for 12 weeks or longer, there was a decrease in glucose, although the reduction was not significant compared to studies where duration was less than 12 weeks. The meta-analysis was problematic from the standpoint of significant heterogeneity in study populations (this included studies with type 2 diabetes, prediabetes, healthy and overweight or obese adults without diabetes). Also, several studies had a small sample size. Due to significant heterogeneity, external validity may be compromised.

Flaxseed administration has also been evaluated in studies assessing blood pressure outcomes. Flaxseed was administered for 6 months to hypertensive patients with peripheral arterial disease (PAD) in a randomized double-blind placebo-controlled trial to determine the impact on blood pressure in a randomized controlled trial.[8] In this study, called the FLAX-PAD study, a total of 58 patients were randomized to 30 g/day of milled flaxseed and 52 to placebo. Systolic blood pressure decreased from 143.3 to 136.2 mm Hg ($P = 0.04$) in the flaxseed group and increased in the placebo group from 142.4 to 145.6 mm Hg, but that increase was not significant. Diastolic pressure decreased from 77 to 71.8 mm Hg in the flaxseed group ($P = 0.004$) and remained the same in the placebo group (79 mm Hg at baseline and 78.5 mm Hg at the end). In the flaxseed group, the systolic pressure was approximately 10 mm Hg lower and diastolic pressure was approximately 7 mm Hg lower than the placebo group.

Two meta-analyses evaluated the impact of flaxseed on blood pressure. In both reports, there was significant heterogeneity in the subject characteristics, types of flaxseed, and duration of evaluation. A 2015 systematic review and meta-analysis by Khalesi et. al., evaluated the impact of flaxseed on blood pressure in 11 studies in 1,004 subjects in studies ranging from 3–24 weeks duration.[13] Overall SBP decreased 1.77 mm Hg ($P = 0.04$) and DBP decreased 1.58 mm Hg ($P = 0.003$). Subgroup analysis found differences based on duration and flaxseed type. For studies longer than 12 weeks, SBP decreased by 1.84 mm Hg ($P = 0.07$) but was not significant, while the impact on DBP was significant with a decrease of 2.17 mm Hg ($P < 0.05$). Subjects that consumed whole flaxseed experienced a decrease in both SBP and DBP, although the result was significant only for DBP. Accordingly, the decreases for SBP and DBP were 3.39 mm Hg ($P = 0.05$) and 1.93 mm Hg ($P < 0.05$), respectively. For flaxseed oil or lignan extract there were no significant differences.

A 2016 systematic review and meta-analysis evaluated flaxseed for blood pressure in 15 studies in in 1,302 subjects, ranging from 4 weeks–6 months.[14] Overall SBP and DBP decreased significantly by 2.85 mm Hg ($P = 0.027$) and 2.39 mm Hg ($P = 0.001$), respectively. Subgroup analyses for duration and flaxseed type also found differences. For studies longer than 12 weeks, SBP decreased by 3.1 mm Hg ($P = 0.072$) although the decrease was not significant. However, DBP decreased significantly by 2.62 mm Hg ($P = 0.003$). The flaxseed powder groups showed a significant SBP and DBP decrease of 1.81 mm Hg ($P < 0.001$) and 1.28 mm Hg ($P = 0.031$), respectively. The flaxseed oil group showed a significant decrease of 4.1 mm Hg ($P = 0.003$) in DBP, but SBP did not decrease significantly ($P = 0.211$). As in the 2015 analysis by Khalesi et. al., there was no significant decrease on blood pressure when lignan extract was used.

Flaxseed has also been studied to assess impact on lipids. One study was an extension of the previously discussed FLAX-PAD hypertension study.[15] Subjects ate foods supplemented with 30 g daily of flaxseed or a whole-wheat placebo for 12 months. Data analyses were done at 1, 6, and 12 months. The LDL and total cholesterol were lower in the flaxseed group compared to whole-wheat placebo after 1 and 6, but not 12, months. However, compared to baseline values, LDL and total cholesterol decreases were significant in the flaxseed group at 6 months ($P \leq 0.001$ and $P = 0.005$, respectively). There were no changes in the placebo group over time. One interesting aspect of this study was the impact on lipids with the combination of flaxseed and lipid lowering medications. At baseline, 74% of subjects were on lipid-lowering medications. In a subgroup analysis of subjects that took flaxseed combined with cholesterol lowering medications, LDL cholesterol was lowered by 8.5% compared to a 3% increase in the whole-wheat-plus-lipid-lowering medications ($P = 0.03$) after 12 months. Compared to baseline, at 12 months, triglycerides increased in both the flaxseed monotherapy and flaxseed plus cholesterol medications group. HDL cholesterol did not change in either group.

Lipid-lowering effects were evaluated in a meta-analysis of 28 trials with 36 comparisons in 1381 subjects that completed the studies.[6] Different flaxseed product types included defatted, whole, ground, and flaxseed oil, ranging from 20–50 g daily and for a median duration of 8.5 weeks. Total cholesterol decreased by 3.867 mg/dL (0.10 mmol/L) in the flaxseed groups but was not significant ($P = 0.06$). The LDL cholesterol decreased significantly by 3.09 mg/dL (0.08 mmol/L) in the flaxseed group ($P = 0.04$). In subgroup analysis, whole flaxseed and lignan extracts significantly decreased total cholesterol by 7.34 mg/dL (0.19 mmol/L; $P = 0.0003$) and 10.82 mg/dL (0.28 mmol/L; $P = 0.04$), respectively. The LDL cholesterol decreased significantly with whole flaxseed and lignan supplements by 6.18 mg/dL (0.16 mmol/L) in both ($P = 0.001$ for whole flaxseed and $P = 0.03$ for lignan). Women had greater decreases than men for total cholesterol (9.2 mg/dL [0.24 mmol/L], $P < 0.0001$; and 3.48 mg/dL [0.09 mmol/L], $P = 0.21$, respectively). There were no significant changes in triglycerides or HDL cholesterol measurements. One important aspect of this meta-analysis is that there was substantial heterogeneity, such as varying products used in the control groups, and potential variation in the quality of flaxseed products used.

Summary

Flaxseed use is very popular to lower glucose, lipids, and blood pressure. There are mixed results in flaxseed studies, and study limitations include small numbers of subjects, limited duration of use, different flaxseed types, and modest benefit. Although thought to decrease inflammation, per a systematic review and meta-analysis, flaxseed did not impact inflammatory markers.[7] Whole flaxseed rather than flaxseed oil or lignan extracts is more effective in lowering glucose. For blood pressure, there is an overall decrease in both SBP and DBP. For glucose, however, results vary according to flaxseed type and duration of the study. The impact on lipids has not been consistent. Although total and LDL cholesterol decrease, HDL does not change, and triglycerides may increase. When added to cholesterol lowering medications, flaxseed lowers LDL cholesterol, per a small study.[15] The fiber content promotes satiety and thus there is interest in possibly helping promote weight loss.[16] Patients should be cautioned regarding use of raw or unripe flaxseed due to possible toxic cyanide ingredients, as well as the possible increased risk for prostate cancer.[9] Doses vary since there are so many forms. For diabetes, whole flaxseed 10–60 g daily is used. For blood pressure lowering, flaxseed powder 28–60 g daily. For lipids, 30–40 g daily of ground flaxseed is used. To suppress appetite, flaxseed drinks prior to a meal are used.[1] While studies providing evidence for its use are fraught with problems, flaxseed remains a highly used product.

References

1. Natural Medicines (Natural Medicines Database search engine). Available from https://naturalmedicines.therapeuticresearch.com. Accessed May 9, 2019

2. Bloedon LT, Szapary PO. Flaxseed and cardiovascular risk. *Nutr Rev* 2004;62:18–27

3. Pan A, Sun J, Chen Y, et al. Effects of a flaxseed-derived lignan supplement in type 2 diabetic patients: a randomized, double-blind, crossover trial. *PLoS One* 2007;2:e1148

4. Mani UV, Mani I, Biswas M, Kumar SN. An open-label study on the effect of flax seed powder (Linum usitatissimum) supplementation in the management of diabetes mellitus. *J Diet Suppl* 2011;8:257–65

5. Hutchins AM, Brown BD, Cunnane SC, Domitrovich SG, Adams ER, Bobowiec CE. Daily flaxseed consumption improves glycemic control in obese men and women with prediabetes: a randomized study. *Nutr Res* 2013;33:367–75

6. Pan A, Yu D, Demark-Wahnefried W, Franco OH, Lin X. Meta-analysis of the effects of flaxseed interventions on blood lipids. *Am J Clin Nutr* 2009;90:288–97

7. Ren GY, Chen CY, Chen GC, et al. Effect of Flaxseed Intervention on Inflammatory Marker C-Reactive Protein: A Systematic Review and Meta-Analysis of Randomized Controlled Trials. *Nutrients* 2016;8

8. Rodriguez-Leyva D, Weighell W, Edel AL, et al. Potent antihypertensive action of dietary flaxseed in hypertensive patients. *Hypertension* 2013;62:1081–9

9. Brouwer IA, Katan MB, Zock PL. Dietary alpha-linolenic acid is associated with reduced risk of fatal coronary heart disease, but increased prostate cancer risk: a meta-analysis. *J Nutr* 2004;134:919–922

10. Caligiuri SP, Aukema HM, Ravandi A, Guzman R, Dibrov E, Pierce GN. Flaxseed consumption reduces blood pressure in patients with hypertension by altering circulating oxylipins via an alpha-linolenic acid-induced inhibition of soluble epoxide hydrolase. *Hypertension* 2014;64:53–9

11. Rodriguez-Leyva D, Dupasquier CM, McCullough R, Pierce GN. The cardiovascular effects of flaxseed and its omega-3 fatty acid, alpha-linolenic acid. *Can J Cardiol* 2010;26:489–96

12. Mohammadi-Sartang M, Sohrabi Z, Barati-Boldaji R, Raeisi-Dehkordi H, Mazloom Z. Flaxseed supplementation on glucose control and insulin sensitivity: a systematic review and meta-analysis of 25 randomized, placebo-controlled trials. *Nutr Rev* 2018;76:125–139

13. Khalesi S, Irwin C, Schubert M. Flaxseed consumption may reduce blood pressure: a systematic review and meta-analysis of controlled trials. *J Nutr* 2015;145:758–765

14. Ursoniu S, Sahebkar A, Andrica F, Serban C, Banach M. Lipid and Blood Pressure Meta-analysis Collaboration (LBPMC) Group. *Clin Nutr* 2016;35:615–625

15. Edel AL, Rodriguez-Leyva D, Maddaford TG, et al. Dietary flaxseed independently lowers circulating cholesterol and lowers it beyond the effects of cholesterol-lowering medications alone in patients with peripheral arterial disease. *J Nutr* 2015;145:749–757

16. Mohammadi-Sartang M, Mazloom Z, Raeisi-Dehkordi H, et al. The effect of flaxseed supplementation on body weight and body composition: a systematic review and meta-analysis of 45 randomized placebo-controlled trials. *Obes Rev* 2017;18:1096–1107

Although there are many ginseng species, Asian or Korean ginseng (*Panax ginseng* CA *Meyer*) and American ginseng (*Panax quinquefolius L*) are the two main ginseng products used for diabetes. The root is the part used. Ginseng has been described as an adaptogen, a product that may increase resistance to adverse influences such as stress and infection. Individuals use both ginseng types as sports performance enhancers, or "ergogenic aids," to help improve physical and athletic stamina. Other uses include psychomotor performance, improved cognitive function, immunomodulation, sexual dysfunction, and diabetes management.[1,2] Panax ginseng is used for prediabetes, and American ginseng is sometimes combined with Panax ginseng to decrease blood pressure.[1] Because of their varied effects both ginseng types are highly used products.[1-3]

Chemical Constituents and Mechanism of Action

Ginseng contains many different chemical ingredients, but the most active ingredients are a family of triterpene saponins called ginsenosides or panaxosides.[1-9] Ginsenosides belong to a steroid family called dammarane-type triterpene glycosides that have either (20S)-protopanaxadiol (PPD) or (20S)-protopanaxatriol (PPT) as the aglycone.[4] Asian and American ginseng may have varying actions due to their varying ginsenoside content. American and Asian ginseng both have PPD ginsenosides, which include Rb1, Rb2, Rc, and Rd. They also both have PPT ginsenosides, including Rg1, Re, and Rf. A higher ratio of PPD to PPT ginsenosides affects glucose lowering potency. Steaming the ginseng may decrease the total ginseng saponins; however, some ginsenosides will increase and others decrease with steaming.[5] Some ginsenosides have opposing effects. For example, ginsenoside Rg1 has hypertensive and central-nervous-system-stimulant effects, while ginsenoside Rb1 has hypotensive and central-nervous-system-depressant effects.[1,9] *In vitro*, Asian ginseng inhibits angiotensin converting enzyme activity.[1] Some ginsenosides inhibit platelets and have analgesic and anti-inflammatory effects. Both Asian and American ginseng may boost the immune system.[2,3] Although it is unknown how ginseng may benefit diabetes, it may decrease the rate of carbohydrate absorption into the portal circulation, increase glucose transport and uptake, promote glucose disposal, enhance β-cell function, and modulate insulin secretion.[3,7,10] American ginseng is most often associated with decreasing postprandial glucose levels.[3,8] Asian ginseng may affect lipid levels by increasing lipoprotein lipase activity.[1,3]

　　White Asian (or Korean) ginseng may be steamed; this causes the roots to turn a red color and possibly alters some of the chemical constituents—this is called Korean red ginseng. Some researchers believe this is a more potent ginseng type.[12]

Nevertheless, it is clear that Asian and American ginseng have distinct ginsenoside content and activity, and researchers have used both types to evaluate ginseng's impact on glycemic parameters in subjects with diabetes.

Adverse Effects and Drug Interactions

Major side effects of both ginseng types include insomnia and restlessness. Worrisome side effects include increased blood pressure or heart rate. However, impact on blood pressure has not always been consistent. Headache is common, and ginseng may also cause mastalgia, mood changes, and nervousness. Ginseng is unsafe in infants and children, and may not be safe in pregnancy.[2] The Rb1 ginsenoside has shown teratogenicity in animals, and there is unreliable information regarding ginseng's effect on lactation.

Ginseng has been reported to decrease the effectiveness of the blood thinner warfarin. However, other reports have not confirmed this effect. Ginseng may decrease the effects of diuretics and hypertension medications. In combination with certain antidepressants, ginseng has resulted in mania. With estrogens, ginseng may produce additive estrogenic effects. Ginseng may inhibit cytochrome P450 (CYP450) 2D6 isoenzymes involved in metabolism of drugs and result in increased effects of drugs such as certain analgesics and some antidepressants.[1] When combined with insulin, sulfonylureas, or other secretagogues, ginseng may cause hypoglycemia.[1,2]

Clinical Studies

Asian and American ginseng have both been extensively studied for diabetes as well as other conditions.[1] A 2012 systematic review of 65 trials in 3,843 subjects evaluated Panax ginseng for various medical disorders.[13] These trials studied ginseng for physical performance, circulatory system problems, glycemic control, quality of life, immunomodulation, and other disorders. The authors noted that further studies are needed because studies used a variety of preparations, which may be problematic. Furthermore, the review included several different disease states. Overall, the review found that results are promising for glucose metabolism and immune response moderation.

Some studies show a benefit for diabetes, while others do not. In a classic study in 36 persons with newly diagnosed type 2 diabetes, ginseng 100 or 200 mg daily was compared with placebo. Although baseline values for glucose and A1C levels were not stated, lower endpoint A1C values were reported.[14] The endpoint A1C level in the 200-mg ginseng group was 6%, and A1C was 6.5% in both the 100-mg and placebo groups. Hence, there may have been an issue with the accuracy of diagnosis or the study population. In two other studies, American ginseng was reported to acutely lower postprandial glucose levels when patients were given a

25-g OGTT.[3,8] In one of these studies, subjects with and without type 2 diabetes were given a 25-g OGTT, with 3 g of ginseng or placebo.[3] Ginseng was given right before or 40 minutes before the OGTT. In subjects without diabetes, there was no difference in postprandial glucose when ginseng was taken right before the OGTT, but when it was taken 40 minutes before, there was a significant decrease in postprandial glucose ($P < 0.05$ vs. placebo). In the participants with diabetes, postprandial glucose decreased whether ginseng was given right before or 40 minutes before the OGTT. The same group of researchers tried the same and higher doses of American ginseng: 3, 6, or 9 g versus placebo.[8] Glucose decreased in all groups, and there was no difference in effect between the three different ginseng doses.

A randomized double-blind placebo-controlled crossover study in 19 persons with type 2 diabetes found that 6 g per day of Korean red ginseng rootlets for 12 weeks did not decrease A1C, but the subjects were at target A1C at baseline (mean A1C of 6.5%).[12] However, some OGTT indices improved, such as peak plasma glucose and peak plasma insulin. Also, fasting insulin sensitivity increased significantly. The authors speculated that ginseng may provide benefits for postprandial carbohydrate metabolism.

A different randomized double-blind placebo-controlled crossover study evaluated 2.2 g per day of Panax ginseng given for 4 weeks to 20 persons with type 2 diabetes.[15] Fasting glucose decreased slightly, but significantly, from 149.4 mg/dL (8.3 mmol/L) to 145.8 mg/dL (8.1 mmol/L; $P < 0.05$). Insulin resistance as measured by homeostatic model of assessment (HOMA-IR) also improved ($P < 0.05$).

In a 4-week double-blind, placebo-controlled trial, 23 subjects with impaired fasting glucose or impaired glucose tolerance and 19 with type 2 diabetes took fermented red ginseng or placebo.[16] The primary outcome was in postprandial glucose; it declined significantly from 167 to 139 mg/dL (9.3 to 7.7 mmol/L) in the ginseng group compared to placebo ($P = 0.008$). Fasting plasma glucose declined significantly from 117 to 110 mg/dL (6.5 to 6.1 mmol/L; $P = 0.039$ vs. baseline), but this was not significant versus placebo.

Another randomized placebo-controlled 30-day trial in 15 overweight or obese subjects (with impaired glucose tolerance or newly-diagnosed type 2 diabetes) found that daily administration of 8 g of ginseng root extract, 250–500 mg of ginsenoside Re, or placebo did not improve β-cell function or insulin sensitivity.[17] The authors theorize that poor systemic bioavailability may have prevented evidence of benefit.

A systematic review evaluated four randomized controlled trials of red ginseng for type 2 diabetes in 76 subjects, with a duration of up to 24 weeks.[18] The weighted mean difference was a decrease in fasting glucose of 7.7 mg/dL (0.43 mmol/L) that was not significant ($P = 0.25$). The A1C weighted mean difference was also not significant (0.14%; $P = 0.32$).

A different 2014 systematic review and meta-analysis of 16 randomized controlled trials in 770 subjects evaluated glycemic control.[19] Fasting glucose was evaluated in all 16 trials, and there was a 5.6 mg/dL (0.31 mmol/L) decrease ($P = 0.03$). Nine trials evaluated A1C, and the decrease was very small and not significant (0.0005%; $P = 0.82$). However, in a subgroup analysis of five parallel trials compared to two crossover trials, there was a small but significant A1C decrease of 0.22% ($P = 0.01$). A limitation noted by the authors of this analysis was that the trials were of short duration. Other problematic issues included use of both Asian and American ginseng and the study populations including persons with and without diabetes. Furthermore, subjects without diabetes in two trials had a baseline median A1C of 5.4% and the median A1C of subjects in seven trials of persons with diabetes indicated good baseline control, since it was 7.1%. The authors of this meta-analysis noted that inconsistencies in inclusion criteria for each study may have led to different outcomes.

A 2016 systematic review and meta-analysis included eight randomized double-blind controlled studies lasting four to 20 weeks in 390 subjects (half assigned to ginseng and half assigned to placebo).[20] Subjects had type 2 diabetes or impaired glucose tolerance. The primary outcome was the change in A1C, and the pooled standard difference in means of three studies did not show a significant difference between the treatment and control groups (0.148 decrease; $P = 0.355$). Subgroup analysis evaluated six studies of fasting glucose and found there was a significant standard difference in means between the ginseng and control groups of 0.306 ($P = 0.01$). There was an improvement in postprandial insulin levels (standard difference in means of 2.132 [$P = 0.008$]). However, the differences for postprandial glucose and fasting insulin were not significant.

Summary

Both Asian and American ginseng may be used by individuals with diabetes. Both ginseng types are complex botanical products containing several ginsenosides with varying effects on blood pressure and the central nervous system. Some estimates indicate that six million Americans use ginseng regularly for a variety of therapeutic reasons, including increased energy.[1] Ginsenoside activity may exhibit considerable variability, and it is important for clinicians to recognize that varying effects may occur. Although ginseng is used for various reasons, it has been frequently studied for diabetes (mostly type 2, but also type 1 diabetes and prediabetes). Since there are two main types, doses vary. Asian ginseng is dosed at 200 mg per day.[1,14] American ginseng is dosed at 3 g per day, right before and up to 2 hours before a meal.[1,3,8] When steamed, white ginseng turns red, and some researchers believe this is a more potent form, but results using this product have been inconsistent. The dose for red ginseng has ranged from 780 mg/day for fermented Korean red ginseng and up to 6 g daily of the Korean red ginseng.[18] Other forms include fresh and dried roots, extracts, solutions, sodas, and teas. Length of use should be limited to 3 months, due to concerns about hormone-like effects.[1] A problematic issue is the inconsistency between the actual amount of active ginsenosides contained in ginseng products and the amount stated on the label.[21] Overall, studies evaluating ginseng have shown very small, if any, decreases in A1C, although there may be decreases in fasting and postprandial glucose. Persons that should avoid ginseng include pregnant and lactating women. Studies where ginseng is added to conventional treatments are emerging. In a small 2019 double-blind randomized crossover trial in 24 subjects, American ginseng or placebo was added to traditional diabetes treatments. In the ginseng group there was a small but significant lowering of A1C of 0.29% ($P = 0.041$) and fasting glucose decreased 12.8 mg/dL (0.71 mmol/L; $P = 0.008$).[22] Although ginseng may provide slight glycemic benefits, it is difficult to definitively specify the appropriate form and dose, and a variety of side effects and drug interactions may occur.

References

1. Natural Medicines (Natural Medicines Database search engine). Available from https://naturalmedicines.therapeuticresearch.com. Accessed May 9, 2019
2. Kiefer D, Pantuso T. Panax ginseng. *Am Fam Physician* 2003;68:1539–1542
3. Vuksan V, Sievenpiper JL, Koo VY, et al. American ginseng (Panax quinquefolius L) reduces postprandial glycemia in nondiabetic subjects and subjects with type 2 diabetes mellitus. *Arch Intern Med* 2000;160:1009–1013
4. Sievenpiper JL, Arnason JT, Leiter LA, Vuksan V. Decreasing, null and increasing effects of eight popular types of ginseng on acute postprandial glycemic indices in healthy humans: the role of ginsenosides. *J Am Coll Nutr* 2004;23:248–258
5. Chen CF, Chiou WF, Zhang JT. Comparison of the pharmacological effects of *Panax ginseng* and *Panax quinquefolium*. *Acta Pharmacol Sin* 2008;29:1103–1108
6. Yuan HD, Kim JT, Kim SH, Chung SH. Ginseng and diabetes: the evidences from in vitro, animal and human studies. *J Ginseng Res* 2012;36:27–39
7. Luo JZ, Luo L. Ginseng on hyperglycemia: effects and mechanisms. *Evid Based Complement Alternat Med* 2009;6:423–427
8. Vuksan V, Stavro MP, Sievenpiper JL, et al. Similar postprandial glycemic reductions with escalation of dose and administration time of American ginseng in type 2 diabetes. *Diabetes Care* 2000;23:1221–1226

9. Raman A, Houston P: Herbal products: ginseng. *Pharm J* 1995;255:150–152

10. Yuan CS, Wu JA, Lowell T, Gu M. Gut and brain effects of American ginseng root on brain-stem neuronal activities in rats. *Am J Chin Med* 1998;26:47–55

11. Mucalo I, Rahelic D, Jovanovski E, et al. Effect of American ginseng (Panax quinquefolius L.) on glycemic control in type 2 diabetes. *Coll Antropol* 2012;36:1435–1440

12. Vuksan V, Sung MK, Sievenpiper JL, et al. Korean red ginseng (Panax ginseng) improves glucose and insulin regulation in well-controlled, type 2 diabetes: results of a randomized, double-blind, placebo-controlled study of efficacy and safety. *Nutr Metab Cardiovasc Dis* 2008;18:46–56

13. Shergis JL, Zhang AL, Zhou W, Xue CC. Panax ginseng in randomised controlled trials: a systematic review. *Phytother Res* 2013;27:949–965

14. Sotaniemi EA, Haapakoski E, Rautio A. Ginseng therapy in non-insulin-dependent diabetic patients. *Diabetes Care* 1995;18:1373–1375

15. Ma SW, Benzie IF, Chu TT, Fok BS, Tomlinson B, Critchley LA. Effect of Panax ginseng supplementation on biomarkers of glucose tolerance, antioxidant status and oxidative stress in type 2 diabetic subjects: results of a placebo-controlled human intervention trial. *Diabetes Obes Metab* 2008;10:1125–1127

16. Oh MR, Park SH, Kim SY, et al. Postprandial glucose lowering effects of fermented red ginseng in subjects with impaired fasting glucose or type 2 diabetes: a randomized double-blind, placebo-controlled trial. *BMC Complement Altern Med* 2014;14:237

17. Reeds DN, Patterson BW, Okunade A, Holloszy JO, Polonsky KS, Klein S. Ginseng and ginsenoside Re do not improve beta-cell function or insulin sensitivity in overweight and obese subjects with impaired glucose tolerance or diabetes. *Diabetes Care* 2011;34:1071–1076

18. Kim S, Shin BC, Lee MS, Lee H, Ernst E. Red ginseng for type 2 diabetes mellitus: a systematic review of randomized controlled trials. *Chin J Integr Med* 2011;17:937–944

19. Shishtar E, Sievenpiper JL, Djedovic V, et al. The effect of ginseng (the genus panax) on glycemic control: a systematic review and meta-analysis of randomized controlled clinical trials. *PLoS One* 2014;9:e107391

20. Gui QF, Xu ZR, Xu KY, Yang YM. The efficacy of ginseng-related therapies in type 2 diabetes mellitus: an updated systematic review and meta-analysis. *Medicine* (Baltimore) 2016;95:e2584

21. Harkey MR, Henderson GL, Gershwin ME, Stern JS, Hackman RM. Variability in commercial ginseng products: an analysis of 25 preparations. *Am J Clin Nutr* 2001;73:1101–1106

22. Vuksan V, Xu ZZ, Jovanovski E, et al. Efficacy and safety of American ginseng (*Panax quinquefolius* L.) extract on glycemic control and cardio-vascular risk factors in individuals with type 2 diabetes: a double-blind, randomized crossover clinical trial. *Eur J Nutr* 2019;58:1237–1245

GYMNEMA (*Gymnema sylvestre R. Br.*)

A member of the milkweed family, gymnema (*Gymnema sylvestre* R.Br.) is a woody climbing plant that is found in the tropical forests of India as well as in Africa and Australia.[1] Used for centuries in Ayurvedic medicine, it is also known as *gurmar*, the "sugar destroyer," because it dulls the tongue's ability to taste "sweetness."[2] The leaves are the part used for medicinal purposes.[3] Gymnema has been used for both type 1 and type 2 diabetes and has a unique history of research and use.[3-8] It also used for metabolic syndrome, weight loss, hyperlipidemia, constipation, infections, asthma, and other conditions.[9]

Chemical Constituents and Mechanism of Action

The chemical constituents are triterpene saponins (also known as gymnemic acids), gymnemasaponins, and gurmarin, a polypeptide. The gymnemic acids and gymnemasaponins are members of oleanane type of saponins, while gymnemasides are dammarane saponins.[9] Other constituents include stigmasterol, betaine, and choline. Gymnemic acid and gurmarin block sweet taste, and this is reputed to mitigate "sugar craving." The exact mechanism of action is unknown, but one thought is that gymnemic acids block glucose absorption in the small intestine.[5] Gymnema also may stimulate pancreatic β-cell function, increase numbers of pancreatic β-cells, and possibly increase insulin release.[3] Thus, the overall mechanism is through stimulation of pancreatic insulin secretion and possible delayed glucose absorption.[9]

Adverse Effects and Drug Interactions

The most relevant potential adverse effect is hypoglycemia, particularly at higher than usual doses.[9] Also, toxic hepatitis has been reported.[1]

Gymnema may enhance the blood glucose lowering effects of certain drugs used to treat diabetes, resulting in hypoglycemia. These drugs include insulin, sulfonylureas, or nonsulfonylurea secretagogues. Gymnema may also affect the Cytochrome P450 system. It may inhibit the CYP 1A2 system; thus, it may increase serum concentrations of some psychiatric meds, such as clozapine (Clozaril®) or fluvoxamine (Luvox®), metabolized through CYP 1A2, although there is contradictory evidence. It may induce or inhibit the CYP 2C9 system and thus affect warfarin or ibuprofen, which are metabolized through CYP 2C9. There is conflicting information on whether gymnema affects CYP 3A4. Some reports indicate that it may inhibit this enzyme and thus increase serum concentrations of medications such as calcium channel blockers and some antibiotics, although other reports state that there is no impact.[1]

Trials conducted in persons with type 1 and type 2 diabetes have reported decreases in A1C, fasting blood glucose, and sometimes postprandial glucose, lipids, and blood pressure.[3,4,6-8] However, some studies omit important details of study design, such as blinding and randomization.

In one of the original studies in 27 patients with type 1 diabetes, gymnema was administered at a dose of 200 mg twice a day for 6–30 months.[3] The researchers tracked A1C, fasting blood glucose, and insulin dose. Average A1C declined from 12.8% at baseline to 9.5% after 6–8 months ($P < 0.001$); and after 16–18 months, 22 individuals continuing to take gymnema had a mean A1C of 9% (P values not stated). At the end of 26–30 months, six patients remaining on gymnema had a further decline to 8.2% (P values not stated). Average fasting glucose declined from 232 mg/dL (12.9 mmol/L) at baseline to 177 mg/dL (9.8 mmol/L) after 6–8 months, 150 mg/dL (8.2 mmol/L) after 16–18 months, and 152 mg/dL (8.4 mmol/L) after 20–24 months (P values not stated). Average insulin dose decreased from 60 units/day to 45 units/day after 6–8 months, and declined further to 30 units/day after 26–30 months (P values not stated). A control group of 37 patients who took only insulin was also followed for 10–12 months, and these individuals had no change in blood glucose or A1C.

In a different study, 22 patients with type 2 diabetes took gymnema at a dose of 400 mg daily for 18–20 months in addition to a sufonylurea.[4] A1C declined from an average baseline of 11.9% to 8.5% ($P < 0.001$), and average fasting glucose decreased from 174 mg/dL (9.7 mmol/L) at baseline to 124 mg/dL (6.9 mmol/L) after 18–20 months ($P < 0.001$). Notably, five individuals were able to discontinue sulfonylurea treatment. Lipids also significantly declined in this study. A control group of 25 patients on sulfonylureas plus placebo had no significant changes in A1C, fasting glucose, or lipids.

An open-label study evaluated 250 mg twice daily of gymnema leaf extract or placebo for three months in 58 persons with type 2 diabetes.[6] A total of 39 took gymnema, and 19 took either placebo or no supplement. A1C decreased approximately 1% in the gymnema group (9.6% to 8.6%; $P < 0.001$). Fasting glucose also decreased significantly from 189 mg/dL (10.5 mmol/L) to 163 mg/dL (9 mmol/L; $P < 0.005$). Post-meal glucose also declined significantly from 275 mg/dL (15.3 mmol/L) to 216 mg/dL (12 mmol/L) (exact P not provided, but authors stated it was significant at $P < 0.001$). There was also a small, significant decrease in systolic blood pressure from 139.1 mm Hg to 132.4 mm Hg ($P < 0.005$). Diastolic pressure also decreased significantly from 84.1 mm Hg to 81.6 mm Hg ($P < 0.05$) Study design was sub-optimal, since it was open label, and there was no statistical analysis comparing active product to the non-active comparator.

A study evaluating gymnema in type 2 diabetes noted a decrease in fasting glucose at 30 days.[7] In this study, *Gymnema sylvestre* (ground herb purchased from a local market) 500 mg twice daily was administered for 30 days to eight subjects who were on oral hypoglycemic drugs. Fasting glucose declined significantly from 219 mg/dL (12.2 mmol/L) to 138 mg/dL (7.7 mmol/L; $P < 0.05$). There was a decrease in lipids as well, although the results were not significant. Gymnema was then stopped for 10 days, and glucose and lipids were re-measured at day 40. The decrease in fasting glucose and lipids was not sustained at day 40. Other botanical products (with hypoglycemic effects in animal research) or placebo were administered as comparators. Eight subjects each were given *Citrullus colocynthis*, *Artemisia absinthium*, or placebo. The decrease from baseline in fasting glucose in the active comparator groups was significant ($P < 0.05$). Lipids decreased in the botanical product groups, but the results were not significant. The authors did not report any results for the placebo group. Additionally, the authors did not state whether randomization or blinding occurred, and did not provide a statistical analysis comparing gymnema to the other groups.

Another article reported the results of 500 mg twice daily of a patented *aqueous alcohol extract* of gymnema leaf administered for 60 days in 11 subjects.[8] Mean fasting glucose decreased from 162 mg/dL (9 mmol/L) to 119 mg/dL (6.6 mmol/L; $P < 0.005$) and postprandial glucose decreased from 291 mg/dL (16.2 mmol/L) to 236 mg/dL (13.1 mmol/L; $P < .02$). Furthermore, serum insulin and C-peptide levels also increased significantly ($P < 0.001$ and $P < 0.05$). Additionally, the researchers evaluated the impact in vitro of the gymnema extract on isolated human islets of Langerhans cells and found an increase in insulin secretion.

A randomized double-blind placebo-controlled trial evaluated 24 overweight individuals with untreated metabolic syndrome.[10] Half the subjects took 300 mg twice daily of gymnema and half took placebo for 12 weeks. In the treatment group body weight decreased significantly from 178.9 lb (81.3 kg) at baseline to 171.4 lb (77.9 kg; $P = 0.02$), and body mass index also decreased significantly from 31.2 kg/m² to 30.4 kg/m² ($P = 0.02$). The placebo group had statistically significant increases in body weight and BMI compared to baseline ($P = 0.01$ and $P = 0.03$, respectively). The treatment group did not have significant changes in insulin secretion or insulin sensitivity, glucose, or lipids, except for a slight decrease in very low density lipoprotein (VLDL) cholesterol from baseline ($P = 0.05$). The main study limitation was the small sample size.

Summary

Gymnema has limited efficacy data in humans. Gymnema has been studied for up to two years in type 1 diabetes and type 2 diabetes. It is sometimes combined with other supplements.[1] The gymnemosides may help stimulate glucose uptake and utilization as well as stimulate β-cell function.[9] Some have speculated that gymnema may help treat obesity since it binds to the same taste buds where sugar binds and thus may help curb sugar craving.[5] A limited systematic review evaluated gymnema for obesity and diabetes management in animal and clinical studies. This review concluded that although gymnema has antidiabetes properties, additional human studies are needed to fully assess its benefits.[11] Typical doses are 400 mg per day, standardized to contain 24% gymnemic acids.[3,4] However, aqueous alcohol extract and ground herb forms are emerging, and varied doses and combinations have been used.[1,7,8] For example, a high molecular weight extract at a dose of 500 mg twice daily has been used.[8] Gymnema should not be used without medical supervision because of potential hypoglycemia and a case report of hepatitis. Doses of secretagogues or insulin may have to be lowered if gymnema is used. Any person taking warfarin should be particularly cautious since gymnema may induce or inhibit its metabolism, and clinicians should carefully monitor its use in this situation. Likewise, monitoring is advised when other medications are used such as calcium channel blockers or certain antibiotics due to inconsistent effects on increasing their serum concentrations. Because hypoglycemia may occur, gymnema should be discontinued 2 weeks prior to elective surgery. The safety of gymnema may also be a concern when combined with other diabetes medications as well as in vulnerable populations, such as children, elderly, and pregnant or lactating women.[1]

References

1. Natural Medicines (Natural Medicines Database search engine). Available from https://naturalmedicines.therapeuticresearch.com. Accessed May 9, 2019
2. Yoshikawa M, Murakami T, Kadoya M, et al. Medicinal foodstuffs. IX. The inhibitors of glucose absorption from the leaves of Gymnema sylvestre R. BR. (Asclepiadaceae): structures of gymnemosides a and b. *Chem Pharm Bull* (Tokyo) 1997;45:1671–1676
3. Shanmugasundaram ER, Rajeswari G, Baskaran K, Rajesh Kumar BR, Radha Shanmugasundaram K, Kizar Ahmath B. Use of Gymnema sylvestre leaf extract in the control of blood glucose in insulin-dependent diabetes mellitus. *J Ethnopharmacol* 1990;30:281–294
4. Baskaran K, Kizar Ahamath B, Radha Shanmugasundaram K, Shanmugasundaram ER. Antidiabetic effect of a leaf extract from Gymnema sylvestre in non-insulin-dependent diabetes mellitus patients. *J Ethnopharmacol* 1990;30:295–300
5. Kanetkar P, Singhal R, Kamat M. Gymnema sylvestre: a memoir. *J Clin Biochem Nutr* 2007;41:77–81
6. Kumar SN, Mani UV, Mani I. An open label study on the supplementation of Gymnema sylvestre in type 2 diabetics. *J Diet Suppl* 2010;7:273–282

7. Li Y, Zheng M, Zhai X, et al. Effect of gymnema sylvestre, citrullus colocynthis and artemisia absinthium on blood gluocse and lipid profile in diabetic human. *Acta Pol Pharm* 2015;72:981–985

8. Al-Romaiyan A, Liu B, Asare-Anane H, et al. A novel Gymnema sylvestre extract stimulates insulin secretion from human islets in vivo and in vitro. *Phytother Res* 2010;24:1370–1376

9. Tiwari P, Mishra BN, Sangwan NS. Phytochemical and pharmacological properties of Gymnema sylvestre: an important medicinal plant. *Biomed Res Int* 2014;2014:830285

10. Zuniga LY, Gonzalez-Ortiz M, Martinez-Abundis E. Effect of Gymnema sylvestre administration on metabolic syndrome, insulin sensitivity, and insulin secretion. *J Med Food* 2017;20:750–754

11. Pothuraju R, Sharma RK, Chagalamarri J, Jangra S, Kumar Kavadi P. A systematic review of Gymnema sylvestre in obesity and diabetes management. *J Sci Food Agric* 2014;94:834–840

HOLY BASIL (*O tenuiflorum L.*; Formerly known as *Ocimum sanctum L.*)

Holy basil is an herb native to India and is regarded as one of the most important plants used in Ayurvedic medicine. It is known by other names, including sacred basil, green holy basil, and hot basil (because of the peppery taste).[1] Another name is *tulsi*, a Hindu word meaning "the incomparable one."[2] It has a pleasant aroma and is available in both red and green varieties. It is planted and grows abundantly around Hindu temples, and it is now widely grown throughout the world. The plant is hairy with multiple branches and small, tender leaves. The leaves, stems, seeds, and oil are used medicinally, but it is a common ingredient in Indian cuisine.[1]

Although holy basil has been used to treat diabetes, it has primarily been used to treat infections, such as colds, influenza, malaria, and tuberculosis.[1,2] It has been used as a mosquito repellant and a topical treatment for ringworm. It has also been used as an antidote for scorpion and snake bites.[1] In animals, it has analgesic and fever-reducing properties and protective effects against the ulcer-producing effects of anti-inflammatory drugs such as aspirin.[3,4] It is also used for stress and obesity.[1,5]

Chemical Constituents and Mechanism of Action

The leaves contain essential oils that yield eugenol, methyl eugenol, and caryophyllene, but also other substances such as ursolic acid and apigenin.[6] It is unknown which of the chemical components may be responsible for the benefit in diabetes, however eugenol is thought to be the most bioactive constituent. Other ingredients with glucose-lowering effects include polyphenols, caffeic acid, chicoric acid, and p-coumaric acid compound.[7] Overall, eugenol and ursolic acid are thought to be the most relevant constituents.[1] Holy basil contains zinc, which may help reduce insulin resistance. It improves the activity of certain enzymes involved in carbohydrate metabolism—glucokinase, hexokinase, and phosphofructokinase.[8] Researchers have theorized that basil leaves may improve pancreatic β-cell function and thus enhance insulin secretion.[6,7]

Adverse Effects and Drug Interactions

In the one major trial for diabetes in humans, no side effects were reported. However, in animals, there are various side effects. It may lower thyroxine (T4) and thus worsen hypothyroidism. It may also have some antiplatelet properties, resulting in bleeding. Holy basil has some anti-androgenic properties and may decrease sperm count and possibly decrease fertility.[1]

There are no reported cases of drug interactions involving holy basil. Theoretical interactions would be possible hypoglycemia when combined with secretagogues or insulin. Holy basil seed oil may increase the risk of bleeding; thus, caution is warranted if combined with anticoagulant and antiplatelet drugs such as aspirin, warfarin, clopidogrel, or CAM supplements that have antiplatelet activity. In theory, holy basil may also interact with sedatives since, per animal data, there is information that it increases pentobarbitone-induced duration of sleep.[1]

Clinical Studies

A small controlled trial evaluated 2.5 g daily of holy basil dried leaf powder and placebo leaf powder in 40 patients with type 2 diabetes.[6] Half the patients had well-established type 2 diabetes and were on oral diabetes medications. Patients were asked to stop their diabetes medications seven days before the start of the trial; then all patients were given holy basil for a run-in period of 5 days. Half were randomly assigned to take the holy basil and 20 were given placebo for 4 weeks and then crossed over to the other treatment group without a washout period for another 4 weeks. Researchers measured fasting and 2-hour postprandial blood glucose as well as total cholesterol. In the first group, mean fasting glucose declined from 134.5 mg/dL (7.5 mmol/L) to 99.7 mg/dL (5.5 mmol/L) after 4 weeks of treatment with holy basil. After patients crossed over to placebo for 4 weeks, fasting glucose increased to 115.6 mg/dL (6.4 mmol/L). In the placebo-first group, mean fasting glucose declined from 132.4 mg/dL (7.4 mmol/L) to 123.2 mg/dL (6.8 mmol/L) after 4 weeks and then declined even further to 97.2 mg/dL (5.4 mmol/L) after they crossed over to holy basil for 4 weeks. Overall, mean fasting blood glucose was 21 mg/dL (1.2 mmol/L) lower in the holy basil group ($P < 0.001$), and postprandial blood glucose decreased during the 4-week treatment with holy basil by 16 mg/dL (0.88 mmol/L; $P < 0.02$). Total cholesterol decreased from 238.2 mg/dL (6.2 mmol/L) to 221.5 mg/dL (5.7 mmol/L). However, the results were not significant. There were no adverse effects reported by those taking holy basil or placebo.

Another 90-day randomized trial compared glibenclamide (glyburide) 5 mg daily to glibenclamide 5 mg daily plus holy basil 250 mg twice daily, with 30 subjects in each group.[9] The researchers measured fasting and postprandial glucose as well as A1C at baseline and 90 days. In the glibenclamide-only group, fasting glucose decreased from 174 mg/dL (9.7 mmol/L) at baseline to 114.5 mg/dL (6.4 mmol/L) at 90 days. Fasting glucose in the glibenclamide plus holy basil group decreased from 171.5 mg/dL (9.5 mmol/L) to 103.5 mg/dL (5.8 mmol/L). Postprandial glucose in the glibenclamide group decreased from 247 mg/dL (13.7 mmol/L) to 152 mg/dL (8.4 mmol/L). Postprandial glucose in the glibenclamide plus holy basil group decreased from 254 mg/dL (14.1 mmol/L) to 143 mg/dL (7.9 mmol/L). All of the decreases were significant ($P < 0.05$ for all groups compared to baseline). The A1C decreased from 7.6% at baseline to 5.3% in the glibenclamide group after 90 days, while A1C decreased in the glibenclamide plus holy basil group from 7.76% to 4.98%. The A1C decrease was significant for both groups ($P < 0.05$ for both groups compared to baseline). However, the authors did not provide a statistical evaluation (P value) comparing the glibenclamide to glibenclamide plus holy basil groups for any of the measurements (fasting or postprandial glucose or A1C). Moreover, the authors did not state whether the subjects were blinded to the treatment provided.

Summary

Holy basil is an important herb used in Ayurvedic medicine. It is used for a variety of ailments such as respiratory disorders, arthritis, and inflammation, as well as stress and diabetes. In patients with type 2 diabetes, a leaf extract was found to reduce fasting blood glucose by 17.6% and postprandial blood glucose by 7.3% as well as to result in a small decrease in total cholesterol.[6] It has also been combined with the sulfonylurea glibenclamide (glyburide) and compared to glibenclamide monotherapy.[9] Although it has been widely studied in animals, there are only a few trials in humans with type 2 diabetes. Caution is warranted, because animal data indicates a potential for increased bleeding risk if combined with anticoagulant or antiplatelet drugs or herbs (ginkgo, garlic, ginger, or others). Thus, it should be discontinued 2 weeks before elective surgery. There is also a possibility of lowered sperm count and decreased fertility. Per animal data, high doses decreased implantation rates and decreased full term pregnancies. There is no adequate information on lactation, and thus it probably should be avoided in nursing women. Holy basil may also augment the effects of sedatives.[1] There is no typical dose, but 2.5 g dried leaf powder once daily to 250 mg twice daily has been used.[6,9] It may be found in combination with other supplements. Holy Basil may be appropriate for people with diabetes as a food, if used in moderation, but is questionable in supplement form.

References

1. Natural Medicines (Natural Medicines Database search engine). Available from https://naturalmedicines.therapeuticresearch.com. Accessed May 9, 2019
2. Cohen MM. Tulsi – Ocimum sanctum: a herb for all reasons. *J Ayurveda Integr Med* 2014;5:251–259
3. Godhwani S, Godhwani JL, Vyas DS. *Ocimum sanctum*: an experimental study evaluating its anti-inflammatory, analgesic and antipyretic activity in animals. *J Ethnopharmacol* 1987;21:153–163
4. Khanna N, Bhatia J. Antinociceptive action of *Ocimum sanctum* (Tulsi) in mice: possible mechanisms involved. *J Ethnopharmacol* 2003;88:293–296

5.   Saxena RC, Singh R, Kumar P, et al. Efficacy of an extract of *Ocimum tenuiflorum* (OciBest) in the management of general stress: a double-blind, placebo-controlled study. *Evid Based Complement Alternat Med* 2012;2012:894509. doi: 10.1155/2012/894509

6.   Agrawal P, Rai V, Singh RB. Randomized placebo-controlled, single blind trial of holy basil leaves in patients with noninsulin-dependent diabetes mellitus. *Int J Clin Pharmacol Ther* 1996;34:406–409

7.   Antora RA, Salleh RM. Antihyperglycemic effect of *Ocimum* plants: a short review. *Asian Pac J Trop Biomed* 2017;7:755–759

8.   Kapoor S. *Ocimum sanctum*: a therapeutic role in diabetes and the metabolic syndrome. *Horm Metab Res* 2008;40:296

9.   Somasundaram G, Manimekalai K, Salwe KJ, Pandiamunian J. Evaluation of the antidiabetic effect of *Ocimum sanctum* in type 2 diabetic patients. *International Journal of Life Science & Pharma Research* 2012;2:75–81

HONEY (Sometimes Known as Manuka Honey)

Honey is a product produced by bees when pollinating different plants. It is a popular sweetener, though due to carbohydrate content, persons with diabetes sometimes use it sparingly. Honey has been used medicinally for thousands of years. Some uses include treatment of asthma, cough, allergic reactions, hyperlipidemia, and diabetes (to lower glucose as well as topically to treat ulcers). Topical honey has also been used for mucositis, an adverse effect of irradiation or chemotherapy.[1] Manuka honey (Medihoney®) is an FDA-approved medical device often used as a wound dressing. Manuka honey is derived from the manuka tree, *Leptospermum scoparium*.[2]

Chemical Constituents and Mechanism of Action

Honey is produced by bees from the nectar of flowers. The source may be monofloral (where bees predominantly forage on one plant type) or multifloral, where the bees use several botanical sources.[2] Honey contains both fructose and glucose.[3] Different honey preparations may vary in the content of fructose and glucose, and some researchers have speculated that the hypoglycemic effect may depend on the fructose content.[4] The fructose to glucose ratio may affect glucose lowering.

In addition to fructose and glucose, honey also contains oligosaccharides, such as palatinose (isomaltulose), as well as phenolic acids, flavonoids, proteins, amino acids, fatty acids, vitamins, and various enzymes.[2,5]

Some theorized mechanisms of action are attributed to fructose—it may stimulate insulin release and glucose uptake. Fructose may enhance hepatic glucose uptake by glucokinase activation, and glycogen synthase activation may promote glycogen synthesis and storage.[3] Oligosaccharides as well as fructose may stimulate pancreatic insulin secretion.[3,5] The glucose-lowering effect of honey may be due to pancreatic antioxidant effects. These antioxidant properties may contribute not only to glucose lowering effects but also to reduced levels of triglycerides and increased HDL cholesterol.[5] Honey may also have prebiotic properties that enhance the effects of *Bifidobacterium* species.[1,5]

Honey may also help decrease weight; the theorized mechanism may be through modulation of appetite regulating hormones, such as ghrelin and peptide YY.[5,6]

Honey has been studied topically in wound care, due to various effects, such as providing a protective barrier and a moist environment that promotes healing and epithelialization, as well as antimicrobial effects.[1,2,7] Honey suppresses inflammatory cell propagation at wound sites, stimulates production of certain inflammatory cytokines that allow healing, and promotes fibroblast and epithelial cell proliferation. Honey also has a 5,8-kDa component that stimulates immune cell activity.[2] These effects may be due to both antioxidant and antimicrobial properties.[2,7] These mechanisms may be critical in promoting foot ulcer healing in persons with diabetes. However, some studies of wound healing benefits have been of low quality.[1]

Adverse Effects and Drug Interactions

The most common side effects are gastrointestinal upset, such as stomach ache, nausea, and vomiting. Honey may be potentially dangerous, since honey made from pollination of certain plants may be toxic. Honey from the rhododendron plant in particular may be toxic, due to presence of grayanotoxins, which may cause adverse cardiac effects. Honey may be contaminated with microorganisms and dust. While most contaminants will not survive, spore-forming organisms associated with botulism may remain; thus, honey should not be given to children under 1 year of age due to the risk of possibly containing botulinum toxin. Medical-grade topical honey is irradiated with gamma rays and thus has low risk for bacterial spores. As a food, honey has not been problematic in pregnant or lactating women, but it is unknown whether medicinal use is appropriate.[1]

Honey may interact with anticoagulants such as warfarin or antiplatelets such as clopidogrel, resulting in possible bleeding reactions. Honey may also impact the pharmacokinetics of the anticonvulsant phenytoin, leading to increased absorption.

Clinical Studies

There are few human studies evaluating honey in diabetes, but murine research supports its use, either alone or in combination with diabetes medications.[5] The following are examples of studies in type 1 and type 2 diabetes.

A complex randomized crossover trial in 20 subjects with type 1 diabetes (aged 4 to 18 years) evaluated the impact of 0.5 mL/kg/day of honey compared to a control group.[8] Subjects were randomized to honey or control for 12 weeks; then they were crossed over to the other group for an additional 12 weeks. The dietary intervention after 12 weeks resulted in a decrease in both fasting plasma glucose (−21.5 mg/dL vs. −0.08 mg/dL [1.19 mmol/L vs. 0.0044 mmol/L]; $P = 0.001$) and 2-hour postprandial plasma glucose (−13.5 mg/dL vs. −0.77 mg/dL [0.75 mmol/L vs. 0.042 mmol/L]; $P = 0.031$) in the group randomized to honey consumption. Moreover, in going from the intervention to control from baseline to 24 weeks, results were significant for the group randomized to honey. At 24 weeks, fasting glucose decreased from 169.5 mg/dL to 142.7 mg/dL (9.4 mmol/L to 7.9 mmol/L; $P = 0.005$). At 24 weeks, postprandial glucose decreased from 210 mg/dL to 167 mg/dL (11.7 mmol/L to 9.3 mmol/L; $P = 0.001$). The A1C also decreased significantly from 7.6% to 6.7% ($P = 0.043$). There was also a significant decrease in lipids.

An open-label study in 97 subjects with type 2 diabetes evaluated the effects of clover honey on an oral glucose tolerance test (OGTT).[9] The study compared two doses of honey and one of glucose: 75 g (Group 1) and 30 g (Group 2) of honey, and 75 g (Group 3) of glucose. The study found that mean rise in blood glucose value at 2 hours was 85 mg/dL (4.7 mmol/L) in Group 1 (75 g of honey), 30 mg/dL (1.67 mmol/L) in Group 2 (30 g of honey), and 170 mg/dL (9.4 mmol/L) in Group 3 (75 g of glucose). The difference between groups was statistically significant ($P < 0.005$). The glucose response for Group 2 (30 g of honey) compared to Group 1 (75 g of honey) or Group 3 (75 g of glucose), was also significant ($P < 0.001$). This study illustrated that there is a lower glycemic response to honey, which can result in a smaller rise in plasma blood glucose following ingestion of honey compared to oral glucose.

An 8-week randomized controlled trial in 48 persons with type 2 diabetes evaluated the impact of increasing doses of natural unprocessed honey compared to control (this group did not take placebo; they simply did not ingest any honey).[10] During the first two weeks, the intervention group ingested 1 g/kg/day, then in the next 2 weeks 1.5 g/kg/day, in the third 2-week period 2 g/kg/day, and in the last 2 weeks 2.5 g/kg/day. In the intervention group, fasting glucose declined from 153 mg/dL to 124 mg/dL (8.5 to 6.8 mmol/L), whereas in the control group the fasting glucose decreased slightly from 136 mg/dL to 132 mg/dL (7.5 to 7.3 mmol/L; $P = 0.01$ for honey vs. control). After adjustment for baseline values the authors reported there was no overall significant difference in fasting glucose ($P = 0.068$). However, A1C increased from 7.1% to 7.7% in the honey group and from 7.1% to 7.3% in the control group ($P = 0.104$ for honey vs. control). Although the difference in A1C between groups was not significant, the increase from baseline in the honey group was significant ($P < 0.01$). Some researchers have theorized that the reason for this was a lower fructose-to-glucose ratio in the type of honey used in this study. However, the honey group did have a significant decrease in weight at eight weeks compared to the control. ($P = 0.000$, per the author). The actual weight decreased from a baseline of 157 lb to 153 lb (71.3 kg to 69.5 kg) at eight weeks in the honey group. In the control group, the weight remained stable at 155 lb (70.3 kg) from baseline to eight weeks.

A randomized anthropometric controlled crossover trial in 53 persons with type 2 diabetes evaluated the impact of milk vetch honey (50 g/day) or no honey (no active comparator; only weight maintenance).[6] There were two 8-week sequences with a 4-week washout, and then subjects were crossed over to the other group. Fasting glucose increased in both groups (135 to 143 mg/dL [7.5 mmol/L to 7.9 mmol/L] in the honey group and 129 to 135 mg/dL [7.2 mmol/L to 7.5 mmol/L] in the control group; $P = 0.71$ between groups). The A1C increased slightly in the honey group and decreased significantly in the control group (6.9% to 7% in the honey group [$P = 0.22$] and 7% to 6.8% in the control group [$P = 0.03$]). The A1C difference was significant between the two groups, favoring the control group ($P = 0.02$). Interestingly, weight decreased slightly in both groups, although the difference was not significant between groups ($P = 0.22$).

Manuka honey has been compared to conventional wound care treatments to treat diabetic foot ulcers.[7] A 16-week prospective randomized control trial evaluated Manuka honey in 32 subjects and conventional treatment in 31 subjects. Manuka honey impregnated dressings were used in the treatment group, and saline soaked dressings were used in the control group. Time to healing in the honey group was 31 days, and 43 days in the control group ($P < 0.05$). Honey dressings also eliminated the need for antibiotics and hospitalization.

Summary

Honey has been theorized to lower glucose in both type 1 and type 2 diabetes, although results may be conflicting. There is much speculation and discussion about potential mechanisms, but overall the fructose content and fructose-to-glucose ratio may be determining factors. The benefit may involve lowering fasting and postprandial glucose as well as weight and some lipid parameters. The impact on A1C has been variable, and even increased in one clinical study, which may have been affected by fructose content.[10] Topical use may be of interest to patients with diabetes since it has successfully treated diabetes-related foot ulcers, accelerating healing time and eliminating need for antibiotic treatment or hospitalization.[7] However, study design evaluating honey for diabetic foot ulcers has not been optimal. Overall, the risks of using honey are not great, but its use should be avoided in young children under one year of age due to the potential for Clostridium botulinum content. Honey from the rhododendron plant is toxic, due to potential adverse cardiac effects such as chest pain, hypotension, and arrhythmias.[1] Doses used have ranged from 50 g daily to 1–2.5 g or 0.5 mL/kg per day for 8-12 weeks.[6,8-10] As a food, honey has not been problematic, but patients with diabetes are encouraged to work with a Diabetes Care and Education Specialist to determine whether honey as a component of a nutrition plan is advisable. Further research is warranted to validate findings from studies presented in this monograph and to help clarify whether fructose content, fructose-to-glucose ratio, or type of honey are key factors for efficacy.

References

1.   Natural Medicines (Natural Medicines Database search engine). Available from https://naturalmedicines.therapeuticresearch.com. Accessed May 9, 2019

2. Alvarez-Suarez JM, Gasparrini M, Forbes-Hernandez TY, Mazzoni L, Giampieri F. The composition and biological activity of honey: a focus on Manuka honey. *Foods* 2014;3:420–432

3. Erejuwa OO, Sulaiman SA, Wahab MS. Fructose might contribute to the hypoglycemic effect of honey. *Molecules* 2012;17:1900–1915

4. Deibert P, Koenig D, Kloock B, Groenefeld M, Berg A. Glycaemic and insulinaemic properties of some German honey varieties. *Eur J Clin Nutr* 2010;64:762–764

5. Erejuwa OO, Sulaiman SA, Wahab MS. Honey--a novel antidiabetic agent. *Int J Biol Sci* 2012;8:913–934

6. Sadeghi F, Salehi S, Kohanmoo A, Akhlaghi M. Effect of natural honey on glycemic control and anthropometric measures of patients with type 2 diabetes: a randomized controlled crossover trial. *Int J Prev Med* 2019;10:3

7. Kamaratos AV, Tzirogiannis KN, Iraklianou SA, et al. Manuka honey-impregnated dressings in the treatment of neuropathic diabetic foot ulcers. *Int Wound J* 2014;11:259–263

8. Abdulrhman MM, El-Hefnawy MH, Aly RH, et al. Metabolic effects of honey in type 1 diabetes mellitus: a randomized crossover pilot study. *J Med Food* 2013;16:66–72

9. Nazir L, Samad F, Haroon W, Kidwai SS, Haroon W, Siddiqi S, Zehravi M. Comparison of glycaemic response to honey and glucose in type 2 diabetes. *J Pak Med Assoc* 2014;64:69–71

10. Bahrami M, Ataie-Jafari A, Hosseini S, Foruzanfar MH, Rahmani M, Pajouhi M. Effects of natural honey consumption in diabetic patients: an 8-week randomized clinical trial. *Int J Food Sci Nutr* 2009;60:618–626

IVY GOURD (*Coccinia indica*, also known as *Coccinia cordifolia* and *Coccinia grandis*)

Ivy gourd is a unique tropical member of the family Cucurbitaceae.[1,2] It grows well in India, Southeast Asia, and the Philippines. It has spread to Australia and has been found in Fiji, Tonga, and Hawaii. Ivy gourd is an aggressive climbing perennial vine that spreads quickly over trees and shrubs. The leaves range from 5–10 cm (about 2–4 inches) in length and have five lobes that vary from a heart to a pentagon shape. Ivy gourd is a dioecious plant, and the white male and female flowers grow separately. The fruit starts out green and turns red when ripe. It has been classified as a medicinal herb in the traditional practice of ancient Thai medicine. For medicinal purposes, several parts of the plant have been used, including the leaves, roots, stems, and whole plant. The juice of the roots, leaves, and fruit are used in diabetes, and the leaves are also used as a poultice for skin eruptions.[1,2]

In Thailand, the young leaves and tips are blanched and prepared in stir-fry dishes, or the leaves are used in curries or for dipping chili paste. Leaves and stems are also added to soup dishes with different meats or noodles. The young leaves are boiled with porridge, then crushed and fed to young children. Other parts of the plant are also used for burns, insect bites, fever, gastrointestinal complaints, and various eye infections.[2]

Chemical Constituents and Mechanism of Action

Ivy gourd contains β-carotene, a major vitamin A precursor from plant sources.[2] As a food, it is thought to be a good source of protein and fiber, and it contains moderate amounts of calcium. As a medicinal agent in diabetes, the definitive active ingredients are unknown. However, the leaves contain triterpenes and the fruit contains pectin.[1] It also contains trace amounts of alkaloids.[3] Per animal studies, it is thought to suppress the activity of certain enzymes involved in glucose production, such as glucose-6-phosphatase and and lactate dehydrogenase. In the lipolytic pathway it may restore lipoprotein lipase activity.[1,4] It may have some insulin-like activity.[3]

Adverse Effects and Drug Interactions

In the limited number of trials evaluating ivy gourd in diabetes, only mild GI upset, headache, and drowsiness may occur. Symptoms of mild hypoglycemia (perspiration, dizziness, and excessive hunger) have been reported.[5] A theoretical side effect may be allergic reactions to some plant constituents. Drug interactions have not been reported, but theoretically, hypoglycemia may occur if ivy gourd is combined with secretagogues or insulin.

A randomized double-blind placebo-controlled trial was conducted in India in 32 patients with type 2 diabetes, many of whom were newly diagnosed.[3] Crushed leaf powder was compounded into 300-mg tablets, and 16 patients took three tablets twice daily for 6 weeks. There were 16 patients randomized to the placebo group (three tablets twice daily). The researchers measured baseline fasting glucose and then administered a 50-g OGTT. The OGTT was repeated at 6 weeks. Ten of the 16 in the ivy gourd group showed significant improvement in OGTT, whereas no one in the placebo group showed improvement. Mean baseline fasting glucose decreased from 179 mg/dL (9.9 mmol/L) at baseline to 122 mg/dL (6.8 mmol/L) at 6 weeks in the ivy gourd group ($P < 0.01$). In the placebo group, mean fasting glucose declined from 195 mg/dL (10.8 mmol/L) at baseline to 181 mg/dL (10.0 mmol/L) at 6 weeks (P value not significant). The 1- and 2-hour OGTT values declined significantly from 268 mg/dL (14.9 mmol/L) and 245 mg/dL (13.6 mmol/L), respectively, at baseline to 225 mg/dL (12.5 mmol/L) and 187 mg/dL (10.4 mmol/L), respectively, at 6 weeks in the ivy gourd group ($P < 0.05$ and $P < 0.01$, respectively). However, OGTT values were unchanged in the placebo group. The researchers reported there were no side effects and noted no adverse effects on hepatic or kidney function.

Another three-arm controlled open-label trial followed 70 subjects with type 2 diabetes for 12 weeks. One group took 6 g daily of dried pellets made from fresh ivy gourd leaves; another group took sulfonylureas; and the third group took placebo.[6] Researchers measured fasting and postprandial glucose. The declines in fasting blood glucose and the OGTT results for those on ivy gourd were similar to the results in those on the sulfonylurea. Fasting glucose declined from 160 mg/dL (8.9 mmol/L) to 110 mg/dL (6.11 mmol/L) after 12 weeks in the ivy gourd group ($P < 0.001$ vs. baseline). Values decreased from 165 mg/dL (9.2 mmol/L) to 120 mg/dL (6.7 mmol/L) after 6 weeks in the sulfonylurea group (P not significant). The 1- and 2-hour OGTT results were similar in the ivy gourd and sulfonylurea groups at 12 and 6 weeks, respectively, and were both significant ($P < 0.001$ and $P < 0.05$, respectively). There were no side effects reported.

Ivy gourd was studied in a 90-day randomized double-blind placebo-controlled trial in 60 persons with newly diagnosed diabetes.[5] Subjects took a daily dose of two 500-mg capsules of ivy gourd alcohol extract or placebo. The authors stated they set the statistical significance level at $P < 0.05$. The A1C decreased significantly in the ivy gourd group, from 6.7% to 6.1%, whereas it remained the same in the placebo group (6.4% at baseline and at 3 months). Fasting glucose decreased significantly from 132 mg/dL (7.3 mmol/L) to 111.4 mg/dL (6.2 mmol/L). Fasting glucose increased nonsignificantly in the placebo group from 125 mg/dL (6.96 mmol/L) to 133 mg/dL (7.4 mmol/L). Postprandial glucose decreased significantly from 183 mg/dL (10.2 mmol/L) to 149 mg/dL (8.3 mmol/L) in the ivy gourd group. Postprandial glucose increased in the placebo group from 155 mg/dL (8.6 mmol/L) to 167 mg/dL (9.3 mmol/L), but the change was not significant. Although cholesterol decreased, there was no significant difference between the groups.

A double-blind phase 1 clinical trial in 61 healthy volunteers used a test meal of 20 g of ivy gourd leaves mixed with scraped coconut and table salt in a fresh salad.[7] The comparison group took a test herb, and then both groups underwent a 75-g OGTT. Postprandial glucose increased in both groups. However, postprandial glucose was significantly lower in the ivy gourd group compared to the comparison group at 1 hour ($P = 0.01$) and 2 hours ($P = 0.03$).

Summary

Ivy gourd is a plant that grows well in India and other tropical areas. It is widely eaten as a vegetable and even fed to young children, and the leaves, fruit, and root juice are used to treat diabetes or digestive disorders. The active ingredients are unknown, and ivy gourd has not been studied well in Western medicine. However, it has been shown to decrease fasting and postprandial glucose, as well as A1C. The main adverse effects are mild gastrointestinal upset. Theoretically, hypoglycemia may occur if ivy gourd is combined with secretagogues or insulin. Doses used have varied from 900 mg twice daily of ground leaves to 1 g daily of alcohol extract and up to 6 g daily of dried pellets.[3,5-6] At this point there is limited evidence for its efficacy in diabetes treatment, but ivy gourd warrants further study.

References

1. Natural Medicines (Natural Medicines Database search engine). Available from https://naturalmedicines.therapeuticresearch.com. Accessed May 9, 2019
2. Wasantwisut E, Viriyapanich T: Ivy gourd (Coccinia grandis Voigt, Coccinia cordifolia, Coccinia indica) in human nutrition and traditional applications. *World Rev Nutr Diet* 2003;91:60–66
3. Azad Khan AK, Akhtar S, Mahtab H: Treatment of diabetes mellitus with Coccinia indica. *Br Med J* 1980;280:1044
4. Kamble SM, Kamlakar PL, Vaidya S, Bambole VD: Influence of Coccinia indica on certain enzymes in glycolytic and lipolytic pathway in human diabetes. *Indian J Med Sci* 1998;52:143–146
5. Kuriyan R, Rajendran R, Bantwal G, Kurpad AV. Effect of supplementation of Coccinia cordifolia extract on newly detected diabetic patients. *Diabetes Care* 2008;31:216–220
6. Kamble SM, Jyotishi GS, Kamlakar PL, Vaidya SM: Efficacy of Coccinia indica S & A in diabetes mellitus. *J Res Ayurveda Siddha* 1996;XVII:77–84

7. Munasinghe MAAK, Abeysena C, Yaddehige IS, Vidanapathirana T, Piyumal KPB. Blood sugar lowering effect of Coccinia grandis (L.) J. Voigt: path for a new drug for diabetes mellitus. *Exp Diab Res* 2011;2011:Article ID 978762

MAGNESIUM

Magnesium is one of the most abundant cations in the body and is used as an antacid, for constipation, and for several medical conditions such as cardiovascular diseases (including hypertension and arrhythmias), migraine headaches, preeclampsia, pregnancy-related leg cramps, and diabetes.[1,2] Furthermore, a 2019 nutritional guidance report from the ADA states that diabetes risk may be associated with magnesium status in persons with prediabetes.[3] Dietary sources include green leafy vegetables, legumes, grains, seeds, nuts, meats, coffee, and dark chocolate.[1,2,4-5]

Magnesium is primarily found in bone, muscle, and soft tissues (99%), and approximately 1% is found in red blood cells and serum. Thus, magnesium levels are measured in the serum, but may not accurately reflect the body's magnesium status.[2] It is estimated that 25–38% of people with type 2 diabetes may have hypomagnesemia.[6] Hyomagnesemia is defined as a serum level of less than or equal to 0.74 mmol/L (1.8 mg/dL). In one meta-analysis, the relative risk of developing type 2 diabetes was decreased by 14% for every 100 mg daily of magnesium intake.[7] Hypomagnesemia has been associated with diabetes-related complications such as neuropathy, retinopathy, coronary heart disease, and foot ulcers.[6,8]

Mechanism of Action

Magnesium is available in numerous forms, such as sulfate, citrate, hydroxide, oxide, and chloride salts. Magnesium is a cofactor for different enzymes in different glucose metabolic pathways and phosphorylation reactions.[2,5,9] Magnesium deficiency may be a factor in several disease states, including diabetes. Furthermore, low dietary magnesium consumption may play a role in insulin resistance and development of type 2 diabetes.[1,2,5,9,10] In a hypomagnesemic state, insulin action is diminished, and insulin resistance is possibly related to reduced tyrosine kinase activity at the insulin receptor. Insulin action may additionally be impaired in the setting of hypomagnesemia, due to impaired insulin signaling.[1,2,4,9-10]

Adverse Effects and Drug Interactions

Adverse effects include gastrointestinal irritation, nausea, vomiting, and diarrhea. In individuals with diminished renal function, hypermagnesemia may occur.[1] There are numerous drug interactions. Many drugs may deplete magnesium, such as diuretics, proton pump inhibitors (PPIs), digoxin, β-2 agonists, steroids, cyclosporine, tacrolimus, and several others.[1,2] Magnesium supplementation may enhance the hypotension effect of calcium-channel blockers or result in hypermagnesemia if used with potassium-sparing diuretics such as spironolactone. Administered concomitantly, magnesium may impair absorption of certain drugs, such as tetracyclines, fluoroquinolones, calcium products, and bisphosphonates. In combination with insulin or insulin secretagogues, hypoglycemia may occur.[1]

Clinical Studies

Several studies have evaluated the relationship between magnesium and diabetes. Decreased magnesium intake as well as lower magnesium levels are associated with prediabetes and diabetes.[1,2] It is unknown whether magnesium levels are directly involved in diabetes development or whether having diabetes reflects magnesium levels. The following studies are examples of research involving magnesium status or supplementation.

A food-frequency questionnaire study gathered data every 2–4 years in a large group of individuals (85,060 women and 42,872 men) followed for 12 or 18 years (men and women, respectively). The investigators found that low dietary magnesium intake was correlated with increased diabetes risk.[5]

A 2011 meta-analysis of 13 prospective cohort studies reported that lower magnesium intake was associated with type 2 diabetes.[7] The analysis involved 536,318 subjects without diabetes at baseline followed for a period of 4–20 years; 24,516 developed diabetes. The relative risk of type 2 diabetes was 22% lower (RR 0.78; 95% CI 0.73–0.84; $P < 0.001$) in the group with the highest magnesium intake compared to the lowest intake. Subgroup analysis found the effect was greater at a BMI higher than 25 kg/m².

The Atherosclerosis Risk in Communities Study (ARIC) was a prospective study in over 12,000 individuals without diabetes at baseline that assessed low magnesium levels as well as magnesium intake and risk of type 2 diabetes.[9] Over a 6-year follow up, low serum magnesium level was predictive of developing type 2 diabetes while there was no association with dietary magnesium consumption. In white subjects, low magnesium concentration was an independent predictor of type 2 diabetes.

Studies evaluating magnesium use in established diabetes range from showing no effect to showing potential benefit. One study that showed no benefit was done in 40 people with type 2 diabetes.[11] Subjects had low magnesium levels and were given magnesium citrate (30 mmol/day) for 3 months. A1C increased slightly, but the change was not significant (7.2% at baseline and 7.4% at study end).

On the same note, a different study in insulin-requiring type 2 patients also showed no improvement in metabolic parameters.[12] A total of 50 patients were administered 15 mmol/day magnesium aspartate hydrochloride or placebo for 3 months. There was no difference in plasma glucose between the treatment and control groups at study end (193 mg/dL [10.7 mmol/L] vs. 209 mg/dL [11.6 mmol/L], respectively; $P = 0.8$), although glucose declined nonsignificantly in the treatment group (212 mg/dL[11.8 mmol/L] at baseline to 193 mg/dL

[10.7 mmol//L] at study end). A1C did not differ in the treatment and control groups (8.9% vs. 9.1%, $P = 0.6$).

On the other hand, a study that describes the benefits of oral magnesium supplementation in type 2 diabetes was a 16-week randomized double-blind placebo-controlled trial in 63 patients with decreased magnesium concentrations who were taking a sulfonylurea.[10] Thirty-two patients took 50 mL of magnesium chloride solution daily (50 g magnesium chloride per 1,000 mL solution), and 31 took placebo. The treatment group had decreased mean fasting glucose and A1C after 16 weeks: 230 mg/dL (12.8 mmol/L) to 144 mg/dL (8.0 mmol/L) and from 11.5% to 8%, respectively ($P < 0.05$ for both). The control group also had significant declines, from 256 mg/dL (14.2 mmol/L) to 185 mg/dL (10.3 mmol/L) and from 11.8% to 10.1% ($P < 0.05$ for both). There was a significant difference favoring the treatment group ($P < 0.05$ for fasting glucose and A1C). A measure of insulin sensitivity, the HOMA-IR (homeostasis model assessment of insulin resistance) index, also improved in the treatment group (4.3 at baseline and 3.8 at treatment end, $P < 0.05$) but not in the control group (4.7 at baseline and 5.0 at study end).

Systematic reviews and meta-analyses are being conducted and published, corroborating the prolific research surrounding the relationship between magnesium and persons with or at risk for diabetes. One 2016 systematic review and meta-analysis by Veronese et al described the impact of magnesium supplementation in 18 randomized controlled trials—12 in persons with type 2 diabetes and six in persons at high risk.[13] In 12 studies, 336 persons with diabetes took magnesium and 334 took placebo for a median of 14 weeks. Nine of these studies reported fasting glucose in 254 subjects on magnesium and 252 on placebo. The significant decrease in standardized mean difference (SMD) in fasting glucose for the diabetes group was −0.4 ($P = 0.049$). The A1C decrease reported for eight studies in 250 subjects in each group was not significant at −0.11 ($P = 0.26$). In the six studies of subjects at risk of diabetes, the decrease in fasting glucose was not significant ($P = 0.14$), but in three studies the decrease in 2-hour OGTT was significant (SMD of −0.35; $P = 0.01$). The researchers also conducted a meta regression analysis to evaluate differences in magnesium levels at follow up between treated and placebo groups. Higher differences were associated with significantly lower A1C in the diabetes group and fasting glucose in the "at risk" for diabetes group (A1C decrease was $\beta = -3.96$ [$P = 0.04$] fasting glucose decrease was $\beta = -4.07$ [$P < 0.0001$]). The insulin sensitivity marker, HOMA-IR, decreased significantly in the "at risk" group ($\beta = -0.382$, $P = 0.003$). The authors stated that although included trials were high quality, magnesium doses and types varied, there were few subjects in the trials, and follow-up time was short. Another limitation was that studies of other diabetes types were not included. However, a three-month prospective cohort trial in 71 children with type 1 diabetes and hypomagnesemia reported that supplementation with 300 mg daily of magnesium oxide resulted in a significant A1C decrease (10.1% to 7.9%; $P < 0.001$).[14]

A different 2016 systematic review and meta-analysis evaluated 21 randomized controlled trials lasting 1–6 months in 1,362 subjects with and without diabetes.[15] A total of 684 subjects took magnesium and 678 were in the control group. Effects were reported as weighted mean differences (WMD). The WMDs for fasting glucose and A1C were not significant (fasting glucose WMD of 0.20 mmol/L [3.6 mg/dL], $P = 0.119$; A1C – WMD of –0.018 mmol/L [0.02%], $P = 0.756$). However, the HOMA-IR improvement was significant (WMD of –0.67; $P = 0.013$). Interestingly, a sub-group analysis determined that for treatment duration longer than 4 months, the WMD was significant for fasting glucose (WMD of –0.73 mmol/L (–13 mg/dL); $P < 0.001$). One limitation of this evaluation was the inclusion of diverse group of individuals—persons with type 1 or type 2 diabetes, prediabetes, metabolic syndrome, insulin resistance, hypertension, or obese individuals. Another limitation was that magnesium type and doses were not consistent - monotherapy or combination products were used.

A 2017 systematic review and meta-analysis evaluated 28 randomized controlled trials in 1,694 subjects with type 2 diabetes or at high risk.[16] This meta-analysis was unique in that the impact of magnesium intake on cardiovascular risk factors was evaluated. Effects were reported as WMD in 834 subjects on magnesium and 860 on placebo. Fasting glucose, certain lipid measures, and systolic blood pressure (SBP) significantly decreased in the magnesium group. The WMD decrease for fasting glucose was –4.64 mg/dL (0.258 mmol/L; $P = 0.002$). The LDL WMD decrease was –10.7 mg/dL (0.276 mmol/L; $P = 0.013$). The SBP WMD decrease was –3.1 mm Hg ($P = 0.015$). The A1C did not decrease significantly. Other parameters that changed significantly were decreased triglycerides and increased HDL ($P = 0.026$ and $P < 0.001$, respectively). In subgroup analysis, there was a significant difference favoring supplementation in the hypomagnesemic versus the normal magnesium group for fasting glucose ($P = 0.001$). Unlike a previous meta-analysis by Veronese et al[13] that found a significant difference when duration of treatment was 4 months or greater, this meta-analysis found that duration of treatment for greater than 3 months had significant effects.

Summary

Magnesium deficiency may result in predisposition to type 2 diabetes or, in those with established type 2 diabetes, diminished metabolic control. However, there are no clear-cut guidelines on when to assess whether a person may have magnesium deficiency, unless they are taking certain medications or have a magnesium-depleting disease. Magnesium-depleting medications may include certain diuretics, steroids, PPIs, cyclosporine, tacrolimus, digoxin, beta-2 agonists, and aminoglycosides. Patients should take tetracyclines, fluoroquinolones, or calcium 2 hours before or 4 hours after magnesium administration.[1]

Use beyond 3 or 4 months may provide the most optimal benefit.[13,16] A previous ADA consensus statement on magnesium indicated that prospective long-term studies are needed to determine whether hypomagnesemia predisposes patients to complication risks and baseline serum magnesium concentrations should be determined in certain hypomagnesemia associated disease states, such as heart failure, coronary artery disease, long-term parenteral nutrition, pregnancy, or ethanol abuse.[17] Many studies report differing results regarding the benefit of magnesium supplementation and the type of magnesium salt, dose, and duration of treatment. In adult males and females over 50, the recommended dietary allowance is 420 and 320 mg, respectively, per day.[18] The tolerable upper intake dose from supplements and pharmacological agents in addition to magnesium intake from food and water is 350 mg daily in adults. Higher doses may result in diarrhea. Clinicians may wish to consider assessing magnesium status to determine which patients would benefit from supplementation. For instance, persons who take diuretics or PPIs long-term should have a baseline level drawn. Periodic testing for hypomagnesemia may be considered at least annually. However, patients with impaired renal function should not routinely take magnesium supplements because of the kidneys' inability to adequately clear magnesium. Overall, the evidence on magnesium is prolific and continues to emerge.

References

1. Natural Medicines (Natural Medicines Database search engine). Available from https://naturalmedicines.therapeuticresearch.com. Accessed May 9, 2019

2. Mooren FC. Magnesium and disturbances in carbohydrate metabolism. *Diabetes Obes Metab* 2015;17:813–823

3. Evert AB, Dennison M, Gardner CD, et al. Nutrition therapy for adults with diabetes or prediabetes: a consensus report. *Diabetes Care* 2019;42:731–754

4. Guerrero-Romero F, Rodriguez-Moran M. Complementary therapies for diabetes: the case for chromium, magnesium, and antioxidants. *Arch Med Res* 2005;36:150–157

5. Lopez-Ridaura R, Willett WC, Rimm EB, et al. Magnesium intake and risk of type 2 diabetes in men and women. *Diabetes Care* 2004;27:134–140

6. Lima MdL, Cruz T, Pousada JC, et al. The effect of magnesium supplementation in increasing doses on the control of type 2 diabetes. *Diabetes Care* 1998;21:682–686

7. Dong J-Y, Xun, P, He K, Qin L-Q. Magnesium intake and risk of type 2 diabetes: meta-analysis of prospective cohort studies. *Diabetes Care* 2011;34:2116–2122

8. Rodriguez-Moran M, Guerrero-Romero F. Low serum magnesium levels and foot ulcers in subjects with type 2 diabetes. *Arch Med Res* 2001;32:300–303

9. Kao WHL, Folsom AR, Nieto FJ, et al. Serum and dietary magnesium and the risk for type 2 diabetes mellitus, the atherosclerosis risk in communities study. *Arch Intern Med* 1999;159:2151–2159

10. Rodriguez-Moran M, Guerrero-Romero F. Oral magnesium supplementation improves insulin sensitivity and metabolic control in type 2 diabetes subjects. *Diabetes Care* 2003;26:1147–1153

11. Eibl NL, Kopp H-P, Nowak HR, et al. Hypomagnesemia in type II diabetes: effect of a 3-month replacement therapy. *Diabetes Care* 1995;18:188–192

12. de Valk HW, Verkaaik R, van Rijn HJM, et al. Oral magnesium supplementation in insulin-requiring type 2 diabetic patients. *Diabet Med* 1998;15:503–507

13. Veronese N, Watutantrige-Fernando S, Luchini C, et al. Effect of magnesium supplementation on glucose metabolism in people with or at risk of diabetes: a systematic review and meta-analysis of double-blind randomized controlled trials. *Eur J Clin Nutr* 2016;70:1354–1359

14. Shahbah D, Hassan T, Morsy S, et al. Oral magnesium supplementation improves glycemic control and lipid profile in children with type 1 diabetes and hypomagnesemia. *Medicine* (Baltimore) 2017;96(11):e6352 doi: 10.1097/MD.0000000000006352

15. Simental-Mendia LE, Sahebkar A, Rodriguez-Moran M, Guerrero-Romero F. A systematic review and meta-analysis of randomized controlled trials on the effects of magnesium supplementation on insulin sensitivity and control. *Pharmacol Res* 2016;111:272–282

16. Verma H, Garg R. Effect of magnesium supplementation on type 2 diabetes associated cardiovascular risk factors: a systematic review and meta-analysis. *J Hum Nutr Diet* 2017;30:621–633

17. American Diabetes Association: Magnesium supplementation in the treatment of diabetes (Consensus Statement). *Diabetes Care* 1992;15:1065–1067

18. NIH Office of Dietary Supplements. Magnesium Fact Sheet for Health Professionals. Available from https://ods.od.nih.gov/factsheets/Magnesium-HealthProfessional/?print=1. Accessed January 6, 2020

MILK THISTLE (*Silybum marianum*)

Milk thistle is a member of the aster family (Asteraceae or Compositae), which also includes daisies and thistles.[1,2] Milk thistle grows well in North America and reaches 5–10 feet (about 2–3 meters) in height, with large prickly leaves that secrete a milk sap when broken.[1,3] It bears pink flowers that are ridged with sharp spines. The fruit, seeds, and leaves of the plant contain the medicinal constituents.

Milk thistle has been used for thousands of years and is noted in ancient Greek and Roman references.[3] It has been used extensively for various hepatic disorders, alcoholic cirrhosis, as well as nonalcoholic steatohepatitis (NASH).[2-6]

Other uses have been to treat *Amanita phalloides* poisoning and to attenuate hepatotoxic effects of certain medications.[1,2] It is also used for menstrual disorders. Milk thistle is consumed as a vegetable and the seeds are roasted as a coffee substitute.[1] Milk thistle is being used to decrease insulin resistance and studied for diabetes complications, such as nephropathy.[7,8] Hyperlipidemia treatment is another use.[1]

Chemical Constituents and Mechanism of Action

Milk thistle contains flavonolignans.[5] Silymarin is a dry mixture of the flavonolignans. Silymarin is extracted with 95% ethyl alcohol, which yields a bright yellow fluid. Silymarin contains silybin A and B, isosilibin A and B, silychristine, isosilychristine, taxifolin, and silidianin.[3,8] Silybin is the constituent thought to have the most potent biological activity.[3]

Milk thistle has various theorized activities in managing hepatic disease.[2] The mechanism of action for diabetes may be antioxidant effects, anti-inflammatory activity, and peroxisome proliferator activated receptor-gamma (PPARγ) agonist properties.[5,9] Additionally, milk thistle may inhibit hepatic gluconeogenesis.[5] Milk thistle is considered a cytoprotectant, and may be of benefit in insulin resistance associated with hepatic damage. One theory is that lipoperoxidation may adversely affect patients with diabetes, and the ability of milk thistle to decrease malondialdehyde (MDA) concentrations (a marker of oxidative stress) may improve diabetes.[7] The antioxidant and anti-inflammatory effects may help diminish diabetes-related complications, such as nephropathy, since these are thought to occur secondary to oxidative stress.[1,9] In nephropathy, milk thistle may help decrease levels of interleukins as well as TNF-α and TNF-β, a marker for fibrosis.[8] Aldose reductase inhibition may also help diminish complications.[5] Milk thistle also benefits hyperlipidemia. Per animal data, milk thistle decreases cholesterol absorption and synthesis. Through free radical scavenging activity it decreases formation of oxidized LDL cholesterol and may diminish the effect of HMG-CoA reductase involved in cholesterol synthesis.[1]

Adverse Effects and Drug Interactions

Side effects of milk thistle include dose-related diarrhea because of increased bile flow.[10] Other adverse effects include intermittent episodes of severe sweating, gastrointestinal upset, and weakness that recurred on rechallenge. Other possible adverse effects include allergic reactions in those sensitive to ragweed, chrysanthemums, marigolds, and daisies. Milk thistle may have estrogenic properties and should probably not be used in hormone sensitive conditions, such as breast, ovarian, or uterine cancer.[1]

Milk thistle may have various drug interactions. Phosphatidylcholine enhances bioavailability, thus allowing for lower doses of milk thistle.[2] Hypoglycemia may theoretically occur in combination with secretagogues, such as sulfonylureas. Since milk thistle inhibits glucuronidation, it may increase serum concentrations of drugs that are glucuronidated, such as haloperidol (Haldol®) or lamotrigine (Lamictal®) or even acetaminophen (Tylenol®). Since it inhibits p-glycoproteins, it may increase absorption of certain drugs that are p-glycoprotein substrates, such as some chemotherapy drugs, cardiac drugs (calcium channel blockers), or certain antibiotics. Milk thistle may also increase the serum concentration of raloxifene or tamoxifen or decrease clearance of sirolimus.[1] On the other hand, milk thistle may decrease serum concentrations of antiretroviral drugs.[11] Information that milk thistle affects CYP 2C9, CYP 2D6, and CYP 3A4 as well as organic anion transporting polypeptides is not consistent.[1]

Clinical Studies

Although milk thistle has been studied in persons with hepatic dysfunction, mortality in high-quality trials has not been diminished.[12] Milk thistle has been studied in several trials in subjects with diabetes. Milk thistle was studied in one randomized, open-label trial in 60 patients with type 2 diabetes and cirrhosis, treated with insulin.[7] One group of 30 subjects received 600 mg/day silymarin, and 30 received placebo for 12 months. In the treatment group, mean fasting glucose declined from 190 mg/dL (10.6 mmol/L) at baseline to 165 mg/dL (9.2 mmol/L) at 12 months ($P < 0.01$ vs. baseline). A1C decreased from 7.9% at baseline to 7.2% at end point ($P < 0.01$ vs. baseline). Moreover, mean daily insulin requirement decreased significantly from 55 units a day to 42 units a day at end point ($P < 0.01$ vs. baseline). Mean malondialdehyde levels also decreased significantly ($P < 0.01$).

In another study of subjects with cirrhosis, 10 subjects on insulin plus milk thistle were compared to 10 subjects on insulin plus L-ornithine and L-aspartate.[4] Measurements of random glucose and liver function tests were done at 3 and 5 months. Certain liver function tests improved, and mean random glucose decreased significantly in both groups ($P < 0.001$ for both versus baseline), but the difference between groups was not significant.

In a 4-month, double-blind study, 25 people were randomized to 200 mg three times daily of silymarin seed extract, and 26 were randomized to placebo.[13] Milk thistle was added to metformin and glibenclamide (glyburide). The A1C decreased significantly in the milk thistle group from 7.8% to 6.8% ($P < 0.001$) and increased significantly in the placebo group from 8.3% to 9.5% ($P < 0.0001$). Fasting blood glucose declined significantly from 156 mg/dL (8.7 mmol/L) to 133 mg/dL (7.4 mmol/L) in the treatment group ($P < 0.001$) but increased significantly in the placebo group ($P < 0.0001$).

In a different 4-month randomized double-blind placebo-controlled trial, milk thistle 200 mg daily of silymarin was added to 18 subjects on glibenclamide and compared to 20 subjects on glibenclamide plus placebo and 21 subjects on glibenclamide monotherapy.[14] In the milk thistle group, A1C decreased significantly from 8.9% at baseline to 7.45% ($P < 0.05$). Fasting glucose decreased significantly in the milk thistle group, from 210 mg/dL (11.7 mmol/L) to 168 mg/dL (9.3 mmol/L; $P < 0.05$). The milk thistle group had a significantly greater decrease than the other groups.

A triple-blind randomized controlled trial evaluated daily doses of 140 mg three times daily of milk thistle or placebo in subjects with type 2 diabetes.[9] Trial duration was 45 days, and there were 40 subjects each in the milk thistle and placebo groups. Fasting glucose decreased significantly by 11% in the milk thistle group, compared to an increase of 8% in the placebo group ($P = 0.009$ for milk thistle versus placebo). Insulin decreased significantly by 14% on milk thistle versus 26% increase on placebo ($P = 0.04$ for milk thistle versus placebo). HOMA-IR also decreased by 26% on milk thistle and increased by 37% on placebo ($P = 0.015$ for milk thistle versus placebo). Triglycerides decreased significantly and HDL cholesterol increased significantly on milk thistle compared to placebo ($P = 0.034$ and $P < 0.05$, respectively), while decreases in total and LDL cholesterol were not significant.

Systematic reviews and meta-analyses evaluating milk thistle have also been published.[15,16] A 2016 analysis of five randomized trials in 270 subjects with a duration of 45 days–4 months reported a significant decrease in A1C of 1.07% and fasting glucose of 26.86 mg/dL (1.5 mmol/L; $P < 0.00001$ and $P = 0.002$, respectively).[15] However, the studies had significant heterogeneity, and the authors stated that the evidence was of low quality. A 2018 systematic review and meta-analysis reported results for seven randomized controlled trials for 370 subjects, with a duration of 45 days–12 months.[16] The A1C and fasting glucose both decreased significantly by 1.4% and 37.9 mg/dL (2.1 mmol/L), respectively ($P < 0.001$ for both). This analysis also reported a significant impact on certain lipid parameters. LDL cholesterol decreased ($P = 0.01$) and HDL cholesterol increased significantly ($P = 0.004$). The authors of this analysis also noted the evaluated trials had significant heterogeneity.

A unique emerging role of milk thistle is decreased proteinuria when added to angiotensin-converting enzyme (ACE) inhibitors in persons with diabetes. A 3-month randomized double-blind placebo-controlled trial of 60 persons with proteinuria and at maximum doses of renin angiotensin system inhibitors evaluated the impact on proteinuria and inflammatory markers.[17] Half were assigned to 420 mg per day of silymarin and half to placebo. Urinary albumin to creatinine ratio (UACR) decreased to a greater extent than placebo in the silymarin group (mean change of 347 mg/g). Serum malondialdehyde levels (a marker for oxidative stress) and urinary tumor necrosis factor-α (TNF-α) also decreased significantly. A measure of fibrosis, transforming growth factor β, also decreased.

Summary

Although milk thistle is an extensively studied agent, there are problems with study design in clinical trials. Nevertheless, it has been safely used for long periods—up to 4 years.[1] There is great interest in its use for diabetes complications such as nephropathy and hepatic disorders. Studies have evaluated the combination of milk thistle with berberine (and other supplements) for diabetes and hyperlipidemia.[1,18] A 2019 meta-analysis of five randomized controlled trials in 497 subjects evaluated berberine-milk thistle combinations and found significant decreases not only in fasting glucose ($P = 0.008$), but also decreased triglycerides, total and LDL cholesterol, and increased HDL cholesterol ($P < 0.001$ for all parameters).[18] Although milk thistle has mostly been studied in type 2 diabetes, it is now being studied in subjects with type 1 diabetes. Moreover, a combination product of milk thistle with berberine was used to treat subjects with type 1 diabetes, with the finding that insulin doses decreased and certain glycemic parameters improved.[19]

Adverse events are rare, although gastrointestinal effects and cross-allergic reactions may occur with members of the daisy and ragweed family. The typical dose of milk thistle for liver disease is 200 mg three times daily. Milk thistle extract should be standardized to contain 70% silymarin (140 mg silymarin).[1] Since phosphatidylcholine enhances oral absorption, preparations containing this ingredient may be dosed at lower doses, such as 100 mg/day.[2] Doses vary in different diabetes studies and have ranged from 200–600 mg/day. Milk thistle has been used extensively to treat a variety of hepatic disorders. However, there is great interest and emerging research for treatment of diabetes and diabetes-related complications, such as nephropathy and NASH.

References

1. Natural Medicines (Natural Medicines Database search engine). Available from https://naturalmedicines.therapeuticresearch.com. Accessed May 9, 2019

2. Pepping J. Alternative therapies: milk thistle: Silybum marianum. *Am J Health-Syst Pharm* 1999;56:1195–1197
3. Flora K, Hahn M, Rosen H, Benner K. Milk thistle (Silybum marinum) for the therapy of liver disease. *Am J Gastroenterol* 1998;93:139–143
4. Jose MA, Abraham A, Narmadha MP. Effect of silymarin in diabetes mellitus patients with liver diseases. *J Pharmacol Pharmacother* 2011;2:287–289
5. Kazazis CE, Evangelopoulos AA, Kollas A, Vallianou NG. The therapeutic potential of milk thistle in diabetes. *Rev Diab Stud* 2014;11:167–174
6. Medina J, Fernandez-Salazar LI, Garcia-Buey L, Moreno-Otero R. Approach to the pathogenesis and treatment of nonalcoholic steatohepatitis. *Diabetes Care* 2004;27:2057–2066
7. Velussi M, Cernigoi AM, De Monte A, et al.: Long-term (12 months) treatment with an anti-oxidant drug (silymarin) is effective on hyperinsulinemia, exogenous insulin need and malondialdehyde levels in cirrhotic diabetic patients. J Hepatol 1997;26:871–879
8. Stolf AM, Campos Cardoso C, Acco A. Effect of silymarin on diabetes mellitus complications: a review. *Phytother Res* 2017;31:366–374
9. Ebrahimpour Koujan S, Gargari BP, Mobasseri M, Valizadeh H, Asghari-Jafarabadi M. Lower glycemic indices and lipid profile among type 2 diabetes mellitus patients who received novel dose of Silybum marianum (L.) Gaertn. (silymarin) extract supplement: a triple-blinded, randomized controlled clinical trial. *Phytomedicine* 2018;44:39–44
10. Luper S. A review of plants used in the treatment of liver disease: part 1. *Altern Med Rev* 1998;3:410–421
11. Jalloh MA, Gregory PJ, Hein D, Cochrane Z R, Rodriguez A. Dietary supplement interactions with antiretrovirals: a systematic review. *Int J STD AIDS* 2017;28:4-15
12. Rambaldi A, Jacobs BP, Iaquinto G, Gluud C: Milk thistle for alcoholic and/or hepatitis B or C liver diseases: a systematic Cochrane Hepato-biliary Group review with meta-analyses of randomized clinical trials. *Am J Gastroenterol* 2005;100:2583–2591
13. Huseini HF, Larijani B, Heshmat R, et al.: The efficacy of Silybum marianum (L.) Gaertn. (silymarin) in the treatment of type II diabetes: a randomized, double-blind, placebo-controlled, clinical trial. *Phytother Res* 2006;20:1036–1039
14. Hussain SA. Silymarin as an adjunct to glibenclamide therapy improves long-term and postprandial glycemic control and body mass index in type 2 diabetes. *J Med Food* 2007;10:543-7

15. Voroneanu L, Nistor I, Dumea R, Apetrii M, Covic A. Silymarin in type 2 diabetes mellitus: a systematic review and meta-analysis of randomized controlled trials. *J Diabetes Res* 2016:5147468,2016
16. Hadi A, Pourmasoumi M, Mohammadi H, Symonds M, Miraghajani M. The effects of silymarin supplementation on metabolic status and oxidative stress in patients with type 2 diabetes mellitus: a systematic review and meta-analysis of clinical trials. *Complement Ther Med* 2018;41:311–319
17. Fallahzadeh MK, Dormanesh B, Sagheb MM, et al. Effect of addition of silymarin to renin-angiotensin system inhibitors on proteinuria in type 2 diabetic patients with overt nephropathy: a randomized, double-blind, placebo-controlled trial. *Am J Kidney Dis* 2012;60:896–903
18. Fogacci F, Grassi D, Rizzo M, Cicero AFG. Metabolic effect of berberine-silymarin association: a meta-analysis of randomized, double-blind, placebo-controlled clinical trials. *Phytother Res* 2019;33:862–870
19. Derosa G, D'Angelo A, Maffioli P. The role of a fixed Berberis aristata/Silybum marianum combination in the treatment of type 1 diabetes. *Clin Nutr* 2016;35:1091–1095

MULBERRY (*Morus alba Linn.*)

White mulberry is a medium size shrub or tree, with fruit that is white or pink.[1,2] The berries and leaves are used medicinally.[3] The fruit is used for constipation and urinary incontinence and to make jams, jellies, and wines. Medicinally, leaves are used for colds and eye infections, whereas mulberry leaf tea and extract have been widely used in Asia for diabetes, as well as hyperlipidemia.[1-3] Mulberry tree wood is very strong and is used to make hockey sticks and tennis rackets, and interestingly, silkworms feed on mulberry leaves.[2,3]

Chemical Constituents and Mechanism of Action

Mulberry leaf contains various active ingredients including 1-deoxynojirimycin, fagomine, and antioxidants. The 1-deoxynojirimycin ingredient has α-glucosidase inhibitor activity; fagomine may induce insulin secretion; and antioxidant ingredients may decrease lipid peroxidation.[3-5] Per animal research, mulberry may decrease atherosclerotic lesions by enhancing resistance of LDL to oxidation.[1] Mulberry may also decrease insulin resistance by activating phosphatidylinositol-3-kinase/protein kinase B, glycogen synthase kinase-3 β signaling pathways, and modulate glucose transporter-4 translocation in skeletal muscle and adipose tissue.[3]

Adverse Effects and Drug Interactions

Theoretical expected side effects would be gastrointestinal upset, similar to α-glucosidase inhibitors. A 2017 meta-analysis that evaluated glycemic and lipid parameters also evaluated adverse effects. The reported effects included headache, nausea, vomiting, fullness, and cough.[6] A different report also noted an increase in serum creatinine.[7] Theoretical drug interactions may be hypoglycemia or additive glucose lowering effects if combined with diabetes medications.[1]

Clinical Studies

Mulberry has been highly researched in the last few years. Unfortunately, many of the studies do not have optimal study design, include only small numbers of individuals, and use varying doses. An early 2007 crossover study compared 10 persons with type 2 diabetes on oral diabetes medications to 10 persons without diabetes.[8] A 1-g dose of mulberry leaf was administered before a 75-g sucrose challenge to evaluate the attenuation of increase in blood glucose. Rise in blood glucose was attenuated in both groups. In subjects with type 2 diabetes, the respective mean glucose increases for mulberry versus placebo over 120 minutes were 42 mg/dL (2.3 mmol/L) and 54 mg/dL (3 mmol/L; $P = 0.002$). For the control group without diabetes, the respective mean glucose increases for mulberry versus placebo over 120 minutes were 15 mg/dL (0.83 mmol/L) and 22 mg/dL (1.2 mmol/L; $P = 0.005$). Carbohydrate malabsorption was evaluated by measuring breath samples for hydrogen (H_2). Carbohydrate malabsorption was greater in those on mulberry versus placebo ($P < 0.01$), which confirmed possible benefit of mulberry.

A 30-day study in 24 persons with T2DM compared 3 g daily of mulberry leaf powder to glibenclamide (glyburide).[9] The A1C decrease was not significant in either the mulberry (12.5% to 11.2%) or glibenclamide (12.5% to 12.4%) groups. Mulberry significantly decreased fasting glucose from 153 mg/dL (8.5 mol/L) to 111 mg/dL (6.2 mmol/L; $P < 0.01$) compared to baseline. Fasting glucose also decreased in the glibenclamide group from 154 mg/dL to 142 mg/dL (8.6 mmol/L to 7.9 mmol/L), but the authors did not provide a P value. In the mulberry group, LDL cholesterol decreased from 102 mg/dL (2.6 mmol/L) to 79 mg/dL (2 mmol/L; $P < 0.01$); triglycerides decreased from 200 mg/dL (2.3 mmol/L) to 168 mg/dL (1.9 mmol/L; $P < 0.01$); and HDL increased from 50 mg/dL (1.3 mmol/L) to 59 mg/dL (1.5 mmol/L; $P < 0.01$). Lipid changes were not significant in the glibenclamide group.

A 3-month randomized placebo-controlled study in 24 subjects with type 2 diabetes evaluated the impact of 1,000 mg mulberry leaf extract MLE administered three times daily compared to placebo.[7] Two parameters measured were A1C and self-monitored postprandial glucose. The A1C decreased nonsignificantly at 3 months from 7.3% at baseline to 6.94% in the mulberry group, and from 7.46% to 7.2% in the placebo group. The difference between groups at endpoint was not significant ($P = 0.44$). Compared to placebo, the decrease in postprandial glucose was 18% in the mulberry group ($P < 0.05$). Of note: there was a significant 15% increase in serum creatinine in the mulberry group compared to baseline ($P = 0.028$) as well as compared to placebo ($P = 0.024$).

A 24-week randomized double-blind study compared the impact of mulberry twig alkaloid (also known as Ramulus Mori or Sangzhi) with acarbose, a prescription α glucosidase inhibitor, in 36 subjects with type 2 diabetes (21 took mulberry and 15 took acarbose).[10] This mulberry twig component contains deoxynojirimycin and has α glucosidase inhibitor activity. The mulberry dose was 50 mg three times daily for 4 weeks then increased to 100 mg three times daily. The acarbose group took 50 mg three times daily for the entire trial. After 24 weeks, A1C decreased significantly by 0.78% (from 8.3%; $P < 0.001$) and by 0.83% (from 8.2%; $P < 0.05$) in the mulberry and acarbose groups, respectively. The difference between groups was not statistically significant ($P = 0.652$). Although 1- and 2-hour postprandial glucose decreased significantly from baseline in each group, the difference between groups was not significant ($P = 0.748$ and $P = 0.558$ for 1- and 2-hour values, respectively). Thus, the mulberry alkaloid had an effect similar to acarbose.

A 2016 systematic review of three randomized controlled trials evaluating mulberry found no improvement in glycemic or lipid parameters.[11] The authors considered but did not include several trials for varying reasons, such as studies that did not include subjects with type 2 diabetes, or trials that included combination products. The authors commented there was a lack of high quality studies to include in the analysis to determine whether mulberry is useful for glycemic or lipid management.

A 2017 meta-analysis of 13 trials evaluated three scenarios of mulberry use in 436 subjects.[6] One scenario considered glycemic parameters. A second scenario considered lipid parameters. The last scenario evaluated adverse effects. Four randomized controlled trials evaluated the impact of mulberry compared to control on A1C and found a small nonsignificant difference of 0.05% (0.05 mmol/L; $P = 0.49$). The pooled mean difference for fasting glucose was a decrease (that was not significant) of 4.5 mg/dL (0.25 mmol/L; $P = 0.10$). The significant postprandial glucose decrease in seven trials was 18.7 mg/dL (1.04 mmol/L) at 30 minutes, 15.7 mg/dL (0.87 mmol/L) at 60 minutes, and 9.9 mg/dL (0.55 mmol/L) at 90 minutes ($P < 0.00001$, $P < 0.0001$, and $P = 0.001$, respectively), compared to placebo. In lipid-lowering trials there were no significant differences in evaluated parameters. Adverse effects noted in the mulberry group were headache, nausea, and fullness, but the symptoms were not significant compared to control. This meta-analysis included heterogeneous populations, ranging from healthy individuals to persons with prediabetes and type 2 diabetes. Moreover, study design was sub-optimal for several studies, including very small numbers of subjects and 1-day evaluations. For instance, some 1-day studies evaluated the impact of mulberry or placebo on glucose measured from 30–120 minutes later. Finally, the analysis also included studies using combination products. Thus, it would be problematic to determine whether any benefit should be attributed to mulberry or the other ingredients. The authors noted there is a need for randomized controlled studies.

Summary

Mulberry has increased in popularity in the last few years. Studied conditions in subjects with type 2 diabetes, prediabetes, or impaired glucose tolerance include glycemic or lipid parameters. Mulberry has not only been used as monotherapy, but also in combination with other natural products, such as ginseng and banaba, or propolis.[12,13] Combinations of black, green, and mulberry tea are also being used. There are several published studies, but study design is not optimal. The impact on lowering A1C is equivocal, but the main benefit may be postprandial glucose lowering, possibly due to α glucosidase inhibitory activity. Although not well characterized, some doses used in studies have ranged from 300 mg daily of a twig formulation and up to 1–3 g daily of oral capsules or tea preparations; important unknowns include the most appropriate dose and formulation. Overall, the benefit may be decreased carbohydrate absorption, due to α glucosidase inhibition from the deoxynojirimycin content. It is feasible that individuals with diabetes may choose to accompany high carbohydrate meals with a mulberry preparation to decrease postprandial glucose. Even though mulberry is popular and studies abound, better designed, long term investigations are necessary to evaluate appropriate use for diabetes.

References

1. Natural Medicines (Natural Medicines Database search engine). Available from https://naturalmedicines.therapeuticresearch.com. Accessed May 9, 2019
2. Moore LM. Plant Guide: White Mulberry. United States Department of Agriculture, Natural Resources Conservation Service. Available from http://plants.usda.gov/plantguide/pdf/pg_moal.pdf. Accessed 2 July 2019
3. Thaipitakwong T, Numhom S, Aramwit P. Mulberry leaves and their potential effects against cardiometabolic risks: a review of chemical compositions, biological properties, and clinical efficacy. *Pharm Biol* 2018;58:109–118
4. Hansawasdi C, Kawabata J. α-glucosidase inhibitory effect of mulberry (Morus alba) leaves on Caco-2. *Fitoterapia* 2006;77:568–573
5. Taniguchi S, Asano N, Tomino F, Miwa I. Potentiation of glucose-induced insulin secretion by fagomine, a pseudo-sugar isolated from mulberry leaves. *Horm Metab Res* 1998;30:679–683
6. Phimarn W, Wichaiyo K, Silpsavikul K, Sungthong B. Saramunee K. A meta-analysis of efficacy of Morus alba Linn. to improve blood glucose and lipid profile. *Eur J Nutr* 2017;56:1509–1521
7. Riche DM, Riche KD, East HE, Barrett EK, May WL. Impact of mulberry leaf extract on type 2 diabetes (Mul-DM): a randomized, placebo-controlled study. *Complement Ther Med* 2017;32:105–108
8. Mudra M, Ercan-Fang N, Zhong L, Furne J, Levitt M. Influence of mulberry leaf extract on the blood glucose and breath hydrogen response to ingestion of 75 g sucrose by type 2 diabetic and control subjects. *Diabetes Care* 2007;30:1274-1274
9. Andallu B, Suryakantham V, Srikanthi BL, Reddy GK. Effect of mulberry (Morus indica L) therapy on plasma and erythrocyte membrane lipids in patients with type 2 diabetes. *Clin Chim Acta* 2001;314:47–53
10. Li M, Huang X, Ye H, et al. Randomized, double-blinded, double-dummy, active-controlled, and multiple-dose clinical study comparing the efficacy and safety of mulberry twig (Ramulus Mori, Sangzhi) alkaloid tablet and acarbose in individuals with type 2 diabetes mellitus. *Evid Based Comple-*

ment Alt Med 2018;Article ID 7121356. Available from http://dx.doi.
org/10.1155/2016/7121356. Accessed 4 July, 2019

11. Shin S-O, Seo H-J, Park H, Song HJ. Effects of mulberry leaf extract on
    blood glucose and serum lipid profiles in patients with type 2 diabetes
    mellitus: a systematic review. *Eur J Integr Med* 2016;8:602–608

12. Kim HJ, Yoon KH, Kang MJ, et al. A six-month supplementation of mul-
    berry, Korean red ginseng, and banaba decreases biomarkers of systemic
    low-grade inflammation in subjects with impaired glucose tolerance and
    type 2 diabetes. *Evid Based Complement Alternat Med* 2012;2012:735191.
    doi: 10.1155/2012/735191

13. Murata K, Yatsunami K, Fukuda E, et al. Antihyperglycemic effects of
    propolis mixed with mulberry leaf extract on patients with type 2 diabe-
    tes. *Altern Ther Health Med* 2004;10:78–79

NOPAL (*Opuntia streptacantha Lemaire*)

Nopal, also known as prickly pear, is a member of the cactus family. There are multiple species known as *Opuntia*, including *O. megacantha*, *O. ficus indica*, and *O. streptacantha* Lemaire. Research has focused on *O. streptacantha* Lemaire for its role in lowering blood glucose. Nopal has been used as a food in Mexico and the Southwestern part of the U.S.[1] The various plant parts have been used for medicinal purposes, including the pad or cladode as well as the fruit.[2] Broiled cladodes (pads) or extracts have been used for diabetes, hyperlipidemia, metabolic syndrome, and obesity.[1-4] Nopal has been used to treat veisalgia (alcohol hangover); in males it has been used to reduce symptoms of bladder fullness or urgency (benign prostatic hyperplasia, or BPH).[1,5]

Chemical Constituents and Mechanism of Action

Nopal contains mucopolysaccharide soluble fibers and phytochemicals (including pectin), phenolic compounds, flavonoids, and betalains (with antioxidant activity).[1,3] The cactus pad contains trivalent chromium.[6]

The mechanism of action is varied and includes slowed carbohydrate absorption and decreased lipid absorption in the digestive tract. Specifically, the pectin and mucilage fibers may increase food viscosity in the digestive tract, thus slowing down glucose absorption.[3,7] Nopal may bind to dietary fat and increase excretion.[3] Nopal has been tested for potential α-glucosidase inhibition but researchers concluded that may not be the mechanism.[8] The high fiber content decreases fat and lipid absorption and thus may be of benefit in hyperlipidemia.[1]

An additional theorized mechanism of action is increased insulin sensitivity, since insulin concentrations decrease with nopal administration.[7] Nopal does not seem to depend on insulin presence, since it has demonstrated hypoglycemic activity in pancreatectomized animals.[9] There is speculation that the high chromium concentrations in the cactus pad may be responsible for improved glucose metabolism.[6]

Adverse Effects and Drug Interactions

The major side effects of nopal include mild diarrhea, nausea, abdominal fullness, increased stool volume, and headache.[1,7] A case report stated that when chlorpropamide (a sulfonylurea) was coadministered with nopal, additive effects on blood glucose and insulin levels occurred, although hypoglycemia did not occur.[10] However, a different case report noted that hypoglycemia might occur if nopal is taken in combination with glipizide (a sulfonylurea) and metformin.[11]

Trials studying nopal are small and mainly published in Spanish, although English language abstracts are available. One trial was done in three groups of type 2 diabetes patients treated with diet alone or in combination with sulfonylureas.[12] Oral medications were discontinued 72 hours before nopal administration. After a 12-hour fast, one group of 16 patients received 500 g broiled nopal, a second group of 10 received 400 mL water as a control, and a third group of six received 500 g broiled zucchini. Subjects had blood drawn at 60, 120, and 180 minutes after receiving the nopal, water, or zucchini. The nopal group had a significant decline from 222 mg/dL (12.3 mmol/L) fasting to 203 mg/dL (11.3 mmol/L), 198 mg/dL (11.0 mmol/L), and 183 mg/dL (10.2 mmol/L), respectively, at 60, 120, and 180 minutes after receiving the treatment ($P < 0.001$ compared with baseline).

Another trial compared the effects of nopal in 14 subjects on sulfonylureas to 14 subjects without diabetes.[13] Individuals in both groups received 500 g broiled nopal or 400 mL water. In the diabetes group, glucose declined by 21 mg/dL (1.2 mmol/L), 28 mg/dL (1.6 mmol/L), and 41 mg/dL (2.3 mmol/L) at 60, 120, and 180 minutes, respectively, after nopal administration ($P < 0.005$ for 60 and 120 minutes vs. baseline; $P < 0.001$ for 180 minutes vs. baseline). Insulin concentrations also declined significantly.

In a study of individuals with type 2 diabetes, 36 subjects were randomly assigned to eat one of three test breakfasts, plus or minus nopales as part of the meal.[14] After the meal, glucose was measured at 30, 45, 60, 90, and 120 minutes with a fingerstick device. When nopal was added to three different Mexican breakfasts consisting of "chilaquiles, burritos, or quesadillas," the glucose incremental area under the curve (IAUC) decreased significantly ($P = 0.013$, $P = 0.011$, and $P = 0.019$, respectively, for the three different meals).

Another complex two-part study evaluated the impact of 300 g of steamed nopal on postprandial glucose.[15] In the first part, the glycemic index was determined for seven subjects without diabetes. The glycemic index was first determined for dried nopal containing 50 g of carbohydrates in part one. In this group, the glucose incremental area under the curve (IAUC) was lower with prickly pear consumption compared to 50 g of glucose consumption (71 vs. 232; $P < 0.001$). The insulin IAUC was also lower after nopal than glucose intake ($P < 0.05$). In the second part, 14 subjects with type 2 diabetes had four evaluations for two different test meals: a high-carbohydrate breakfast (HCB) and a high soy–protein breakfast (HSPB). The test meals were each administered without or with nopal and the researchers measured postprandial glucose every 15 minutes until 120 minutes passed. For the HCB in the diabetes group, postprandial glucose without nopal was 183.8 mg/dL (10.2 mmol/L) and with nopal, it was 36 mg/dL (2 mmol/L) lower ($P < 0.01$). The glucose IAUC was lower in the group that consumed the high-carbohydrate breakfast with nopal than without (287 vs. 443, $P < 0.001$). Both glucose values and glucose IAUC were higher in the diabetes group compared to the subjects without diabetes. In the diabetes group, insulin IAUC was also lower when the HCB was taken with nopal (5,953 uU/mL vs. 7,313 uU/mL; $P < 0.05$). For the HSPB there was no difference in glucose or insulin IAUC when the meal did or did not include nopal. Postprandial glucose dependent insulinotropic peptide (GIP) index was also measured. In the HSPB plus nopal group, GIP was lower at 30 and 45 minutes ($P < 0.01$) but did not decrease significantly in the HCB plus nopal group. Overall, nopal attenuated postprandial glucose elevations when given with a high-carbohydrate breakfast. The biggest issue with this study was the small sample size.

A 200-mg capsule consisting of a mixture of the cladode and fruit skin extract was studied in a 16-week randomized double-blind placebo-controlled trial in 29 persons with prediabetes.[16] Patients underwent two different OGTT challenges—one without nopal to determine baseline values and one administered 30 minutes after a double dose (two capsules). When nopal was administered acutely before the start of the OGTT, glucose decreased significantly at 60, 90, and 120 minutes ($P < 0.05$). Half of the patients took the supplement daily, and half took placebo for 16 weeks. At the end of 16 weeks, there was no difference in blood chemistry values (insulin, proinsulin, hsCRP, or adiponectin levels as well as A1C) between the supplement and placebo groups. Thus, the main impact was on post glucose load.

A 2015 systematic review and meta-analysis of five blinded randomized clinical trials evaluated the impact of nopal on body weight and composition as a primary outcome and cardiovascular risk factors as secondary outcomes.[4] The trials included 382 subjects in evaluations ranging from 6 weeks–2 years. The control groups included cellulose, placebo, calcium caseinate complex, and one study included low-dose dehydrated nopal. Daily doses ranged from 400 mg–15 g. Meta-analysis of four trials found a nonsiginificant mean decrease (MD) in body weight for nopal versus control (MD –0.83 kg [1.83 lb], $P = 0.33$). Meta-analysis of three trials found a significant decrease in body mass index for nopal versus control (MD –0.69 kg/m²; $P = 0.0003$). Meta-analysis of four trials found a significant decrease in percentage body fat for nopal versus control (MD –1.02%; $P < 0.00001$). Meta-analysis of two trials found a significant MD in systolic blood pressure of –0.88 mm/Hg ($P = 0.05$) and a significant MD in diastolic blood pressure of 1.14 mm Hg ($P < 0.00001$) for nopal versus control. Total cholesterol also decreased significantly in a meta-analysis of two trials. The MD for nopal versus control was 4.77 mg/dL (0.124 mmol/L; $P = 0.04$). There was no significant impact on LDL or HDL cholesterol, or triglycerides. The authors acknowledged that problematic issues included having only a few studies to evaluate with a low number of subjects, heterogenous study design, and a wide range in doses used.

Summary

Nopal may help lower blood glucose when cooked or consumed as a dietary supplement. Various forms are used, including raw (in smoothies with vegetables and fruit), cooked (broiled or grilled), and as powders, juices, capsules, and products, such as tortillas that include the cladode.[2,15] Some researchers believe the benefit is greater when nopal is cooked.[12] Different plant parts have been evaluated, and a systematic review concluded that the cladode may be more relevant in glycemic control than the fruit.[3]

There are no long-term studies evaluating nopal for diabetes treatment. Nopal has been shown to slightly but significantly decrease body mass index, percentage body fat, blood pressure, and total cholesterol.[4] The dose in diabetes ranges from 300 g of steamed nopal with a high-carbohydrate meal to 500 g of broiled nopal.[15,17] An extract containing 1,500 IU taken prior to drinking large quantities of alcohol decreased hangover symptoms.[5] For BPH, the dose used was 500 mg of powdered nopal flowers three times a day.[1] Optimal doses of extracts have not been established to treat diabetes, although a 200-mg capsule of the cladode and fruit skin extract has been studied. Standardized capsules and other forms are emerging. Caution should be exercised regarding recommendation of nopal in supplement form. As a food, however, it appears quite safe.

References

1. Natural Medicines (Natural Medicines Database search engine). Available from https://naturalmedicines.therapeuticresearch.com. Accessed May 9, 2019

2. Gouws CA, Georgousopoulou EN, Mellor DD, McKune A, Naumovski N. Effects of the consumption of prickly pear cacti (Opuntia spp.) and its products on blood glucose levels and insulin: a systematic review. *Medicina* (Kaunas) 2019;55:pii: E138. doi: 10.3390/medicina55050138

3. Santos Diaz MdS, Barba de la Rosa A-P, Helies-Toussaint C, Gueraud F, Negre-Salvayre A. Opuntia spp.: characterization and benefits in chronic diseases. *Oxid Med Cell Longev* 2017;2017:8634249. doi: 10.1155/2017/8634249

4. Onakpoya IJ, O'Sullivan J, Heneghan CJ. The effect of cactus pear (Opuntia ficus-indica) on body weight and cardiovascular risk factors: a systematic review and meta-analysis of randomized clinical trials. *Nutrition* 2015;31:640–646

5. Wiese J, McPherson S, Odden MC, Shlipak MG. Effect of Opuntia ficus indica on symptoms of the alcohol hangover. *Arch Intern Med* 2004;164:1334–1340

6. Diaz-Medina E, Martin-Herrera D, Rodriguez-Rodriguez E, Diaz-Romero C. Chromium (III) in cactus pad and its possible role in the anti-hyperglycemic activity. *J Funct Foods* 2012;4:311–314

7. Rayburn K, Martinez R, Escobedo M, et al. Glycemic effects of various species of nopal (Opuntia sp.) in type 2 diabetes mellitus. *Texas J Rural Health* 1998;26:68–76

8. Becerra-Jimenez J, Andrade-Cetto A. Effect of Opuntia streptacantha Lem. on alpha-glucosidase activity. *J Ethnopharmacol* 2012;139:493–496

9. Ibanez-Camacho R, Roman-Ramos R. Hypoglycemic effect of Opuntia cactus. *Arch Invest Med* (Mex) 1979;10:223–230

10. Meckes-Lozyoa M, Roman-Ramos R. Opuntia streptacantha: a coadjutor in the treatment of diabetes mellitus. *Am J Chin Med* 1986;14:116–118

11. Sobieraj DM, Freyer CW. Probable hypoglycemic adverse drug reaction associated with prickly pear cactus, glipizide, and metformin in a patient with type 2 diabetes mellitus. *Ann Pharmacother* 2010;44:1334–1337

12. Frati-Munari AC, Gordillo BE, Altamirano P, Ariza CR. Hypoglycemic effect of Opuntia streptacantha Lemaire in NIDDM. *Diabetes Care* 1988;11:63–66

13. Frati AC, Gordillo BE, Altamirano P, Ariza CR, Cortes-Franco R, Chavez-Negrete A. Acute hypoglycemic effect of Opuntia streptacantha Lemaire in NIDDM (Letter). *Diabetes Care* 1990;13:45–46

14. Bacardi-Gascon M, Duenas-Mena D, Jimenez-Cruz A. Lowering effect on postprandial glycemic response of nopales added to Mexican breakfasts. *Diabetes Care* 2007;30:1264–1265

15. Lopez-Romero P, Pichardo-Ontiveros E, Avila-Nava A, et al. The effect of nopal (Opuntia ficus indica) on postprandial blood glucose, incretins, and antioxidant activity in Mexican patients with type 2 diabetes after consumption of two different composition breakfasts. *J Acad Nutr Diet* 2014;114:1811–8

16. Godard MP, Ewing BA, Pischel I, Ziegler A, Benedek B, Feistel B. Acute blood glucose lowering effects and long-term safety of OpunDia supplementation in pre-diabetic males and females. *J Ethnopharmacol* 2010;130:631–634

PROBIOTICS

Millions of microbes in the gut constitute what is known as the human microbiome.[1,2-5] The role of the human microbiome is being researched and evaluated in obesity, insulin resistance, and diabetes (including gestational diabetes).[6-8] A dysfunctional microbiome is characterized by a disrupted intestinal barrier that results in increased production of inflammatory lipopolysaccharides that leak to the systemic circulation and promote release of inflammatory cytokines. There is a decrease in beneficial short-chain fatty acids such as butyrate, activation of the endocannabinoid system, and a decrease in beneficial bacteria such as *Akkermansia muciniphila*.[9,10] Altered gut microbiota may correlate with suppression of beneficial incretins such as glucagon-like peptide-1 (GLP-1), increased inflammation, increased triglyceride production, inhibition of insulin signaling, and energy harvesting changes.[5,11] Microbiome dysfunction is thus associated with different inflammatory states, obesity, and possibly diabetes. One species of microbe, *Lactobacillus*, may possibly be effective for treating hyperlipidemia.[1]

Chemical Constituents and Mechanism of Action

Probiotics are "live microorganisms that, when administered in adequate amounts, confer a health benefit on the host."[12] They are used to manage microbiome dysfunction. There is an increase in the study of probiotics to examine their benefits in diabetes. Four types of probiotics are mainly used: *Lactobacillus* and *Bifidobacterium* species, *Saccharomyces boulardii*, and *Streptococcus thermophilus*. The theoretical mechanism of action is complex and involves release of beneficial organic and free fatty acids that act against pathogenic microbes associated with obesity and insulin resistance. Other actions include possible enhanced incretin activity, decreased inflammation, decreased insulin resistance, and antioxidant activity.[2-5] There is increasing interest in *Akkermansia muciniphila*, since it promotes mucin production and thus strengthens the intestinal mucus layer to prevent pathogens from transitioning from the intestine to the systemic circulation. Metformin use is associated with increased *Akkermansia muciniphila*, and it is theorized that this may contribute to its benefit in treatment of type 2 diabetes.[10]

Adverse Effects and Drug Interactions

The most common side effects include gastrointestinal upset, constipation, and possibility of systemic infections due to microbial migration from the digestive tract into the bloodstream, and possible transfer of antibiotic resistance to pathogenic bacteria.[2,9] Immunocompromised individuals, such as those on chemotherapy, radiation treatment, or other immunocompromised states are especially vulnerable to infections. Increased mortality occurred in persons with pancreatitis who were given probiotics.[13]

Possible drug interactions are mostly with antimicrobials. If antimicrobials are coadministered at the same time, probiotic efficacy may be attenuated. Individuals taking immunosuppressive medications such as cyclosporine or tacrolimus or methotrexate or biologic agents may be susceptible to microbial infections caused by the probiotics.[2] A pharmacodynamics interaction reported in murine research is increased systemic absorption of gliclazide, a sulfonylurea.[14]

Clinical Studies

There are numerous studies of probiotics used in diabetes, but only a few will be presented here. One study found that gut microbiota changes may help identify persons who are at risk for diabetes.[15] An evaluation of 36 individuals with and without type 2 diabetes found that certain gram-negative bacteria are found in persons with diabetes.[16] In one small 4-week study, 45 males with type 2 diabetes and either impaired glucose tolerance or normal glucose tolerance were randomized to receive treatment with a probiotic or placebo. After 4 weeks, probiotics enhanced insulin sensitivity.[17]

The literature regarding probiotics in gestational diabetes mellitus (GDM) has been conflicting, since some studies show benefit, while others do not. A study in 238 pregnant women randomized to intensive dietary counseling plus probiotics, intensive dietary counseling plus placebo, or standardized dietary counseling, found that probiotic use resulted in fewer gestational diabetes cases.[18] However, the SPRING trial, a double-blind randomized controlled trial in overweight and obese women, found that probiotics administered from the second trimester onward did not prevent GDM.[19] A 2017 systematic review and meta-analysis of four randomized controlled trials involving 288 women with GDM found that probiotics did not decrease fasting glucose significantly.[20] However, insulin resistance, per HOMA-IR measurement, did decrease significantly ($P = 0.01$) A 2019 double-blind randomized placebo-controlled trial comparing probiotics to placebo evaluated 57 women with GDM in the late second and early third trimester.[21] Compared to placebo, women on probiotics had a significant mean difference decrease in fasting plasma glucose of 4 mg/dL (0.22 mmol/L; $P = 0.034$). The probiotic group also had a lower plasma insulin and homeostasis model assessment-estimated insulin resistance (HOMA-IR) ($P = 0.001$ for both).

A 2016 meta-analysis of randomized, placebo-controlled trials evaluated multiple forms of probiotics used for diabetes and related conditions (such as metabolic syndrome or obesity) in 614 subjects.[22] The main outcomes evaluated were changes in glycemic parameters, insulin, and HOMA-IR. Study quality was evaluated using the Physiotherapy Evidence Database (PEDro) scale, and 11 high-quality studies were selected for evaluation. Study duration ranged from 3–12 weeks.

Pooled mean differences and effect sizes using a 95% confidence interval were used to evaluate the data. The pooled mean difference in glucose between the probiotics group compared to placebo in all 614 subjects was a significant decrease of 9.4 mg/dL (0.52 mmol/L; $P = 0.01$). In six studies of 348 subjects, A1C also decreased significantly by 0.32% ($P = 0.01$). For insulin or HOMA-IR there was no significant mean difference between the probiotics and placebo groups. Subgroup analyses were also done for trials involving only patients with type 2 diabetes. In five trials that evaluated 252 subjects with only diabetes, the pooled mean difference in glucose between the probiotics and placebo groups was a significant decrease of 26.3 mg/dL (1.46 mmol/L; $P < 0.001$). Subgroup analysis for A1C in four trials of 218 subjects with only diabetes was a decrease of 0.52% ($P < 0.001$). Per subgroup analysis, effects of probiotics on glucose was significant when used in capsule form compared to probiotic diets ($P < 0.05$). Another subgroup analysis also found the effects were significant for multiple probiotic strains, rather than single strains. The authors noted that a noteworthy limitation was that probiotics strains were not homogeneous across studies.

A 2016 systematic review and meta-analysis of studies ranging in duration from 4–8 weeks evaluated randomized controlled trials of probiotics.[23] Five trials involved only type 2 diabetes and a sixth included type 2 diabetes, prediabetes, and healthy subjects. Six trials were evaluated in the systematic review, and five were included in the meta-analysis. Fasting plasma glucose and A1C were the two main outcomes. The five trials of 252 subjects evaluated fasting glucose. Mean difference in fasting glucose for the probiotics versus placebo groups was a significant decrease of 17.6 mg/dL (0.98 mmol/L; $P < 0.00001$). Four studies of 218 subjects evaluated A1C. The decrease in A1C for the probiotics versus placebo groups was not significant (0.11%, $P = 0.81$). Other findings were a difference between groups in HOMA-IR and fasting insulin concentrations that were not significant. Limitations of the analysis included small sample size and short duration.

A 2017 systematic review and meta-analysis evaluated the impact of probiotics on diabetes and related disorders (including GDM, overweight/obesity, and metabolic syndrome).[24] Pooled standardized mean difference on glucose and A1C reduction were 11 mg/dL (0.61 mmol/L) and 0.39% ($P = 0.001$ and $P = 0.0001$, respectively). Of 18 trials involving 1056 subjects ranging from three to 12 weeks, 10 trials evaluated glucose in type 2 diabetes. There were 268 subjects on probiotics and 270 not on probiotics. Subgroup analysis in subjects with type 2 diabetes found the standardized mean difference in glucose between the probiotics group compared to control was a significant decrease of 7.7 mg/dL (0.43 mmol/L; $P = 0.008$). Subgroup analysis of five studies evaluated A1C in 258 subjects with type 2 diabetes comparing probiotics to control. Standardized mean difference was significant, favoring the probiotics group with a value of 0.51% ($P < 0.0001$). The authors noted that subgroup analysis found significant effects in studies longer than 8 weeks. The authors noted that limitations included multiple species used, variable doses, variable forms ranging from capsules to fermented milk, and study duration.

Summary

Persons with diabetes have an altered microbiome which may start with changes that are correlated with obesity and insulin resistance. Theoretical mechanisms of benefit are release of beneficial organic and free fatty acids that act against pathogenic microbes associated with obesity and insulin resistance. Probiotics may also enhance incretin effects, decrease inflammation, enhance insulin sensitivity, and have antioxidant effects.[2-5] Four types of probiotics are mainly used: *Lactobacillus* and *Bifidobacterium* species, *Saccharomyces boulardii*, and *Streptococcus thermophiles*. There is emerging research on *Akkermansia muciniphila*, and it is noteworthy that metformin use is associated with increased levels of this organism.

Other probiotic strains have recently been studied in combination with *Akkermansia muciniphila* and include *Clostidrium beijerinckii*, *Clostridium butyricum*, *Bifidobacterium infantis*, and *Anaerobutyricum hallii*.[25] A 12-week randomized, placebo-controlled, double-blind proof of concept study was conducted in 76 individuals with type 2 diabetes. The individuals were treated with lifestyle or metformin alone or in combination with a sulfonylurea. Subjects were randomized to placebo, a probiotic proprietary blend consisting of the prebiotic inulin, the two Clostridium species and the Bifidobacterium species, or a blend of inulin plus all five probiotic strains. The primary endpoint was the change at 12 weeks in area under the curve during a standard 3-hour meal tolerance test ($AUC_{0-180\,min}$). Other secondary outcomes included A1C and change at 12 weeks from baseline in incremental glucose AUC ($AUC_{0-180\,min}$). The results for the five strain probiotic group were notable for a significant decrease in glucose total area under the curve (−36.1 mg/dL [2 mmol/L; $P = 0.05$]). The A1C decrease was 0.6% ($P = 0.054$), and the incremental glucose decrease was −28.6 mg/dL (1.6 mmol/L; $P = 0.0066$).

However, probiotic supplementation is not without adverse effects, and problems may occur. For example, increased mortality in persons with pancreatitis who were given probiotics has been reported.[13] Other effects have included GI upset, constipation, possible microbe migration from the digestive tract into the bloodstream, and transfer of antibiotic resistance to pathogenic bacteria. In immunocompromised patients, infections may occur. Drug interactions may occur with different antimicrobials. With antibiotics or antifungals the probiotic benefit may be diminished. Antibiotics should be administered separately from probiotics, at least by 2 hours. Caution should be exercised in persons on immunosuppressants since the probiotic may cause an infection.[2] There are many unknowns, such as what is the most appropriate probiotic or combination of probiotic species to use for specific diseases. Another unknown is the most appropriate form, since they are available in various formulations (yogurt, fermented milk, powders, capsules, etc.). Also, some have queried whether prebiotics should be used instead of probiotics. These are nondigestible food constituents that help the host organism stimulate growth or activity of gut bacteria and have been shown to enhance incretin secretion in animals.[26,]

It is important for individuals with diabetes to learn how to read a probiotic label for information such as the strain, expiration dates, dosing, and storage information. Two documents from the International Probiotics Association provide consumer guidance.[27,28] Moreover, the Council for Responsible Nutrition and the International Probiotics Association have published a document on best practices guidelines for probiotics that may help clinicians guide patients in appropriate product selection.[29] The research on probiotics for diabetes has increased exponentially; however, study design may be flawed and thus results are not definitive. Some studies find benefit and others do not. An editorial regarding systematic reviews and meta-analyses of probiotics has suggested that researchers conduct subgroup analyses of specific species and strains and specific combinations.[30] More research is needed, with long-term double-blind randomized design using consistent product ingredients. Currently, evidence of long-term benefit on morbidity and mortality is absent.

References

1. Natural Medicines (Natural Medicines Database search engine). Available from https://naturalmedicines.therapeuticresearch.com. Accessed May 9, 2019
2. Williams NT. Probiotics. *Am J Health Syst Pharm* 2010;67:449-58
3. Diamant M, Blaak EE, de Vos WM. Do nutrient-gut-microbiota interactions play a role in human obesity, insulin resistance and type 2 diabetes? *Obes Rev* 2011;12:272–281
4. Musso G, Gambino R, Cassader M. Obesity, diabetes, and gut microbiota: the hygiene hypothesis expanded? *Diabetes Care* 2010;33:2277–2284
5. Cani PD, Possemiers S, Van de Wiele T, et al. Changes in gut microbiota control inflammation in obese mice through a mechanism involving GLP-2-driven improvement of gut permeability. *Gut* 2009;58:1091–1103
6. Turnbaugh PJ, Ley RE, Mahowald MA, Magrini V, Mardis ER, Gordon JI. An obesity-associated gut microbiome with increased capacity for energy harvest. *Nature* 2006;444:1027–1031
7. Turnbaugh PJ, Hamady M, Yatsunenko T, et al. A core gut microbiome in obese and lean twins. *Nature* 2009;457:480–484
8. Qin J, Li Y, Cai Z, et al. A metagenome-wide association study of gut microbiota in type 2 diabetes. *Nature* 2012;490:55–60

9. Bordalo Tonucci L, Dos Santos KM, De Luces Fortes Ferreira CL, et al. Gut microbiota and probiotics: Focus on diabetes mellitus. *Crit Rev Food Sci Nutr* 2017;57:2296–2309

10. Patterson E, Ryan PM, Cryan JF, et al. Gut microbiota, obesity and diabetes. *Postgrad Med J* 2016;92:286–300

11. Baggio LL, Drucker DJ. Biology of incretins: GLP-1 and GIP. *Gastroenterology* 2007;132:2131–2157

12. Hill C, Guarner F, Reid G, et al. Expert Consensus Document. The International Scientific Association for Probiotics and Prebiotics consensus statement on the scope and appropriate use of the term probiotic. *Nat Rev Gastroenterol Hepatol* 2014;11:506–514

13. Besselink MG, van Santvoort HC, Buskens E, et al. Probiotic prophylaxis in predicted severe acute pancreatitis: a randomised, double-blind, placebo-controlled trial. *Lancet* 2008;371:651–659

14. Al-Salami H, Butt G, Fawcett JP, et al. Probiotic treatment reduces blood glucose levels and increases systemic absorption of gliclazide in diabetic rats. *Eur J Drug Metab Pharmacokinet* 2008;33:101–106

15. Karlsson FH, Tremaroli V, Nookaew I, et al. Gut metagenome in European women with normal, impaired and diabetic glucose control. *Nature* 2013;498:99–103

16. Larsen N, Vogensen FK, van den Berg FW, et al. Gut microbiota in human adults with type 2 diabetes differs from non-diabetic adults. *PLoS One* 2010;5:e9085

17. Andreasen AS, Larsen N, Pedersen-Skovsgaard T, et al. Effects of Lactobacillus acidophilus NCFM on insulin sensitivity and the systemic inflammatory response in human subjects. *Br J Nutr* 2010;104:1831–1838

18. Luoto R, Laitinen K, Nermes M, Isolauri E. Impact of maternal probiotic-supplemented dietary counselling on pregnancy outcome and prenatal and postnatal growth: a double-blind, placebo-controlled study. *Br J Nutr* 2010;103:1792–1799.

19. Callaway LK, McIntyre HD, Barrett H, et al. Probiotics for the prevention of gestational diabetes mellitus in overweight and obese women: findings from the SPRING double-blind randomized controlled trial. *Diabetes Care* 2019; 42:364–371

20. Taylor BL, Woodfall GE, Sheedy KE, et al. Effect of probiotics on metabolic outcome in pregnant women with gestational diabetes: a systematic review and meta-analysis of randomized controlled trials. *Nutrients* 2017;995:pii:E461. doi: 10.3390/nu9050461

21. Kijmanawat P, Panburana P, Reutrakul S, Tangshewinsirikul S. Effects of probiotic supplements on insulin resistance in gestational diabetes melli-

tus: a double-blind randomized controlled trial. *J Diabetes Investig* 2019;10:163–170

22. Sun J, Buys NJ. Glucose- and glycaemic factor-lowering effects of probiotics on diabetes: a meta-analysis of randomized placebo-controlled trrials. *Br J Nutr* 2016;115:1167–1177

23. Samah S, Ramasamy K, Lim SM, Neoh CF. Probiotics for the management of type 2 diabetes mellitus: a systematic review and meta-analysis. *Diabetes Res Clin Pract* 2016;118:172–182

24. Wang X, Juan Q-F, He Y-W, et al. Multiple effects of probiotics on different types of diabetes: a systematic review and meta-analysis of randomized, placebo-controlled trials. *J Pediatr Endocrinol Metab* 2017;30:611–622

25. Perraudeau F, McMurdie P, Bullard J, et al. Improvements to postprandial glucose control in subjects with type 2 diabetes: a multicenter, double blind, randomized placebo-controlled trial of a novel probiotic formulation. *BMJ Open Diab Res Care* 2020;8:e001319. doi:10.1136/bmj-drc-2020-001319.

26. Cani PD, Dewever C, Delzenne NM. Inulin-type fructans modulate gastrointestinal peptides involved in appetite regulation (glucagon-like peptide-1 and ghrelin) in rats. *Br J Nutr* 2004;92:521–526

27. International Scientific Association for Probiotics and Prebiotics. The P's and Q's of Probiotics: A consumer guide for making smart choices. Available from https://www.bifantis.com/pdf/Ps_and_Qs_of_probiotics.pdf. Accessed July 17, 2019

28. International Scientific Association for Probiotics and Prebiotics. Probiotics: A consumer guide for making smart choices. Available from https://4cau4jsaler1zglkq3wnmje1-wpengine.netdna-ssl.com/wp-content/uploads/2016/02/Consumer-Guidelines-probiotic.pdf. Issued May 3, 2016. Accessed July 17, 2019

29. Council for Responsible Nutrition, International Probiotics Association. Best practices guidelines for probiotics. Available from https://www.crnusa.org/sites/default/files/pdfs/CRN-IPA-Best-Practices-Guidelines-for-Probiotics.pdf. Accessed July 17, 2019

30. Whelan K. Editorial: The importance of systematic reviews and meta-analyses of probiotics and prebiotics. *Am J Gastroenterol* 2014;109:1563–1565

PSYLLIUM (*Plantago ovata*)

Psyllium is also known by several other names, including blonde psyllium, plantago psyllium, ispaghula husk, or simply psyllium.[1,2] The plant grows in various parts of the world and bears flowers and fruit, but the relevant part of the plant so far is the seed and seed husk. Although primarily used as a bulk-forming laxative and for diarrhea and irritable bowel syndrome, psyllium is also used for diabetes, hypertension, and hyperlipidemia.[1]

Chemical Constituents and Mechanism of Action

Psyllium is a nonfermented soluble viscous gel-forming fiber.[3] It is a mixture of acidic and neutral polysaccharides with galacturonic acid. The polysaccharides are composed of monomers of D-xylose and L-arabinose and pentosanes.[2] The mechanism of action is probably similar to that of other soluble fibers or gel-forming substances.[4,5] In aqueous solution, psyllium forms a viscous gel that slows glucose absorption into the small intestine and thereby allows a decrease in postprandial peak glucose values.[4] Another potential mechanism is a delay in gastric emptying that diminishes postprandial hyperglycemia. Carbohydrate sequestering is yet another possible mechanism, slowing carbohydrate access to digestive enzymes. Some studies have demonstrated a "second-meal effect," possibly because the soluble fiber may elicit a lower postprandial increase in insulin concentrations with a smaller counterregulatory meal response.[4] Lipid-lowering effects may be due to various mechanisms.[5,6] One is prevention of reabsorption of bile salts and enhanced elimination in fecal bile acids. Another is reduced insulin stimulation of hepatic cholesterol synthesis secondary to decreased glucose.[6] Psyllium may help obesity by decreasing appetite.

Adverse Effects and Drug Interactions

Allergic reactions including cough and sinusitis have been reported, as well as adverse gastrointestinal effects, including flatulence. The inner seed parts may be responsible for the allergic reactions. Swallowing disorders may occur due to possible esophageal obstruction.[1] Individuals with phenylketonuria may have problems if the supplement is sweetened with aspartame. Some products contain sugars that may increase blood glucose.

There are varieties of drug interactions, mainly due to binding and thus decreased absorption of medications taken at the same time as psyllium. This includes decreased carbamazepine, lithium, metformin, iron, and riboflavin absorption. Additive effects may occur with hypoglycemics, antihypertensives, and lipid-lowering agents. Additive effects with certain statins and other antihyperlipidemics have led to improved lipid profiles.[1]

Several small studies demonstrate the benefit of psyllium in reducing postprandial glucose and lipids. One frequently quoted study had a randomized placebo-controlled crossover design in 18 patients with type 2 diabetes.[4] Subjects received 6.8 g of twice-daily psyllium or placebo before a standardized breakfast and supper in two study phases that lasted 15 hours each. Glucose was measured at baseline, and postprandial values were measured every 15 minutes for 2 hours, then once after 30 minutes and hourly thereafter for 2.5 more hours. After a week-long washout, subjects were crossed over to the opposite treatment and the test was repeated. Peak postprandial glucose value elevations were 14% lower than with placebo after breakfast (109 mg/dL [6.0 mmol/L] vs. 126 mg/dL [7.0 mmol/L]) and 20% lower after dinner (54 mg/dL [3.0 mmol/L] vs. 68 mg/dL [3.8 mmol/L]). These numbers did not achieve statistical significance ($P = 0.08$ and $P = 0.06$ after breakfast and dinner, respectively). Post-lunch numbers were reduced significantly by 31% compared to placebo ($P = 0.01$), and the authors speculated that this was a "second-meal" or residual effect of the psyllium.

One of the largest studies was a 6-week double-blind placebo-controlled trial in 125 patients with type 2 diabetes that took 5 g psyllium or placebo three times daily.[5] Mean plasma glucose values declined 6 weeks after diet treatment (values not stated but shown in a graph). After an additional 6 weeks of psyllium, mean plasma glucose declined even further (no values given, only a graph showing that end point values were ~140 mg/dL [7.8 mmol/L] and ~175 mg/dL [9.7 mmol/L] 6 weeks earlier). The authors stated that there was a significant difference between the psyllium and placebo groups ($P < 0.01$). Mean LDL cholesterol also declined from 6–12 weeks of psyllium use (141 mg/dL [3.7 mmol/L] to 118 mg/dL [3.1 mmol/L]; $P < 0.01$).

A 10-week randomized double-blind placebo-controlled trial assessed 34 men with type 2 diabetes: 18 and 16 in the psyllium and placebo groups, respectively.[7] Following a dietary stabilization phase, subjects were randomized to 5.1 g of psyllium or placebo twice daily. Evaluations were done twice weekly on an outpatient basis and also in a metabolic ward at "0" and 8 weeks. Compared to baseline in the metabolic ward, the all-day postprandial glucose declined 4.2% in the psyllium group but rose 6.8% in the placebo group ($P < 0.05$). Post-lunch glucose decreased 6.5% in the psyllium group and increased 12.7% in the placebo group ($P < 0.01$). Thus, all-day and post-lunch postprandial glucose were 11% and 19.2% lower in the psyllium groups, respectively ($P < 0.05$ for all-day and $P < 0.01$ for post-lunch values). LDL cholesterol decreased by 4.7% in the psyllium group and increased by 8.3% in the placebo group (a 13% nonsignificant difference with $P = 0.07$). Total cholesterol decreased by 2.1% in the psyllium group and increased by 6.9% in the placebo group (a significant 9% difference, $P < 0.05$).

An 8-week randomized controlled study in 36 subjects with type 2 diabetes found that 10.5 g daily of psyllium compared to usual diet (control) resulted in a significant decrease in A1C and fasting glucose.[8] In the psyllium group, A1C decreased from 8.5% to 7.5% and remained at 8.5% in the control group ($P < 0.001$ for psyllium vs. control). Fasting glucose decreased from 163 mg/dL (9.1 mmol/L) to 120 mg/dL (6.7 mmol/L) in the psyllium group and decreased slightly in the control group by 5 mg/dL (0.28 mmol/L), but the results significantly favored psyllium ($P < 0.001$ for psyllium vs. control). Another significant finding was that BMI also decreased significantly for psyllium vs. control ($P < 0.001$).

A 2015 meta-analysis evaluated the impact of psyllium in subjects with type 2 diabetes as well as those who were euglycemic or at risk for type 2 diabetes.[3] The authors identified 35 randomized controlled trials and distilled this down to eight meta-analyses. Seven were aggregate-data meta-analyses and one was an individual subject data meta-analysis. Fasting glucose, A1C, peak postprandial glucose and peak postprandial insulin were evaluated in the seven aggregate data meta analyses. The remaining three analyses were in euglycemic and at-risk subjects. Mean fasting glucose decreased significantly in four studies, ranging from 6–12 weeks by 37 mg/dL (2.1 mmol/L; $P < 0.001$). In three studies that evaluated A1C, the mean decrease was 0.97% and was significant ($P = 0.048$). In six studies that evaluated peak postprandial glucose, the mean decrease was 29 mg/dL (1.6 mmol/L) and was significant ($P < 0.001$). Mean peak postprandial insulin decrease was not significant. In euglycemic subjects, mean fasting glucose did not decrease significantly ($P = 0.075$) although decrease in mean peak postprandial glucose was significant (12.4 mg/dL [0.69 mmol/L]; $P < 0.001$). Mean peak postprandial insulin decrease was also significant in euglycemic subjects ($P = 0.007$). The authors also noted that benefit of psyllium correlated with glycemia, and the greatest benefit was in those with type 2 diabetes.

A 2019 systematic review and meta-analysis of randomized controlled trials of viscous fiber supplements included not only psyllium but also guar gum, β-glucan, konjac (glucomannan), and other fiber products.[9] In this analysis of supplements added to standard care treatment in subjects with diabetes, 27 studies and 28 trial comparisons were evaluated. For A1C, 20 trial comparisons reported results for 1,148 subjects. Compared to control A1C decreased significantly by 0.58% ($P = 0.0002$) in the viscous fiber group, using a median dose of 10.9 g/day for a median duration of eight weeks. For fasting glucose, 28 trial comparisons reported results for 1,394 subjects. Compared to control fasting glucose decreased significantly by 14.8 mg/dL (0.82 mmol/L; $P = 0.001$) at a median dose of 13.1 g/day of viscous fiber for a median duration of 8 weeks. Fasting insulin did not decrease significantly in the nine trials that reported results in 228 subjects. Eleven trials reported results for HOMA-IR in 652 subjects, which decreased significantly ($P = 0.02$). The authors noted that the most viscous fiber, konjac (glucomannan), had the greatest postprandial glucose reduction. The authors concluded that viscous fiber supplements should be considered as part of the management for type 2 diabetes.

Summary

Psyllium is a mainstream product that is available to treat constipation. A commonly used form is the nonprescription product Metamucil®. Although readily available as a nonprescription medication, it is not approved for glucose-lowering effects; however, it is often used empirically to lower postprandial glucose, improve hyperlipidemia, or aid in obesity management. As with all nonprescription products, clinicians should counsel persons with diabetes that products may be sweetened, or may contain sugar substitutes, and those with phenylketonuria should avoid the aspartame-containing products. The FDA has allowed the claim that psyllium products containing at least 1.7 g of soluble fiber per reference amount may reduce coronary heart disease risk.[10] The Metamucil® label further states that "low saturated fat and low cholesterol diets that include daily intake of 7 g of soluble fiber from psyllium husk (as in Metamucil®) may reduce risk of heart disease by lowering cholesterol." The label also states, this product "helps maintain healthy blood sugar levels as part of your diet." However, the FDA has concluded there is "little evidence that psyllium husk may help prevent type 2 diabetes."[11] Emerging research is evaluating the impact of dietary soluble fiber such as psyllium (and others) on microbiome health.[12] Psyllium may potentially have a beneficial effect on gut microbiota. The dose used to lower lipids has been 3–20 g daily in divided doses. The dose for diabetes has ranged from 10.2–22 g per day, in divided doses.[1]

References

1. Natural Medicines (Natural Medicines Database search engine). Available from https://naturalmedicines.therapeuticresearch.com. Accessed May 9, 2019
2. Sierra M, Garcia JJ, Fernandez N, et al. Therapeutic effects of psyllium in type 2 diabetic patients. *Eur J Clin Nutr* 2002;56:830–842
3. Gibb RD, McRorie JW, Russell DA, Hasselblad V, D'Alessio DA. Psyllium fiber improves glycemic control proportional to loss of glycemic control: a meta-analysis of data in euglycemic subjects, patients at risk of type 2 diabetes mellitus, and patients being treated for type 2 diabetes mellitus. *Am J Clin Nutr* 2015;102:1604–1614
4. Pastors JG, Blaisdell PW, Balm TK, et al. Psyllium fiber reduces rise in postprandial glucose and insulin concentrations in patients with non-insulin-dependent diabetes. *Am J Clin Nutr* 1991;53:1431–1435

5. Rodriguez-Moran M, Guerrero-Romero F, Lazcano-Burciaga G. Lipid and glucose lowering efficacy of plantago psyllium in type II diabetes. *J Diabetes Complications* 1998;12:273–278

6. Rudkowska I. Lipid lowering with dietary supplements: Focus on diabetes. *Maturitas* 2012;72:113–116

7. Anderson JW, Allgood LD, Turner J, et al.: Effects of psyllium on glucose and serum lipid responses in men with type 2 diabetes and hypercholesterolemia. *Am J Clin Nutr* 1999;70:466–473

8. Abutair AS, Naser IA, Hamed AT. Soluble fibers from psyllium improve glycemic response and body weight among diabetes type 2 patients (randomized control trial). *Nutr J* 2016;15:86

9. Jovanovski E, Khayyat R, Zurbau A, et al. Should viscous fiber supplements be considered in diabetes control? Results from a systematic review and meta-analysis of randomized controlled trials. *Diabetes Care* 2019;42:755–766

10. U.S. Food and Drug Administration. CFR – Code of Federal Regulations Title 21. Part 101 – Food Labeling. Subpart E – Specific Requirement for Health Claims. Health Claims: Soluble fiber from certain foods and risk of coronary heart disease. Available from https://www.accessdata.fda.gov/scripts/cdrh/cfdocs/cfcfr/CFRSearch.cfm?fr=101.81. Accessed July 24, 2019

11. U.S. Food and Drug Administration. Summary of Qualified Health Claims Subject to Enforcement Discretion. Qualified Claims about Diabetes. Available from https://wayback.archive-it.org/7993/20180423202320/https:/www.fda.gov/Food/LabelingNutrition/ucm073992.htm#diabetes. Accessed August 25, 2019

12. Makki K, Deehan EC, Walter J, Backhed F. The impact of dietary fiber on gut microbiota in host health and disease. *Cell Host Microbe* 2018; Jun 13;23(6):705–715. doi: 10.1016/j.chom.2018.05.012

TEA (*Camellia sinensis*)

Camellia sinensis is a woody plant, and the leaves and leaf buds are used to make the beverage known as tea.[1] Tea is produced by steeping the leaves and has been popularly consumed for thousands of years. A member of the Theaceae family, the tea plant is an evergreen shrub or tree that may grow several feet tall but is usually pruned to 2 to 5 feet (below 2 meters) when cultivated. The leaves are dark green with serrated edges, and the tree bears white fragrant blossoms.[2] Three types of tea—oolong, black, and green—are produced from the leaves of the tea plant, depending on the processing technique.[3-5] Oolong tea is partially fermented, black tea is completely fermented, and green tea is not fermented.[5] Oolong and green tea are closely related.

Medicinally, tea has been used to prevent or treat cardiovascular disease (including hypertension and hyperlipidemia), diabetes, obesity, NAFLD, and other disease states such as cancer. It is also used for promoting mental alertness, solar radiation protection, topically to treat genital warts, and its anti-aging effects.[1,2-6] Green tea has been widely used, but oolong tea is also used. Various observational studies have noted that tea consumption is inversely related to diabetes risk. One often-quoted study indicated that regular consumption of ≥6 cups/day of green tea may lower the risk of developing of diabetes.[7]

Chemical Constituents and Mechanism of Action

Tea contains caffeine (in its natural state) and polyphenols.[2-3,5,8] The major active components are the polyphenols, collectively known as catechins.[1-3,5] The most significant polyphenols are epigallocatechin gallate, epicatechin gallate, tannins, epigallocatechin, epicatechin, and gallocatechin gallate.[1-2,5,8] The most significant catechin is epigallocatechin gallate (EGCG). Unfermented tea (green) contains more catechins, while semi-fermented (oolong) and fermented (black) tea contain theaflavins and thearubigins.[5]

Tea has varying mechanisms in diabetes. The mechanism of action of EGCG includes complex and varying effects. These include inhibition of hepatic gluconeogenesis, tyrosine phosphorylation of the insulin receptor and insulin receptor substrate. It also suppresses gene expression of the gluconeogenic enzyme phosphoenolpyruvate carboxykinase, modulates glucose-6-phosphatase, and improves insulin sensitivity.[5] Specific polyphenols are thought to enhance insulin activity, which may be responsible for some of the benefit in diabetes.[8] Also, EGCG regulates gene expression involved in insulin signal transduction pathways and glucose uptake.[5] Other mechanisms include antioxidant effects, α-glucosidase and α–amylase inhibition, improved endothelial dysfunction, protection of β-cells against cytokine induced injuries, possible insulin secretion stimulation, decreased insulin resistance, and decreased glucose absorption.[5]

The mechanism for cardiovascular protection may be a result of decreased LDL oxidation by some of the components in tea.[4] Green tea catechins may enhance gene expression of certain enzymes in hepatic cells that may stimulate bile acid production and decrease hepatic cholesterol concentrations. Another possible mechanism is diminished intestinal lipid absorption and upregulation of hepatic LDL receptors. Blood pressure lowering may be due to suppression of NADPH oxidase activity and reducing reactive oxygen species in the vascular system.[9] Green tea is the type primarily used for obesity. The catechins may stimulate thermogenesis, decrease carbohydrate absorption, inhibit catechol-o-methyltransferase enzymes that catalyze norepinephrine breakdown thus stimulating the sympathetic nervous system, and suppress appetite.[10] Green tea may also suppress ghrelin and increase adiponectin.[11] The caffeine content has varying effects, including increased resting energy expenditure and cellular thermogenesis, increased or decreased blood glucose, and varying effects on blood pressure.[1]

Adverse Effects and Drug Interactions

The most serious potential adverse effect of tea is hepatotoxicity. This has been mostly associated with green tea extracts that are often more concentrated, rather than with beverage consumption.[1,12] Higher EGCG content has a greater possibility of inducing hepatic damage. Gastrointestinal upset may occur with tea, including nausea, vomiting, and dyspepsia. Due to caffeine content, certain effects such as insomnia, anxiety, restlessness, and tachycardia may occur.[1] In pregnancy, daily caffeine intake greater than 300 mg may be associated with miscarriage.

There are many potential drug interactions with either green or oolong tea. Adding milk (including soy milk) or creamers to tea decreases the insulin potentiation, although adding lemon has no effect.[8] The caffeine content may result in toxicity when tea is combined with sympathomimetics, amphetamines, or with CAM supplements that cause stimulant effects, particularly ephedra and bitter orange. In combination with monoamine oxidase (MAO) inhibitors, increased blood pressure and heart rate may occur. Although tea has been reported to have antiplatelet effects, green tea may antagonize the antiplatelet effects of warfarin because of its vitamin K content. The calming effect of certain drugs, such as pentobarbital, may be negated by tea consumption. There is a theoretical additive hypoglycemic effect if combined with insulin or secretagogues. Green tea may also greatly decrease serum concentrations of nadolol, a beta blocker. Tea may diminish absorption of iron and folic acid.[1]

Clinical Studies

Although there is a plethora of studies involving various types of tea, only a few studies will be discussed. Epidemiological studies report that increased tea consumption may decrease risk of diabetes.[7] In one trial evaluating oolong tea in type 2 diabetes, 20 individuals on diabetes agents were assigned in a randomized crossover fashion to drink 1,500 mL (~6.25 cups) of oolong tea or water daily (consumed five times per day) for 1 month.[3] Following a 2-week washout from tea consumption, patients were randomized to tea or water for 1 month, followed by another 2-week washout and crossover to the other group for 30 days. Plasma glucose was measured after each washout and treatment period. Mean plasma glucose decreased from 229 mg/dL (12.7 mmol/L) at baseline to 162 mg/dL (9.0 mmol/L; $P < 0.001$) in the tea group. Fructosamine also decreased from 410 μmol/L at baseline to 323 μmol/L after treatment ($P < 0.01$).

In another randomized crossover trial, oolong tea was administered to 22 patients with type 2 diabetes.[11] Twelve patients had a history of myocardial infarction, and 10 had angina. After a 2-week washout, patients were randomized to 4 weeks of water or 1,000 mL/day (4.5 cups) of oolong tea for 4 weeks. Patients then also had another 2-week washout and were crossed over to the other group for 4 weeks. A1C levels decreased from a baseline of 7.23% to 6.99% ($P < 0.05$), and glucose decreased from 173 mg/dL (9.6 mmol/L) to 156 mg/dL (8.7 mmol/L). However, the difference was not significant. LDL cholesterol decreased slightly (123 mg/dL [3.2 mmol/L] to 117 mg/dL [3.0 mmol/L]), although the results were not significant. Total cholesterol decreased significantly (209 mg/dL [5.4 mmol/L] to 197 mg/dL [5.1 mmol/L]; $P < 0.01$). Adiponectin increased significantly (6.26 μg/mL to 6.88 μg/mL; $P < 0.05$). Another study showed that when 240 subjects with hyperlipidemia were given a green tea extract for 12 weeks, total and LDL cholesterol decreased significantly (11.3% and 16.4%, respectively; $P = 0.01$ for both).[13]

Several small studies such as those described above have discussed the benefit of tea in subjects with diabetes. Conversely, some studies have reported there is no benefit. For instance, one such randomized double-blind placebo-controlled study in 49 subjects compared A1C outcome after 3 months of administration of 375 or 750 mg of a tea extract containing green and black tea with placebo.[14] After 3 months, A1C increased, although not significantly, by 0.4% in the placebo group, 0.3% in the 375-mg group, and 0.5% in the 750-mg group, and there was no significant difference between the groups ($P = 0.83$ for analysis of covariance between the groups).

The preponderance of literature regarding tea has focused on various meta-analyses, but results are inconsistent. A 2013 meta-analysis of 17 randomized controlled trials lasting 2 weeks–6 months of green tea administered to 1,133 subjects reported benefit.[15] In this analysis, only four studies were conducted in subjects with type 2 diabetes, two in subjects with borderline diabetes, nine focused on overweight to obese subjects, and two were in healthy individuals. The 17 trials reported that fasting glucose decreased significantly in the green tea groups by

1.62 mg/dL (0.09 mmol/L; P < 0.01). Seven trials reported that A1C decreased significantly by 0.30% ($P \leq 0.01$). There were no significant differences in HOMA-IR, but a subgroup analysis of studies with high Jadad scores noted a significant decrease in fasting insulin of 1.16 µ U/mL (P = 0.03). A limitation of this analysis was heterogeneity in study populations, and only four trials included persons with type 2 diabetes.

A 2016 meta-analysis evaluated 10 randomized controlled trials ranging from 4–16 weeks in 608 subjects.[16] The included studies evaluated a variety of different tea types—oolong, green tea, green tea extract, black tea extract, and green plus black tea extracts. Significant effects reported were an amelioration in decrease of fasting serum insulin of 1.3 U/L (P = 0.005) in seven studies and decreased waist circumference of 2.7 cm (P = 0.009) in five studies. The authors analyzed results for green tea or green tea extract and found a decrease in fasting glucose that was not significant of 1.26 mg/dL (0.07 mmol/L; P = 0.81) and also an A1C decrease of 0.28% (P = 0.08) that was not significant. A notable limitation was that trials included in the analysis used varying types of tea products. However, the authors did calculate results for green tea products for fasting glucose and A1C.

A controversy surrounding green tea has been whether caffeine content may affect results on glucose or other parameters. A 2013 meta-analysis evaluated 22 randomized controlled trials with 25 comparisons using green tea with or without caffeine in 1,584 subjects.[17] The trials included subjects mostly diagnosed as overweight/obese, but some trials were in subjects with type 2 diabetes, prediabetes, or metabolic syndrome. A few trials were in healthy subjects. Trial duration was 3–24 weeks, with a median of 12 weeks. Sixteen trials included tea products with caffeine and six without caffeine. Overall results of trials with or without caffeine reported a significant decrease in fasting glucose of 1.48 mg/dL (0.008 mmol/L; P = 0.008). Seven trials evaluated A1C and the decrease was not significant (decrease of 0.04%; P = 0.54). The change in fasting insulin and HOMA-IR were also not significant (P = 0.83 and P = 0.74, respectively).

Green tea has also been evaluated for cardiovascular disease, such as hypertension and hyperlipidemia. A 2014 systematic review and meta-analysis of 20 double-blind randomized trials lasting at least 2 weeks in 1,536 subjects evaluated the impact of green tea versus placebo (or identical controls).[9] In 18 trials of 1,342 subjects, the mean difference between tea and placebo for systolic blood pressure was a significant decrease of 1.94 mm Hg (P = 0.0002) although diastolic pressure did not decrease significantly. In 19 trials of 1,487 subjects, mean difference for total cholesterol was a significant decrease of 5.03 mg/dL (0.13 mmol/L; P < 0.0001). In 17 trials of 1,422 subjects, mean difference for LDL cholesterol was a significant decrease of 7.35 mg/dL (0.19 mmol/L; P = 0.0004). There were no significant changes in HDL or triglycerides. Notably this analysis included some studies in patients with type 2 diabetes.

A 2013 Cochrane Systematic Review evaluated the impact of green and black tea in 821 subjects for cardiovascular disease.[18] There were 11 trials evaluated—four of black tea and seven of green tea. There was a significant impact on blood pressure and certain lipid parameters. For black tea, LDL cholesterol decreased significantly by 16.6 mg/dL (0.43 mmol/L [95% CI of −0.56 to −0.31]) but there was no impact on total or HDL cholesterol or triglycerides. Systolic blood pressure (SBP) decreased significantly by 1.85 mm Hg (95% CI of −3.21 to −0.48) and although diastolic pressure (DBP) decreased by 1.27 mm Hg, the decrease was not significant. For green tea, LDL and total cholesterol both decreased significantly. LDL cholesterol decreased 24.7 mg/dL (0.64 mmol/L [−0.77 to −0.52]). Total cholesterol decreased 23.9 mg/dL (0.62 mmol/L [95% CI of −0.77 to −0.46]). In the green tea group, SBP decreased significantly by 3.18 mm Hg (95% CI of −5.25 to −1.11) and DBP decreased by 3.42 mm Hg (95% CI of −4.54 to −2.3). Decreases in triglycerides and increases in HDL cholesterol for green tea were not significant. This evaluation was characterized by considerable heterogeneity. Notably, the researchers excluded trials where more than 25% of subjects had diabetes.

Although green tea has been widely used for weight loss, evidence to support this use has been inconsistent. Some studies show a small benefit while others do not. A 2020 systematic review and meta-analysis evaluated the efficacy of green tea for obesity.[19] Twenty two studies evaluated the impact of daily doses of 99–20,000 mg of green tea in trials ranging from 2 weeks–5 months in 2,357 persons. There were 1,197 subjects on green tea and 1,160 on control. The random-effects model results found that subjects on green tea had a significant weighted mean difference (WMD) decrease of −1.78 kg [3.9 lb]; ($P = 0.001$). For trials lasting longer than 12 weeks, the WMD decrease was a bit greater, at −2.63 kg (5.8 lb; 95% CI of −3.85 to −1.42). Decrease in BMI was also significant with a WMD decrease of −0.65 kg/m² ($P = 0.001$).

Summary

Next to water, tea is the most highly consumed beverage in the world. Some types used in diabetes include oolong, green, and black tea. There are many reasons why patients may drink tea for health-related purposes; however, numerous drug, herb, nutrient, and disease interactions are possible. Pregnant women should consider caffeine content in tea and avoid daily doses higher than 300 mg, since this may be associated with increased risk of miscarriage.[1] Pregnant women also may be vulnerable since tea may inhibit folate absorption, an important nutrient necessary to diminish neural tube defects. Persons with iron deficiency anemia should also be aware that tea may diminish iron absorption. As a beverage, tea may not be problematic unless consumed in excessive quantities, and then adverse effects of caffeine may predominate. Green tea extracts, particularly in high doses, may result in hepatotoxicity.[1,12] For persons with established diabetes, tea may not have much effect on lowering glucose. However, tea may have more of an impact on decreasing diabetes onset. For example, a 5-year observational study found that consumption of ≥6 cups/day of green tea was associated with a decreased risk of type 2 diabetes.[7] Overall, evidence supporting green tea for diabetes, cardiovascular effects, and obesity are inconsistent at best, and only modest benefit may be achieved. Doses are quite variable and catechin content may vary considerably. For green tea extract supplements, catechin content may not be listed on the label, thus it would be difficult for consumers to determine whether the product is a low or high dose. Doses used in studies have been quite variable, and there is no typical dose for either the beverage or extracts. Certainly, in beverage form, individuals may enjoy tea, as it has been enjoyed for thousands of years. However, evidence does not support safe use of tea in supplement form.

References

1. Natural Medicines (Natural Medicines Database search engine). Available from https://naturalmedicines.therapeuticresearch.com. Accessed May 9, 2019
2. Anonymous. Green tea. *Altern Med Rev* 2000;5:372–375
3. Hosoda K, Wang MF, Liao ML, et al. Antihyperglycemic effect of oolong tea in type 2 diabetes. *Diabetes Care* 2003;26:1714–1718
4. Cabrera C, Artacho R, Gimenez R. Beneficial effects of green tea: a review. *J Am Coll Nutr* 2006;25:79–99
5. Fu Q-Y, Li Q-S, Lin X-M, et al. Antidiabetic effects of tea. *Molecules* 2017; 22(5). pii: E849. doi: 10.3390/molecules22050849
6. Han LK, Takaku K, Li J, et al. Anti-obesity action of oolong tea. *Int J Obes Relat Metab Disord* 1999;23:98–105
7. Iso H, Date X, Wak ai K, et al. The relationship between green tea and total caffeine intake and risk for self-reported type 2 diabetes among Japanese adults. *Ann Intern Med* 2006;144:554–562
8. Anderson RA, Polansky MM. Tea enhances insulin activity. *J Agric Food Chem* 2002;50:8182–8186
9. Onakpoya I, Spencer E, Heneghan C, Thompson M. The effect of green tea on blood pressure and lipid profile: A systematic review and meta-analysis of randomized clinical trials. *Nutr Metab Cardiovasc Dis* 2014;24:823–836
10. Rains TM, Agarwal S, Maki KC. Antiobesity effects of green tea catechins: a mechanistic review. *J Nutr Biochem* 2011;22:1–7
11. Shimada K, Kawarabayashi T, Tanaka A, et al. Oolong tea increases plasma adiponectin levels and low-density lipoprotein particle size in patients with coronary artery disease. *Diab Res Clin Pract* 2004;65:227–234
12. Roytman MM, Poerzgen P, Navarro V. Botanicals and hepatotoxicity. *Clin Pharmacol Ther* 2018;104:458–469

13. Maron DJ, Lu GP, Cai NS, et al. Cholesterol-lowering effect of a theaflavin-enriched green tea extract: a randomized controlled trial. *Arch Intern Med* 2003;163:1448–1453

14. MacKenzie T, Leary L, Brooks WL. The effect of an extract of green and black tea on glucose control in adults with type 2 diabetes mellitus: double-blind randomized study. *Metabolism* 2007;56:1340–1344

15. Liu K, Zhou R, Wang B, et al. Effect of green tea on glucose control and insulin sensitivity: a meta- analysis of 17 randomized controlled trials. *Am J Clin Nutr* 2013;98:340–348

16. Li Y, Wang C, Huai Q, et al. Effects of tea or tea extract on metabolic profiles in patients with type 2 diabetes mellitus: a meta-analysis of ten randomized controlled trials. *Diabetes Metab Res Rev* 2016;32:2–10

17. Zheng XX, Xu YL, Li SH, et al. Effects of green tea catechins with or without caffeine on glycemic control in adults: a meta-analysis of randomized controlled trials. *Am J Clin Nutr* 2013;97:750–762

18. Hartley L, Flowers N, Holmes J, et al. Green and black tea for the primary prevention of cardiovascular disease. *Cochrane Database Syst Rev* 2013;(6):CD009934.

19. Lin Y, Shi D, Su B, et al. The effect of green tea supplementation on obesity: a systematic review and dose-response meta-analysis of randomized controlled trials. Phytother Res 2020;34:2459-2470.

TURMERIC (*Curcuma longa Linn*)

Turmeric is a member of the Zingiberaceae ginger family and a frequently used culinary spice. It is a perennial herb and the rhizomes or roots are the parts used. Turmeric powder has a characteristic bright yellow hue used to color foods and cosmetics.[1] Turmeric is highly popular and, due to pleiotropic effects, it is used medically for several diverse disorders, including osteoarthritis, gastrointestinal inflammatory disorders, depression, different cancers, nonalcoholic liver disease, hyperlipidemia, and diabetes.

Chemical Constituents and Mechanism of Action

Curcumin (diferuloyolmethane) is the yellow, most active constituent of turmeric, and is found in curry powder.[1,2] Additional constituents include demethoxycurcumin, bisdemethoxycurcumin, and cyclocurcumin. Curcumin has the greatest antioxidant effects, while bisdemethoxycurcumin has the most potent anti-inflammatory effects.[2]

Turmeric has a plethora of multimodal actions in addition to antioxidant properties. It may improve β-cell function and decrease insulin resistance.[4] Turmeric also exhibits α-glucosidase inhibitor activity.[5] Turmeric has numerous anti-inflammatory effects.[2,3,6] It is thought to inhibit tumor necrosis factor α (TNFα) as well as plasma free fatty acids. It also inhibits nuclear factor-κ B (NF-κB) activation, lipid peroxidation, and protein carbonyl and lysosomal enzyme activities. It can lower levels of thiobarbiturate acid reactive substance (TBARS) and decrease activity of sorbitol dehydrogenase.[4] It also may induce peroxisome proliferator-activated receptor-γ (PPARγ) activation, increase lipoprotein lipase activity, and activate hepatic enzymes involved with gluconeogenesis, glycolysis, and other metabolic processes.[4] Turmeric may stimulate glucagon-like peptide 1 secretion.[7] Emerging research has provided evidence that curcumin may exert some of its effects through modulation of the microbiome. For obesity, turmeric may downregulate Janus kinase.[1]

Animal research has found that turmeric may have a beneficial role in nephropathy, neuropathy, and retinopathy. In nephropathy, turmeric may diminish renal inflammation by suppressing NF-kB and IxBa action, reducing regulation of TGF-B1, monocyte chemoattractant protein-1, and ICAM-1. These actions decrease macrophage infiltration. For neuropathy, turmeric diminishes neuroinflammatory and lipid peroxidation that cause oxidative neural tissue damage. In retinopathy, turmeric stops retinal expression of proinflammatory cytokines, TNFα, VEGF and ICAM-1. Human research is emerging that addresses the possibility that turmeric may diminish inflammatory eye disorders, and ongoing trials are being conducted.[3]

Adverse Effects and Drug Interactions

Side effects are mostly gastrointestinal upset and constipation, pruritus, and allergic dermatitis. Turmeric root products may contain higher concentrations of lead than curcuminoid extracts, per a study that evaluated randomly selected products in the United States.[9]

Turmeric may have antiplatelet properties and thus possibly cause bleeding. If co-administered with anticoagulant or antiplatelet agents, such as warfarin, clopidogrel, or aspirin, bleeding may occur. Also, additive hypoglycemia may occur if taken with insulin or insulin secretagogues.[1] In vitro research has shown that curcuminoids may inhibit some Cytochrome P450 enzyme systems, such as CYP1A2, 2B6, 2C19, 2C9, 2D6, 2E1, and 3A4. Thus, turmeric may increase concentrations of several drugs such as sulfonylureas, some statins, warfarin, or other agents. Turmeric may also inhibit organic anion transporting polypeptides and thus lower clearance of medications that use these transporters, such as pioglitazone or repaglinide.[2] High doses of turmeric may bind iron and inhibit its absorption.[1] Turmeric is poorly absorbed, and is sometimes manufactured in formulations using nanoparticles and lipid/liposome particles, complexed with zinc, or coadministered with piperidine to improve absorption and bioavailability.[1,2,6,10]

Clinical Studies

Turmeric has been used for metabolic disorders including prediabetes, diabetes, and hyperlipidemia. The results show inconsistent benefit. Only a few of these studies will be presented here.

A unique study determined that turmeric might have benefit in preventing type 2 diabetes.[11] In a 9-month randomized double-blind placebo-controlled trial, 240 patients with prediabetes were given 1,500 mg/day of turmeric or placebo. At the study's end, 16.4% of patients on placebo had developed type 2 diabetes, whereas there were no cases in those on turmeric ($P < 0.001$). There was also an overall lowering in A1C when compared to the placebo group (A1C 5.6% vs. 6.02%, $P < 0.01$). Furthermore, turmeric improved β-cell function with higher HOMA-IR, lower C-peptide, and higher adiponectin levels.

A 3-month randomized double-blind placebo-controlled trial compared a curcuminoid capsule (150 mg by mouth twice daily) to placebo in 100 persons with type 2 diabetes.[12] In the curcuminoid group, fasting glucose decreased from 154 mg/dL (8.6 mmol/L) at baseline to 131 mg/dL (7.3 mmol/L), and decreased from 151 mg/dL (8.4 mmol/L) to 147 mg/dL (8.2 mmol/L) in the placebo group (the decrease was significant for the intervention versus placebo, $P < 0.01$). In the curcuminoid group, A1C decreased from 7.8% to 7.02%, and in the placebo group it increased from 7.7% to 7.99% ($P = 0.031$ for curcuminoid compared to placebo). In the curcuminoid group, triglycerides decreased from 198 mg/dL (2.23 mmol/L) to 158 mg/dL (1.78 mmol/L), and in the placebo group from 194 mg/dL (2.2 mmol/L) to 187 mg/dL (2.1 mmol/L). The decrease was significant in the curcuminoid group compared to placebo ($P = 0.018$). HOMA-IR also decreased significantly in the curcuminoid group compared to placebo ($P < 0.01$).

A 2019 systematic review and meta-analysis evaluated four trials of 508 subjects with prediabetes and eight trials of 646 subjects with type 2 diabetes.[13] The duration of prediabetes studies ranged from 8 weeks–9 months. For prediabetes studies, fasting glucose decreased nonsignificantly by 10.8 mg/dL (0.6 mmol/L; $P = 0.08$ for curcumin versus placebo) in four trials. Three studies of 370 subjects with prediabetes showed a significant decrease in A1C of 0.89% ($P = 0.03$ for curcumin versus placebo). The duration of type 2 diabetes studies ranged from 8 weeks–6 months. For eight trials, fasting glucose decreased significantly by 11.7 mg/dL (0.65 mmol/L; $P = 0.03$ for curcumin versus placebo). Six studies of 546 subjects with type 2 diabetes showed a significant decrease in A1C of 0.49% ($P = 0.04$ for curcumin versus placebo). There were no significant changes in lipids in either the prediabetes or the diabetes studies.

Lipid-lowering studies investigating curcumin have shown variable effects. A 2014 systematic review and meta-analysis of five randomized controlled studies in 243 subjects ranging from 7 days–6 months reported that curcumin did not lower total or LDL cholesterol, decrease triglycerides, or increase HDL cholesterol.[14]

A 2017 meta-analysis evaluated seven randomized controlled trials of turmeric or curcumin in 649 subjects, ranging from 4 weeks–6 months.[15] In this analysis, three studies were in subjects with metabolic syndrome and four studies were in persons with type 2 diabetes. Compared to control, turmeric and curcumin significantly decreased LDL cholesterol and triglycerides ($P < 0.0001$ and $P = 0.007$, respectively). There was no benefit to total or HDL cholesterol. However, subgroup analysis of two metabolic syndrome studies reported a significant decrease in total cholesterol ($P < 0.0001$). Subgroup analysis for the type 2 diabetes studies did not show a significant decrease in total cholesterol ($P = 0.612$).

A 2019 systematic review and meta-analysis evaluated 20 trials in 1,427 subjects, ranging from 7 days–6 months.[16] The studies included a diverse group of different populations including trials in healthy individuals. The analysis included five trials in persons with type 2 diabetes. There was a significant decrease in weighted mean difference (WMD) for triglycerides (–21.4 mg/dL [0.24 mmol/L]; $P < 0.001$) and a significant increase in HDL cholesterol (1.42 mg/dL [0.04 mmol/L]; $P = 0.046$). Although there was a decrease in LDL cholesterol of 5.82 mg/dL (0.15 mmol/L), it was not significant ($P = 0.253$). Similarly the decrease in total cholesterol of 9.6 mg/dL (0.25 mmol/L) was not significant ($P = 0.098$).

Another 2019 systematic review and meta-analysis evaluated 14 randomized controlled trials with 16 arms in persons with metabolic disorders.[17] For 12 trials of 592 on curcuminoids and 591 on controls, triglycerides decreased 19.1 mg/dL

(0.22 mmol/L; $P = 0.003$). For 14 trials of 632 on curcuminoids and 634 on controls, total cholesterol decreased 11.4 mg/dL (0.295 mmol/L; $P < 0.0001$). For 13 trials of 582 on curcuminoids and 584 on controls, LDL cholesterol decreased 9.8 mg/dL (0.253 mmol/L; $P = 0.002$). For 16 trials of 726 on curcuminoids and 727 on controls, HDL cholesterol increased 1.9 mg/dL (0.049 mmol/L; $P = 0.02$). Limitations of this analysis are the greater than 50% heterogeneity in the trials and issues with randomization. The authors stated that more than half of the trials did not clearly state random sequence generation. Moreover, varying doses of curcuminoids were used in trials. However, the authors noted that daily doses higher than 300 mg and treatment longer than 8 weeks were associated with better results.

Summary

Turmeric is a popular culinary spice that has been used for a variety of medical conditions. It has pleiotropic effects with many potential mechanisms of action, but generally modulates several cell signaling pathways.[18] It has garnered interest for the many potential therapeutic benefits in diabetes and its co-morbidites. The evidence is inconsistent, with some studies showing a benefit for fasting glucose and A1C, while others do not. The same is true for hyperlipidemia—some studies show benefit while others do not. Evidence supports curcumin use for the treatment of many diabetes-related complications, including hepatic disorders, neuropathy, retinopathy, and nephropathy.[3,18-20] In 40 type 2 diabetes patients with nephropathy, a 2-month randomized controlled trial showed that turmeric 1,500 mg daily versus placebo improved urinary protein excretion.[19] In a lecithinized system, turmeric was given to 38 persons with diabetic microangiopathy and retinopathy.[20] Benefits included improved venoarterial response, decreased retinal edema, and improved visual acuity.

Turmeric is usually well tolerated but may cause gastrointestinal upset and bleeding. Patients should be counseled to use curcumoid extracts and avoid products containing turmeric root due to possible lead content.[1] It has the potential to interact with many prescription medications. Doses used have been quite variable, with no established dose due to the many different formulations, ranging from powders to emulsions, capsules, tablets, and standardized extracts. Commonly used doses range from 1,500–2,000 mg daily in divided doses, although up to 6 g daily has been used. Absorption of the active ingredient may be optimized when taken with food or combined with piperine.[10] Clinicians should consider that coadministration with piperine (to increase bioavailability) may increase serum concentrations of conventional drugs, and thus doses of these medications may require adjustment. Due to the antiplatelet activities, patients should be counseled to stop the supplement 2 weeks before surgery due to possible bleeding.[1]

References

1. Natural Medicines (Natural Medicines Database search engine). Available from https://naturalmedicines.therapeuticresearch.com. Accessed May 9, 2019
2. Rivera-Mancia S, Trujillo J, Pedraza Chaverri J. Utility of curcumin for the treatment of diabetes mellitus: Evidence from preclinical and clinical studies. *J Nutr Intermed Metab* 2018;14:29–41. Available from https://doi.org/10.1016/j.jnim.2018.05.001. Accessed August 5, 2019
3. Parsamanesh N, Moossavi M, Bahrami A, Butler AE, Sahebkar A. Therapeutic potential of curcumin in diabetic complications. *Pharmacol Res* 2018;136:181–193
4. Zhang D-W, Fu M, Gao S-H, Liu J-L. Curcumin and diabetes: a systematic review. *Evid Based Complement Alternat Med* 2013;2013:636053
5. Lekshmi PC, Arimboor R, Indulekha PS, Menon AN. Turmeric (Curcuma longa L.) volatile oil inhibits key enzymes linked to type 2 diabetes. *Int J Food Sci Nutr* 2012;63:832–834
6. Maradana MR, Thomas R, O'Sullivan BJ: Targeted delivery of curcumin for treating type 2 diabetes. *Mol Nutr Food Res* 2013;57:1550–1556 doi 10.1002/mnfr.201200791.
7. Takikawa M, Kurimoto Y, Tusda T: Curcumin stimulates glucagon-like peptide-1 secretion in GLUTag cells via Ca2+/calmodulin-dependent kinase II activation. *Biochem Biophys Res Commun* 2013;435:165–170
8. Peterson CT, Vaughn AR, Shama V, et al. Effects of turmeric and curcumin dietary supplementation on human gut microbiota: A double-blind, randomized placebo-controlled pilot study. *J Evid Based Integr Med* 2018;23:2515690
9. Skiba MB, Luis PB, Alfafara C, et al. Curcuminoid content and safety-related markers of quality of turmeric dietary supplements sold in an urban retail marketplace in the United States. *Mol Nutr Food Res* 2018;62:1800143
10. Meghwal M, Goswami TK. Piper nigrum and piperine: an update. *Phytother Res* 2013;27:1121–1130
11. Chuengsamarn S, Rattanamongkolgul S, Luechapudiporn R, Phisalaphong C, Jirawatnotai S. Curcumin extract for prevention of type 2 diabetes. *Diabetes Care* 2012;35:2121–2127
12. Na LX, Li Y, Pan H-Z, et al. Curcuminoids exert glucose-lowering effect in type 2 diabetes by decreasing serum free fatty acids: a double-blind, placebo-controlled trial. *Mol Nutr Food Res* 2013;57:1569–77
13. Poolsup N, Suksomboon N, Kurnianta PDM, Deawjaroen K. Effects of curcumin on glycemic control and lipid profile in prediabetes and type 2

diabetes mellitus: A systematic review and meta-analysis. *PLoS One* 2019;14:e0215840

14. Sahebkar A. A systematic review and meta-analysis of randomized controlled trials investigating the effects of curcumin on blood lipid levels. *Clin Nutr* 2014;33:406–414

15. Qin S, Huang L, Gong J, et al. Efficacy and safety of turmeric and curcumin in lowering blood lipid levels in patients with cardiovascular risk factors: a meta-analysis of randomized controlled trials. *Nutr J* 2017;16:68

16. Simental-Mendia LE, Pirro M, Gotto AM Jr., et al. Lipid-modifying activity of curcuminoids: A systematic review and meta-analysis of randomized controlled trials. *Crit Rev Food Sci Nutr* 2019;59:117801187

17. Yuan F, Dong H, Gong J, et al. A systematic review and meta-analysis of randomized controlled trials on the effects of turmeric and curcuminoids on blood lipids in adults with metabolic diseases. *Adv Nutr* 2019; pii: nmz021. doi: 10.1093/advances/nmz021

18. Gupta SC, Patchva S, Aggarwal BB. Therapeutic roles of curcumin: Lessons learned from clinical trials. *AAPS J* 2013;15:195–218

19. Khajehdehi P, Pakfetrat M, Javidnia K, et al: Oral supplementation of turmeric attenuates proteinuria, transforming growth factor-b and interleukin-8 levels in patients with overt type 2 diabetic nephropathy: a randomized, double-blind and placebo-controlled study. *Scan J Urol Nephrol* 2011;45:365–70

20. Steigerwalt R, Nebbioso M, Appendino G, et al; Meriva®, a lecithinized curcumin delivery system, in diabetic microangiopathy and retinopathy. *Panminerva Med* 2012;54(1 Suppl 4):11–16

VINEGAR (*Acetic acid*)

Vinegar is a product derived from various crushed fermented fruits, such as apples.[1] Other fermented carbohydrates that are a source of vinegar include pears, grapes, melons, beets, berries, and potatoes. Vinegar is used as a folk remedy and food preservative. It has also been used as an antiseptic, and was used by Hippocrates in 420 BC to clean ulcers and treat sores. It was also combined with honey to treat coughs. In the early history of the United States, it was used for many purposes, such as poison ivy, croup, stomachache, and "dropsy." Before hypoglycemic agents were developed, vinegar "teas" were sometimes used to manage diabetes.[2] Vinegar has been used for various medical reasons, including diabetes, hyperlipidemia, weight loss, detoxification, and other purposes.[1]

Chemical Constituents and Mechanism of Action

Acetic acid is a short-chain fatty acid that is the main active chemical ingredient in vinegar, but it also contains mineral salts, amino acids, and polyphenols.[2-3] The polyphenols include galic acid, catechin, caffeic acid, ferulic acid, and organic acids (tartaric, citric, malic, and lactic acid). The mechanism of action of vinegar in diabetes is multimodal. Vinegar may delay gastric emptying, suppress disaccharidase activity, and promote muscle glucose uptake.[3] It may also suppress hepatic glucose production, increase peripheral tissue glucose utilization, enhance flow-mediated vasodilation, and facilitate insulin secretion.[4] Other researchers have also described the varied mechanisms in modulating glucose.[5] These mechanisms include binding to and activating free fatty acid receptors located in the intestinal lumen L-cells, which may lead to increased glucagon like peptide l (GLP-1) secretion. Moreover, the short chain fatty acids may stimulate AMP-activated protein kinase (AMPK) activation, which may increase peripheral glucose utilization and GLUT4 mobilization to increase glucose uptake. Due to alteration of the glycolysis and hepatic gluconeogenesis cycle, vinegar may benefit individuals with the "dawn phenomenon."[6]

In hyperlipidemia, vinegar may inhibit hepatic cholesterol production and lipogenesis through AMPK activation, which may then lead to a decrease in sterol regulatory element-binding protein-1. Vinegar may affect weight as well as visceral fat accumulation, and mechanisms include decreased lipogenesis, increased lipolysis, increased oxygen consumption via AMPK activation, increased energy expenditure via peroxisome proliferator-activated receptor α gene, and increased satiety.[4] Satiety may occur due to the increase in the satiety hormones, Peptide Y-Y (PYY) and oxyntomodulin, as well as a decrease in the appetite stimulant, ghrelin.[5]

Adverse Effects and Drug Interactions

The main adverse effect is gastrointestinal upset.[1,7] However, hypoglycemia in type 1 diabetes patients with gastroparesis has been reported.[8] Oropharyngeal inflammation and caustic esophageal injury has also been reported.[9] Hypokalemia is possible per a case report with ingestion of large amounts of vinegar.[10] Drug interactions are mainly theoretical related to the mechanism of action of vinegar and could involve additive hypoglycemia with secretagogues or insulin or problems with agents where hypokalemia may pose a risk, such as digoxin, certain diuretics that lower potassium (such as furosemide), or even supplements that deplete potassium (such as licorice rhizome).[1,10]

Clinical Studies

Vinegar has been studied in healthy individuals, type 1 and type 2 diabetes, and prediabetes. There are numerous studies, but only a few will be highlighted here. Initial studies have been mostly in small numbers of subjects and have focused on acute vinegar ingestion and impact on postprandial glucose. For instance, a small randomized study of 10 patients with well-controlled type 1 diabetes evaluated the impact of vinegar on postprandial glucose. The study showed that vinegar significantly decreased postprandial glucose by 20% after a standardized meal.[11] Another small randomized crossover study in 11 well-controlled persons with type 2 diabetes found that vinegar given for a few days with a standardized bedtime meal decreased fasting glucose by 4.7 mg/dL (0.26 mmol/L; $P = 0.033$).[6]

A complicated, randomized double-blind crossover study of 38 patients with and without diabetes consisted of four sub-trials.[12] The overall findings were that approximately 2 teaspoons of vinegar taken with meals decreased postprandial glucose by about 20%. Vinegar did not decrease postprandial glucose when taken with a monosaccharide (dextrose beverage), and glucose was greater when compared to placebo.

Some studies have not shown benefit. For instance, in a randomized controlled crossover trial, 12 subjects with type 2 diabetes drank a 75-g glucose beverage with or without 25 g of white vinegar (4% acetic acid).[13] When vinegar was co-administered with the glucose beverage, it did not alter postprandial glucose or postprandial insulin. Equivocal efficacy was shown in a different study in type 2 diabetes.[14] In this small study of 16 subjects, vinegar decreased postprandial glucose only in response to a high-glycemic but not a low glycemic–index meal. These results are equivocal since glycemic index reliability is still controversial.

A 12-week study of 14 subjects with prediabetes assessed 750 mg of acetic acid as a vinegar drink or 40 mg of acetic acid (considered a control) twice daily with meals.[15] Fasting glucose decreased significantly by 16.4 mg/dL (0.91 mmol/L) in the vinegar group versus a decrease of 4.7 mg/dL (0.26 mmol/L) in the control group ($P = 0.05$). However, there was no significant decrease in postprandial glucose or A1C.

A 12-week randomized trial in 24 patients with well controlled type 2 diabetes compared twice daily ingestion of 300-mg tablets (containing 15 mg of acetic acid), 2 tablespoons of liquid vinegar (1,400 mg), and one dill pickle (700 mg acetic acid).[3] Liquid vinegar resulted in a small but significant 0.16% decrease in A1C whereas A1C increased 0.06% and 0.22% for the vinegar pills and pickles, respectively ($P = 0.018$).

A 2017 systematic review and meta-analysis evaluated the impact of vinegar versus control on postprandial glucose and insulin responses in studies where glucose incremental area under the curve and insulin area under the curve were considered primary and secondary outcomes.[16] Eleven crossover studies in 204 subjects were assessed for impact on glucose area under the curve (AUC). Seven trials studied white vinegar, two studied apple cider vinegar, one studied wine vinegar, and one studied grape vinegar. The outcome studied was the pooled estimated standard mean difference (SMD) between vinegar and control groups for glucose and insulin AUC. The SMD for vinegar versus control showed a significant mean glucose AUC reduction of 0.60 ($P = 0.01$) in 11 studies (20 comparisons). For eight studies (14 comparisons) of insulin AUC, the SMD for vinegar versus control was a significant mean reduction of 1.3 ($P < 0.001$).

A 2018 review evaluated the impact of vinegar on fasting glucose, postprandial glucose, and A1C.[17] Studies that were 8 weeks or longer were assessed using standard meta-analysis methodology. Short-term studies with less than 3 hours of follow-up were evaluated using repeated measures meta regression. Twelve articles reporting 11 studies in 278 subjects were evaluated. For short-term outcomes, postprandial glucose was evaluated at 30, 60, 90, and 120 minutes. In five studies at 30 minutes, pooled mean difference of postprandial glucose for vinegar versus control was 15.8 mg/dL (0.88 mmol/L) and was significant (95% CI of 0.51–1.25). Pooled mean differences decreased, but not significantly, at 60, 90, and 120 minutes. For long-term outcomes of three studies at 8 weeks or longer in 147 subjects, A1C decreased significantly by 0.39% ($P = 0.0003$). Fasting glucose decreased in long term studies (8 weeks or longer) in 161 subjects by 2.2 mg/dL (0.12 mmol/L; $P = 0.78$), although the change was not significant. Postprandial glucose in long-term studies (8 weeks or longer) in 72 subjects also decreased, but not significantly, by 8.3 mg/dL (0.46 mmol/L; $P = 0.38$).

Summary

Vinegar has been used throughout the ages as a food and a medicinal agent. Vinegar has multimodal effects that may affect glucose, but the evidence is mixed and not all studies show benefit; however, this variability may be due to the study participants that included healthy subjects as well as those with prediabetes, type 1, and type 2 diabetes. Most studies have assessed glycemic impact on a short-term basis, while emerging studies are evaluating longer use. In addition, its utility for hyperlipidemia and weight loss are being researched. One small study in 39 subjects used 15 mL twice daily of apple cider vinegar or control for 12 weeks along with calorie restriction. The investigators reported a significant decrease in total cholesterol, triglycerides, and an increase in HDL cholesterol as well as decreased appetite and body weight ($P < 0.05$ for apple cider vinegar versus control); however, there was no decrease in LDL cholesterol.[18] It is used in the liquid form primarily as either apple cider or white vinegar as well as in tablet form. Doses used in studies have varied, as does the acetic acid content in different products. A dose used for glucose lowering has been 20 g with meals.[1] Some authors have suggested that as little as two teaspoonfuls of vinegar used in a salad, for instance, may attenuate increased postprandial glucose.[12] Overall, many patients have expressed interest in using vinegar for glycemic control, but they should be advised to avoid ingesting large quantities.

References

1. Natural Medicines (Natural Medicines Database search engine). Available from https://naturalmedicines.therapeuticresearch.com. Accessed May 9, 2019
2. Johnston CS, Gaas CA. Vinegar: medicinal uses and antiglycemic effect. *MedGenMed* 2006;8:61
3. Johnston CS, White AM, Kent SM. Preliminary evidence that regular vinegar ingestion favorably influences hemoglobin A1c values in individuals with type 2 diabetes mellitus. *Diabetes Res Clin Pract* 2009;84:e15–17
4. Petsiou EI, Mitrou PI, Raptis SA, Dimitriadis GD. Effect and mechanisms of action of vinegar on glucose metabolism, lipid profile, and body weight. *Nutr Rev* 2014;72:651–661
5. Lim J, Henry CJ, Haldar S. Vinegar as a functional ingredient to improve postprandial glycemic control – human intervention findings and molecular mechanisms. *Mol Nutr Food Res* 2016;60:1837–1849
6. White AM, Johnston CS. Vinegar ingestion at bedtime moderates waking glucose concentrations in adults with well-controlled type 2 diabetes. *Diabetes Care* 2007;30:2814–2815
7. Johnston CS, White AM, Kent SM. A preliminary evaluation of the safety and tolerance of medicinally ingested vinegar in individuals with type 2 diabetes. *J Med Food* 2008;11:179–83
8. Hlebowicz J, Darwiche G, Bjorgell O, Almer L. Effect of apple cider vinegar on delayed gastric emptying in patients with type 1 diabetes: a pilot study. *BMC Gastroenterol* 2007;7:46

9. Wrenn K. The perils of vinegar and the Heimlich maneuver. *Ann Emerg Med* 2006;47:207–208

10. Lhotta K, Hofle G, Gasser R, Finkenstedt G. Hypokalemia, hyperreninemia and osteoporosis in a patient ingesting large amounts of cider vinegar. *Nephron* 1998;80:242–243

11. Mitrou P, Raptis AE, Lambadiari V, et al. Vinegar decreases postprandial hyperglycemia in patients with type 1 diabetes. *Diabetes Care* 2010;33:e27

12. Johnston CS, Steplewska I, Long CA, et al. Examination of the antiglycemic properties of vinegar in healthy adults. *Ann Nutr Metab* 2010;56:74–79

13. van Dijk JW, Tummers K, Hamer HM, van Loon LJ. Vinegar co-ingestion does not improve oral glucose tolerance in patients with type 2 diabetes. *J Diabetes Complications* 2012;26:460–461

14. Liatis S, Grammatikou S, Poulia KA, et al. Vinegar reduces postprandial hyperglycaemia in patients with type II diabetes when added to a high, but not to a low, glycaemic index meal. *Eur J Clin Nutr* 2010;64:727–732

15. Johnston CS, Quagliano S, White S. Vinegar ingestion at mealtime reduced fasting blood glucose concentrations in healthy adults at risk for type 2 diabetes. *J Funct Foods* 2013;5:2007–2011

16. Shishehbor F, Mansoori A, Shirani F. Vinegar consumption can attenuate postprandial glucose and insulin responses; a systematic review and meta-analysis of clinical trials. *Diabetes Res Clin Pract* 2017;127:1–9

17. Siddiqui FJ, Assam PN, de Souza NN, et al. Diabetes control: Is vinegar a promising candidate to help achieve targets? *J Evid Based Integr Med* 2018;23:1–12

18. Khezri SS, Saidpour A, Hosseinzadeh N, Amiri Z. Beneficial effects of apple cider vinegar on weight management, visceral adiposity index and lipid profile in overweight or obese subjects receiving restricted calorie diet: A randomized clinical trial. *J Funct Foods* 2018;43:95–102

ZINC

Zinc is an essential trace element. It is associated with over 300 enzymes and is a necessary cofactor for DNA, RNA, and protein synthesis. Zinc is also needed for various metabolic functions associated with the immune system, growth, reproduction, neurobehavioral development, wound healing, and insulin action. The body does not store zinc, so humans must regularly consume zinc-containing foods, such as whole grains, nuts, legumes, poultry, seafood, red meat, and dairy products. Zinc supplements are widely used for various medical conditions such as common colds, macular degeneration, Alzheimer's Disease, attention deficit hyperactivity disorder, acne, and other dermatologic disorders. There is emerging evidence that zinc supplements may benefit persons with diabetes, prediabetes, gestational diabetes, and hyperlipidemia.[1]

Chemical Constituents and Mechanism of Action

Zinc is available in several different forms, such as zinc sulfate, zinc gluconate, zinc chloride, and zinc acetate. Zinc is often combined with other substances, such as magnesium, manganese, lysine, vitamin C, or vitamin D.[1]

Zinc has extensive and very complex roles in glucose regulation and β-cell function. Hypozincemia and hyperzincuria may occur in persons with diabetes, and zinc supplementation may help restore normal body stores.[2] One mechanism that may explain how zinc affects glucose is its antioxidant activity. Supplementation decreases elevated levels of a marker of oxidative stress, Plasma Thiobarbituric Acid Reactive Substances (TBARS). Supplementation also may increase levels of antioxidant enzymes that are depleted, such as glutathione peroxidase (GPx), super-oxide dismutase (SOD), and catalase. Zinc may inhibit gluconeogenesis and enhance glycolysis by increasing glycolytic enzyme activity (phosphofructose and pyruvate kinase). Zinc may stimulate phosphorylation reactions to help activate the insulin signaling cascade and mobilize GLUT4 transporters in muscle and adipose tissue to promote glucose uptake. Zinc also protects β-cell function by inhibiting activity of destructive amyloid polypeptides. Zinc also helps protect β-cells by suppressing proinflammatory molecules. Zinc transporters (such as ZnT8) have important roles in pancreatic islet cells, and Zinc Influx Transporters (ZIPs) also help regulate insulin production. Zinc may inhibit α-glucosidase activity. Overall, zinc maintains glucose homeostasis, protects and promotes the role of β-cell function, and facilitates insulin activity. Furthermore, due to its antioxidant properties, zinc may help attenuate diabetes-related microvascular complications that are associated with increased production of reactive oxygen species.[2]

Zinc supplements may cause stomach upset (nausea or vomiting) and a disagreeable metallic taste. Toxic side effects may occur with daily doses higher than 40 mg. At higher doses, zinc may cause copper deficiency and affect iron levels, resulting in anemia. High dose zinc may cause diarrhea and actually weaken—instead of boost—the immune system. At high doses (> 50 mg/day) it may lower HDL, a beneficial lipid. Another dose-related side effect is the possibility of worsening prostate function; it may even lead to prostate cancer when consumed at very high doses for several years.[1]

Zinc may compete with the absorption of certain beneficial minerals such as chromium. Also, zinc and iron supplements may interfere with each other's absorption. However, taking zinc and iron with food will make this interference negligible. High doses of zinc may interfere with magnesium balance, and conversely, high magnesium intake may decrease zinc absorption. Taking zinc supplements with black coffee instead of water may decrease zinc absorption by half.

Zinc may also interfere with absorption of some antibiotics, such as ciprofloxacin, cephalexin, or certain tetracyclines, and thus lower their efficacy. Some medications may decrease zinc levels, such as the ACE inhibitor lisinopril, which is commonly taken by persons with diabetes. Other medications may possibly decrease zinc levels, such as the cholesterol-lowering medication cholestyramine, steroids such as prednisone, certain estrogens, certain acid-lowering drugs such as proton pump inhibitors, or some anticonvulsants such as phenytoin or divalproex sodium.[1]

Clinical Studies

Zinc supplementation in gestational diabetes (GDM), prediabetes, or diabetes, has improved glycemic parameters. One small 6-week randomized double-blind placebo-controlled study in 58 women with GDM evaluated the impact of zinc supplements on fasting glucose.[3] Half the women took 30 mg daily of zinc and half took placebo. After 6 weeks, the fasting glucose decreased significantly by 6.6 mg/dL (0.37 mmol/L; $P = 0.005$). A 6-month double-blind randomized placebo-controlled study in 55 subjects with prediabetes evaluated the impact of zinc supplementation on fasting glucose and homeostatic model assessment (HOMA) parameters of insulin resistance, insulin sensitivity, and β-cell function.[4] Half the subjects took 30 mg of zinc sulfate once daily and half took placebo. In the zinc group, fasting glucose decreased from 104.4 mg/dL (5.8 mmol/L) to 96.7 mg/dL (5.37 mmol/L), and in the placebo group fasting glucose decreased slightly from 104.4 mg/dL (5.8 mmol/L) to 102.4 mg/dL (5.69 mmol/L). The decrease was statistically significant for zinc versus placebo ($P < 0.001$). There was also a statistically significant improvement in HOMA parameters for the zinc versus placebo group ($P < 0.001$ for β-cell function; $P = 0.01$ for insulin sensitivity, and $P = 0.002$ for insulin resistance).

A different 12-month randomized double-blind placebo-controlled study evaluated the impact of zinc supplementation in 200 subjects with prediabetes on fasting glucose, 2-hour glucose levels in an oral glucose tolerance test (OGTT), HOMA-IR, and lipids.[5] Half the subjects took 20 mg daily of elemental zinc and half took placebo. The primary outcomes were change in fasting glucose and 2-hour OGTT, and one of the secondary outcomes was development of diabetes in the follow-up period. In the zinc group, fasting glucose decreased from 115.9 mg/dL (6.4 mmol/L) to 95.1 mg/dL (5.3 mmol/L; $P < 0.05$ compared to baseline) at 12 months. In the placebo group, fasting glucose decreased slightly from 113.9 mg/dL (6.3 mmol/L) to 112.4 mg/dL (6.2 mmol/L). The 2-hour OGTT In the zinc group decreased from 169 mg/dL (9.4 mmol/L) to 149 mg/dL (8.3 mmol/L; $P < 0.05$ compared to baseline) at 12 months. In the placebo group, 2-hour OGTT increased significantly from 160 mg/dL (8.9 mmol/L) to 171.4 mg/dL (9.5 mmol/L; $P < 0.05$). HOMA-IR decreased significantly in the zinc group ($P < 0.05$ versus baseline). Total and LDL cholesterol also decreased significantly in the zinc group ($P < 0.05$ versus baseline). An important finding in this study was that the number of new diabetes cases was lower in the zinc than the placebo group (11% versus 25%, $P = 0.016$). However, the authors noted the study was not powered to detect whether differences in rate of progression to diabetes was significant.

Several meta-analyses have evaluated the impact of zinc supplementation on glycemic parameters in various populations. A 2012 systematic review and meta-analysis evaluated 25 studies in 1,362 subjects—22 studies were in type 2 and three in type 1 diabetes.[6] Nine studies evaluated zinc in combination with other nutrients, and 16 evaluated zinc monotherapy. Study duration lasted from 3 weeks–5 years. Twelve studies in 580 subjects compared the impact of zinc versus placebo on fasting glucose and found that the pooled mean difference was a decrease of 18.13 mg/dL (1 mmol/L); this difference was significant ($P = 0.02$). Four studies in 170 subjects evaluated 2-hour postprandial glucose and found a nonsignificant decrease of 34.87 mg/dL (1.94 mmol/L; $P = 0.09$). Eight studies in 430 subjects found a significant decrease in A1C of 0.54% ($P = 0.001$). There was a significant decrease in pooled mean difference for total and LDL cholesterol for zinc versus placebo. Total cholesterol decreased by 32.4 mg/dL (0.84 mmol/L; $P = 0.01$) and LDL cholesterol decreased by 11.2 mg/dL (0.29 mmol/L; $P = 0.03$). Changes in triglycerides and HDL were not significant. There were decreases in systolic and diastolic blood pressure noted in some studies. Although there may have been heterogeneity in studies due to varying zinc doses, study duration, small sample sizes, and serum levels, beneficial effects were shown.

A 2013 meta-analysis of randomized placebo-controlled trials evaluated the impact of zinc on glycemic values in varying populations (type 1 or type 2 diabetes, metabolic syndrome, obesity, and healthy individuals).[7] Fourteen trials in 3,978 subjects evaluated 18 interventions. Eleven interventions evaluated zinc monotherapy, whereas seven interventions evaluated zinc in combination with other micronutrients. Study duration ranged from 1.5–390 weeks, and the median dose of zinc used was 30 mg daily as monotherapy (20 mg when used in combination with other nutrients). Fasting glucose decreased significantly with zinc supplementation in the overall group by 3.4 mg/dL (0.19 mmol/L; $P = 0.013$). In the combined subgroup with diabetes, obesity, or metabolic syndrome, fasting glucose decreased to a greater extent, by 8.8 mg/dL (0.49 mmol/L; $P = 0.001$), compared to healthy individuals. Although there was a decrease in A1C in individuals supplemented with zinc, it was not significant (–0.64%; $P = 0.072$).

A 2019 systematic review and meta-analysis of randomized placebo-controlled trials ranging from 1–12 months evaluated the impact of zinc supplementation on glycemic control in individuals with prediabetes or diabetes, and in pregnant women with prediabetes or gestational diabetes.[8] There were 32 randomized controlled trials from 36 publications in 1,700 subjects. In 10 studies, zinc was used in combination with other supplements, and in 22 interventions in 26 studies, zinc was used as monotherapy. The mean daily dose of the various zinc salts used was 35 mg. For the overall analysis, the weighted mean decrease (WMD) in fasting glucose was –14.15 mg/dL (–0.79 mmol/L) and was significant (95% CI –17.4 to –10.9). The WMD decrease of 2-hour plasma glucose was –36.85 mg/dL (–2.05 mmol/L) and was significant (95% CI of –62.1 to –11.65). Overall, the decrease in A1C was a significant WMD decrease of –0.55% and was significant (95% CI –0.84 to –0.27). Impact on fasting glucose, postprandial glucose, and A1C was significant in studies when zinc was used as monotherapy or in combination with other nutrients. Some limitations of this meta-analysis included small numbers of subjects in individual studies, high heterogeneity with dose variability, varying disease states, and the fact that most trials were conducted in Asian countries.[8]

Another 2019 meta-analysis evaluated the impact of zinc monotherapy or in combination with other nutrients on glycemic and lipid values.[9] There were 20 studies using various zinc salts and ranging from 3 weeks–6 months with varying daily doses ranging from 7.5–660 mg. The co-nutrients included magnesium, vitamin C, and vitamin E. The authors rated study quality according to Jadad scores, and stated that six studies were of good quality and 14 were not. Fasting glucose in 16 trials with 764 subjects decreased by a WMD of 19.7 mg/dL (1.09 mmol/L) and was significant ($P = 0.006$). The WMD for A1C in 13 trials of 654 subjects was 0.43% ($P = 0.02$). The WMD for total cholesterol in 13 trials of 551 subjects was 18.5 mg/dL (0.48 mmol/L) and was significant ($P < 0.00001$). The LDL cholesterol significant decrease was 4.8 mg/dL (0.12 mmol/L; $P < 0.00001$). The HDL cholesterol significant increase was 1.45 mg/dL (0.04 mmol/L;

$P < 0.00001$). Triglycerides did not decrease significantly. Subgroup analysis based on zinc combination treatment showed improvement in almost all parameters, except A1C. However, zinc monotherapy showed significant improvement only in HDL cholesterol and fasting glucose. Limitations of this study were heterogeneity among studies and results that may vary according to intervention strategies (differing doses and use as monotherapy or in combinations).

An 8-week randomized double-blind placebo-controlled trial evaluated the effects of 25 mg twice daily of zinc gluconate and placebo in overweight persons with type 2 diabetes.[10] Each group had 35 subjects. Along with studying the impact of zinc on glycemic parameters, lipids, and weight, the researchers were also trying to determine whether zinc supplementation affects superoxide dismutase activity (SOD), a molecule that facilitates conversion of superoxides to harmless products. At the end of the study, the increase in SOD gene expression and enzyme activity was statistically significant ($P < 0.001$ and $P < 0.01$, respectively). In the zinc group, A1C decreased from 7.7% to 7.35% and increased from 7.51% to 7.56% in the placebo group ($P < 0.001$ in favor of zinc). Fasting glucose decreased from 161 mg/dL (8.9 mmol/L) to 122 mg/dL (6.8 mmol/L) in the zinc group and increased from 148.3 mg/dL (8.2 mmol/L) to 149.4 mg/dL (8.3 mmol/L) in the placebo group ($P < 0.001$). Weight decreased from 172 lb (78.2 kg) to 166 lb (75.5 kg) in the zinc group and increased from 174.7 lb (79.4 kg) to 176.4 lb (80.2 kg) in the placebo group ($P < 0.001$). Total and LDL cholesterol, as well as triglycerides, decreased significantly compared to placebo ($P = 0.04$, $P = 0.01$, $P = 0.01$, respectively). The increase in HDL cholesterol for the treatment group compared to placebo was also statistically significant ($P < 0.001$). The investigators concluded that zinc was a potentially beneficial supplement in type 2 diabetes.

As in some of the meta-analyses discussed previously, zinc is being studied either as monotherapy or in combination with other nutrients. A 12-week randomized double-blind placebo-controlled pilot study used zinc in combination with lysine and vitamin C in 67 subjects with diabetes.[11] Subjects were randomized to daily doses of placebo, 2.2 g of the zinc, lysine, and vitamin C combination, or 3.3 g of the zinc combination product. The primary outcome was to evaluate A1C at the end of 12 weeks. The lower-dose combination group had a significant decrease in A1C of 0.3%, and the higher-dose combination product had a significant decrease in A1C of 0.97% ($P < 0.02$ and $P < 0.004$, respectively, versus placebo). Other parameters that also improved were a significant decrease in systolic and diastolic blood pressure as well as total cholesterol and triglycerides in the higher dose group.

Summary

Zinc is a key essential nutrient involved in several metabolic actions in the human body and is used for multiple medical conditions. It helps maintain glycemic control by modulating the action of different enzymes involved in antioxidant activity. It may help insulin signaling and protect pancreatic β-cells by decreasing the activity of harmful cytokines. Several studies have evaluated the impact of zinc supplementation in diabetes, reporting improvement of various glycemic and lipid parameters. Some studies used zinc monotherapy while others combined zinc with other nutrients. Emerging planned studies of zinc in combination with other nutrients will evaluate whether zinc may help prevent type 2 diabetes in persons with prediabetes.[12] A 6-month randomized, double-blind placebo controlled trial in 110 subjects with prediabetes found that the combination product containing zinc, lysine, and vitamin C decreased diabetes onset. In the treatment group 7.3% developed diabetes compared to 25.4% on placebo (P = 0.018).[13] If persons choose to take zinc, they should be cautioned about possible interactions with certain other nutrients, such as magnesium or chromium, and the possibility of decreased iron levels. Patients should be advised to take zinc and iron supplements with food. Also, zinc levels may decrease in persons taking some prescription antihypertensives, steroids, acid reducing drugs, or anticonvulsants. Moreover, zinc may decrease absorption of certain antibiotics. Recommended daily zinc intake varies depending on age and health. Women older than 19 should consume daily doses of 8 mg, while males age 14 and older should consume 11 mg. However, pregnant and lactating women may require higher doses. The upper tolerable recommended daily dose in people 19 and older who are not medically supervised is 40 mg.[1] Daily doses used in diabetes studies are variable, but common doses range from 20–50 mg. Future research may help shed more light on the role of zinc in diabetes, including appropriate doses and optimal co-nutrients.

References

1. Natural Medicines (Natural Medicines Database search engine). Available from https://naturalmedicines.therapeuticresearch.com. Accessed May 9, 2019

2. Ranasinghe P, Pigera S, Galappatthy P, Katulanda P, Constantine GR. Zinc and diabetes mellitus: understanding molecular mechanisms and clinical implications. *DARU* 2015;23:44

3. Karamali M, Heidarzadeh Z, Seifati SM, et al. Zinc supplementation and the effects on metabolic status in gestational diabetes: A randomized, double-blind, placebo-controlled trial. *J Diabetes Complications* 2015;29:1314–1319

4. Islam MR, Attia J, Ali L, et al. Zinc supplementation for improving glucose handling in prediabetes: A double-blind randomized placebo-controlled pilot study. *Diabetes Res Clin Pract* 2016;115:39–46

5. Ranasinghe P, Wathurapatha WS, Galappatthy P, et al. Zinc supplementation in prediabetes: A randomized double-blind placebo-controlled clinical trial. *J Diabetes* 2018;10:386–397

6. Jayawardena R, Ranasinghe P, Galappatthy P, et al. Effects of zinc supplementation on diabetes mellitus: a systematic review and meta-analysis. *Diabetol Metab Syndr* 2012;4:13

7. Capdor J, Foster M, Petocz P, Samman S. Zinc and glycemic control: A meta-analysis of randomised placebo-controlled supplementation trials in humans. *J Trace Elem Med Biol* 2013;27:137–142

8. Wang X, Wu W, Zheng W, et al. Zinc supplementation improves glycemic control for diabetes prevention and management: a systematic review and meta-analysis of randomized controlled trials. *Am J Clin Nutr* 2019;110:76–90

9. Jafarnejad S, Mahboobi S, McFarland LV, Taghizadeh M, Rahimi F. Meta-analysis: Effects of zinc supplementation alone or with multi-nutrients, on glucose control and lipid levels in patients with type 2 diabetes. *Prev Nutr Food Sci* 2019;24:8–23

10. Nazem MR, Asadi M, Jabbari N, Allameh A. Effects of zinc supplementation on superoxide dismutase activity and gene expression, and metabolic parameters in overweight type 2 diabetes patients: a randomized, double-blind, controlled trial. *Clin Biochem* 2019;69:15–20

11. Burd JF, Noetzel V, Gonzalez A, Alvarez Melero FA. Lysulin®: A double-blind placebo-controlled pilot study of daily oral supplementation in people with type 2 diabetes. *Diabetes Manag* 2018;8:154–162

12. Ranasinghe P, Jayawardena R, Chandrasena L, Noetzel V, Burd J. Effects of Lysulin™ supplementation on prediabetes: study protocol for a randomized controlled trial. *Trials* 2019;20:171. doi: 10.1186/s13063-019-3269-8

13. Ranasinghe P, Jayawardena R, Chandrasena L. Effects of the Lysulin™ supplementation on prediabetes: a randomized double-blind, placebo-controlled clinical trial. *Diabetes Metab Syndr* 2020;14:1479-1486

Botanical and Nonbotanical Products Used for Diabetes Comorbidities

α-Lipoic Acid   160

Benfotiamine   166

Coenzyme Q10   170

Fish Oil   180

Garcinia   189

Garlic   193

Ginkgo   198

Glucomannan   204

Hibiscus   208

Pine Bark Extract   214

Red Yeast Rice   219

St. John's Wort   225

Vitamin D   229

α-LIPOIC ACID

α-lipoic acid (ALA), also known as thioctic acid, is a vitamin-like disulfide compound synthesized in the liver that functions similarly to B-complex vitamins in the body.[1] Plant sources (from highest to lowest content) include greens such as spinach or broccoli, tomatoes, peas, brussel sprouts, and rice bran. It is also found in organ meats such as liver.[2]

ALA has been widely used in Germany to treat peripheral neuropathy.[1] It has also been used for retinopathy, nephropathy, and obesity. Other clinical applications include ischemic reperfusion injury, cataracts, glaucoma, and *Amanita phalloides* poisoning. ALA has also been used for neurological disorders such as Parkinson's and Alzheimer's disease.[3]

Chemical Constituents and Mechanism of Action

ALA is readily converted to the reduced form—dihydrolipoic acid (DHLA). The supplement is mostly found as a mixture of both R and S enantiomers.[3-5] However, the naturally occurring form is the R enantiomer.[2] ALA is a catalytic agent associated with pyruvate dehydrogenase and α-ketoglutarate dehydrogenase enzyme complexes. In carbohydrate metabolism, it functions as a cofactor and interacts with pyrophosphatase to convert pyruvic acid to acetyl-coenzyme A (in the Krebs cycle) and to produce energy in the form of adenosine triphosphate.[1,3,6]

ALA and DHLA are both potent antioxidants.[2,6] Superoxide anion and peroxynitrite are oxidative-stress markers that are increased in diabetes and implicated in neuropathy pathogenesis.[7] ALA augments and maintains cellular glutathione (GSH) levels, an endogenous antioxidant. It increases levels of Nrf2, a substance that modulates antioxidant/detoxification genes modulated by antioxidant response element (ARE). ALA directly scavenges reactive oxygen species and reactive nitrogen species, thus protecting cells against oxidative stress. It also helps regenerate the endogenous antioxidants, vitamins E and C. It also inhibits NF-κB activation.[5] Since ALA may decrease oxidative stress, it may help to minimize symptoms of neuropathy and other microvascular complications.[7]

For glucose lowering, ALA plays a role in tyrosine phosphorylation of insulin receptor substrate and thus enhances glucose uptake by promoting activity of the glucose transporters GLUT1 and GLUT4.[4,5] For obesity, ALA may increase energy expenditure by suppressing hypothalamic AMP-activated protein kinase.[1]

Cytokine-induced inflammation may be attenuated by ALA supplementation with resultant decreases in inflammatory markers such as tumor necrosis factor α (TNF-α), interleukin-6, and the acute phase reactant, C-reactive protein.[8]

Adverse Effects and Drug Interactions

To date, no serious side effects have been reported, even though ALA has been used in long-term trials. However, ALA may produce dose-related gastrointestinal side effects, including nausea and vomiting, as well as vertigo.[1] Allergic skin conditions are also possible. When used intravenously, headache, pain, and injection site reactions may occur. Malodorous urine odor is also possible.[2]

Hypoglycemia may occur when ALA is combined with insulin or insulin secretagogues. The benefit of chemotherapy drugs may be attenuated by antioxidants such as ALA. Since antacids may bind to ALA, administration should be spaced at least a few hours apart.[1] Food decreases bioavailability, so it should be taken on an empty stomach.[2] ALA may decrease the conversion of thyroxine to the active T3 form; therefore, thyroid function should be monitored in persons taking thyroid replacement therapy.[1]

Clinical Studies

ALA has been extensively studied for a variety of clinical reasons, and although there are numerous studies, this review will focus on only a few trials for peripheral neuropathy. A series of four randomized double-blind placebo-controlled trials of 1,258 subjects where ALA was administered intravenously (IV) at a daily dose of 600 mg for 3 weeks were included in a meta-analysis of ALA.[9] The trials were the Alpha Lipoic Acid in Diabetic Neuropathy (ALADIN I and III) trials, the Symptomatic Diabetic Neuropathy (SYDNEY) Study, and the Neurological Assessment of Thioctic Acid in Neuropathy (NATHAN II) trials. The meta-analysis found that 52.7% of patients on ALA versus 36.9% on placebo had improved total symptom scores (TSS) consisting of pain, burning, paresthesiae, and numbness. The TSS score was significant for ALA vs. placebo ($P < 0.05$). A limitation was that one of the trials (NATHAN II) had not been published when the meta-analysis was published. However, a positive finding was that to decrease TSS, the number needed to treat was only 6.3.

A different trial was the NATHAN I (Neurological Assessment of Thioctic Acid in Neuropathy) trial.[10] It was a long-term randomized placebo-controlled multicenter trial that assessed the role of administration of a daily dose of oral 600 mg of ALA in 460 subjects with mild to moderate distal symmetric sensorimotor polyneuropathy (DSPN). The primary outcome was a composite score of the Neuropathy Impairment Score (NIS), the Neuorpathy Impairment Score-Lower Limbs (NIS-LL), and seven other neurophysiologic tests. There was no change in the primary endpoint at the end of 4 years ($P = 0.105$). However, certain secondary outcomes significantly improved. These included the NIS ($P = 0.028$), the NIS-LL ($P = 0.05$), and NIS-LL muscular weakness subscore ($P = 0.045$). Notably, more subjects showed clinically significant improvement, and fewer had progression of NIS (P = 0.013) and NIS-LL (P = 0.025). The authors noted that the lack of improvement in the primary outcome was mostly due to lack of progression in nerve conduction deficits in the placebo-treated group. An interesting finding was that subjects on placebo did not deteriorate, because glucose and triglycerides improved. Since this study evaluated subjects with mild to moderate DSPN, the results may not be extrapolated to those with severe disease.

A post hoc analysis of the NATHAN I trial found other interesting findings.[11] Improvement and prevention of progression of the NIS-LL score by ≥ 2 points from baseline to four years was predicted by several factors—older age, lower BMI, male gender, normal blood pressure, history of cardiovascular disease, insulin treatment, longer neuropathy and diabetes duration, and more advanced neuropathy stage. Subjects who received ACE inhibitors and ALA had improved cardiac autonomic function.

A 2012 meta-analysis of 15 randomized controlled trials in 1,058 subjects evaluated 300–600-mg daily doses of intravenous (IV) ALA for 2–4 weeks.[12] ALA was compared to other active substances (Ginkgo biloba injection, Methylcobalamin, vitamin B1, Prostaglandin E1, cilostazol, ligustrazine). The primary endpoints were efficacy (symptom improvement, nerve conduction velocities, and tendon reflex). The specific nerve conduction velocity (NCV) evaluations were median motor nerve conduction velocity (MNCV), median sensory nerve conduction velocity (SNCV), peroneal MNCV, and peroneal SNCV. Outcomes were assessed using Odds Ratio (OR) for efficacy and weighted mean differences (WMD) for other parameters. The analysis determined that the overall efficacy of ALA compared to control was a significant OR of 4.03 (P <0.00001). The WMD for median MNCV in 10 trials for 756 subjects was 4.63 (P < 0.00001). The WMD for median SNCV in 10 trials of 754 subjects was 3.17 (P < 0.0001). For peroneal MNCV, the WMD in eight trials of 613 subjects was 4.25 (P < 0.00001). The WMD for peroneal SNCV for six trials in 462 subjects was 3.65 (P = 0.0009). Overall, the investigators concluded that ALA improves neuropathic symptoms and nerve conduction velocity.

A different 2012 meta-analysis of four randomized controlled trials in 653 subjects compared ALA to placebo in reducing symptoms of preexisting diabetes-related peripheral neuropathy.[13] The primary outcome measure was Total Symptom Score (TSS), consisting of pain, burning, paresthesias, and numbness. Two trials used the IV form of ALA, and two used the oral form, with multiple dose comparisons ranging from 100–1,800 mg daily. The IV studies had a duration of 3 weeks, whereas the oral trials ranged from 3 weeks–6 months. The researchers considered that a 30% change in TSS (or at least a two point change for patients with a baseline score of ≤ 4) was considered clinically relevant. The overall analysis showed a significant decrease in TSS with a Standardized Mean Difference (SMD) of –2.26 (P = 0.00001) for all trials. Subgroup analysis of two trials of 600-mg daily

IV ALA for 3 weeks showed decreased neuropathy symptoms with a SMD of –2.8 ($P = 0.0001$). Subgroup analysis of oral ALA had a SMD of –1.78 ($P = 0.00001$). Thus, for the oral treatment, the TSS improvement did not meet the criteria for clinical significance (a decrease in score of at least two points).

ALA may decrease glucose, and studies have emerged that evaluate the impact on glycemic parameters. A 2018 systematic review and meta-analysis evaluated ALA administration on glucose and lipid values in persons with metabolic diseases.[14] Twenty-four studies evaluated Standardized Mean Difference (SMD) using doses ranging from 200–1,800 mg of daily ALA for a duration of 2–51 weeks. ALA significantly decreased fasting glucose by a SMD of –0.54 ($P = 0.003$) and A1C by –1.22 ($P = 0.002$). The SMD for triglycerides was –0.58 ($P = 0.006$); for total cholesterol the SMD was –0.64 ($P = 0.001$); and for LDL cholesterol the SMD was –0.44 ($P = 0.008$). The change in HDL cholesterol was not significant. A major limitation of this meta-analysis is that only seven of the included studies were in subjects with diabetes—other studies included individuals with other conditions such as metabolic syndrome, prediabetes, and heart disease, among others. Thus, this analysis had a very heterogeneous population.

A more focused evaluation of the impact of ALA on glycemic and lipid parameters was reported in a 2019 systematic review and meta-analysis of 280 subjects who had experienced a stroke.[15] This analysis evaluated three studies of fasting glucose in 185 subjects. There were 93 subjects on daily doses of 600 mg of ALA, and 92 on control, for a duration of 2–12 weeks. The pooled WMD for fasting glucose was a significant decrease of 36.9 mg/dL (2.05 mmol/L) in the ALA group compared to control ($P = 0.01$). There was no significant change in lipid parameters. However, this study had only a few studies with limited number of subjects.

Another 6-month trial that used varying doses of ALA evaluated impact on glucose as well as oxidative status.[16] In this study, 38 subjects were randomized to daily doses of 300, 600, 900, or 1,200 mg of ALA or placebo. The most important finding in this study was that fasting glucose and A1C decreased in a dose-dependent manner. The decreases were greater in the 900- and 1,200-mg dose groups. Furthermore, ALA demonstrated suppression of lipid peroxidation per decreased urinary isoprostanes.

Summary

ALA has been called the "universal antioxidant" due to its pleiotropic effects in diminishing many physiologic oxidative processes. However, it has not universally shown benefit for some diabetes-related complications, such as macular edema.[17] Although ALA has been used for several years in Germany for neuropathy, long-term trials are needed to determine whether ALA truly slows progression or only improves neuropathy symptoms. A Cochrane Review of ALA for diabetes-related neuropathy is planned and hopefully will shed more light in the near future.[18]

Emerging information shows that ALA may have a dose-related impact on glycemic parameters and possibly lipid values, and per a meta-analysis shows a small decrease in weight and body mass index.[19] Clinicians should monitor thyroid function tests in persons receiving thyroxine, since ALA may decrease the conversion to active T3 levels. Because ALA is a chelating agent, individuals who use antacids should space ALA doses a few hours apart from an antacid. Persons with cancer should be advised that, due to antioxidant properties, ALA might diminish the benefit of chemotherapy. Also, ALA should be taken on an empty stomach. Typical doses of oral ALA have been 600–1,200 mg/day. ALA has been evaluated for peripheral neuropathy, glycemic parameters, lipids, and obesity. A plethora of research is still emerging, and although much is still unknown, ALA is a benign agent that has been taken by patients for many years.

References

1. Natural Medicines (Natural Medicines Database search engine). Available from https://naturalmedicines.therapeuticresearch.com. Accessed May 9, 2019
2. Singh U, Jiatal I. Alpha-lipoic acid supplementation and diabetes. *Nutr Rev* 2008;66:646-657
3. Nichols TW: Alpha-lipoic acid: biological effects and clinical implications. *Altern Med Rev* 1997;2:177–183
4. Shay KP, Moreau RF, Smith EJ, Smith AR, Hagen TM. Alpha-lipoic acid as a dietary supplement: Molecular mechanisms and therapeutic potential. *Biochim Biophys Acta* 2009;1790:1149–1160
5. Rochette L, Ghibu S, Muresan A, Vergely C. Alpha-lipoic acid: molecular mechanisms and therapeutic potential in diabetes. *Can J Physiol* 2015;93:1021–1027
6. Evans JL, Goldfine ID. Alpha-lipoic acid: a multi-functional antioxidant that improves insulin sensitivity in patients with type 2 diabetes. *Diabetes Technol Ther* 2000;2:401–413
7. Ziegler D Thioctic acid for patients with symptomatic diabetic polyneuropathy: a critical review. *Treat Endocrinol* 2004;3:173–189
8. Akbari M, Ostadmohammadi V, Tabrizi R, et al. The effects of alpha-lipoic acid supplementation on inflammatory markers among patients with metabolic syndrome and related disorders: a systematic review and meta-analysis of randomized controlled trials. *Nutr Metab* 2018;15:39
9. Ziegler D, Nowak H, Kemplert P, et al. Treatment of symptomatic diabetic polyneuropathy with the antioxidant a-lipoic acid: a meta-analysis. *Diabet Med* 2004;21:114–121

10. Ziegler D, Low PA, Litchy WJ, et al. Efficacy and safety of antioxidant treatment with a–lipoic acid over 4 years in diabetic polyneuropathy. *Diabetes Care* 2011,34:2054–2060

11. Ziegler D, Low PA, Freeman R, Tritschler H, Vinik AI. Predictors of improvement and progression of diabetic polynueuropathy following treatment with a–lipoic acid for 4 years in the NATHAN 1 trial. *J Diabetes Complications* 2016;30:350–356

12. Han T, Bai J, Liu W, Hu Y. A systematic review and meta-analysis of a-lipoic acid in the treatment of diabetic peripheral neuropathy. *Eur J Endocrinol* 2012;67:465–471

13. Mijnhout GS, Kollen BJ, Alkhalaf A, Kleefstra N, Bilo HJG. Alpha lipoic acid for symptomatic peripheral neuropathy in patients with diabetes: A meta-analysis of randomized controlled trials. *Int J Endocrinol* 2012;2012:456279

14. Akbari M, Ostadmohammadi V, Lankarani KB, et al. The effects of alpha-lipoic acid supplementation on glucose control and lipid profiles among patients with metabolic diseases: A systematic review and meta-analysis of randomized controlled trials. *Metabolism* 2018;87:56–69

15. Tabrizi R, Borhani-Haghighi A, Mirhosseini N, et al. The effects of alpha-lipoic acid supplementation on fasting glucose and lipid profiles among patients with stroke: a systematic review and meta-analysis of randomized controlled trials. J Diabetes Metab Disord 2019;18:585–595

16. Porasuphatana S, Suddee S, Nartnampong A, et al. Glycemic and oxidative status of patients with type 2 diabetes mellitus following oral administration of alpha-lipoic acid: a randomized double-blind placebo-controlled study. *Asia Pac J Clin Nutr* 2012;21:12–21

17. Haritoglou C, Gerss J, Hammes HP, Kampik A, Ulbig MW, and RETIPON Study Group. Alpha-lipoic acid for the prevention of diabetic macular edema. *Ophthalmologica* 2011;226:127–137

18. Baicus C, Purcarea A, von Elm E, Delcea C, Furtunescu FL. Alpha-lipoic acid for diabetic peripheral neuropathy (Protocol). *Cochrane Database Syst Rev* 2018; Issue 2. Art No: CD012967

19. Namazi N, Larijani B, Azadbakht L. Alpha-lipoic acid supplement in obesity treatment: a systematic review and meta-analysis of clinical trials. *Clin Nutr* 2018;37:419–428

BENFOTIAMINE (also known as Vitamin Bl, Allithiamines)

Persons with neuropathy may have thiamine deficiency. Thiamine deficiency may result in neurological disorders, including diabetes and alcohol-related neuropathy. These disorders are treated with vitamin B1 (thiamine); however, it is not well absorbed, and high doses are necessary for successful treatment. Another name for this group of B vitamins is allithiamines because they are found in the *Allium* vegetable family, including garlic and onions.[1,2] Benfotiamine has been used for diabetes-related neuropathy in both type 1 (T1DM) and type 2 diabetes (T2DM) as well as nephropathy.

Chemical Constituents and Mechanism of Action

Benfotiamine, a fat-soluble form of thiamine, provides much higher blood and tissue levels than thiamine and thus may be the more effective form.[1,2] Benfotiamine enhances transketolase activity (the rate-limiting enzyme of the pentose phosphate pathway) and thus may inhibit three major pathways possibly involved in vascular damage such as the diacylglycerol-protein kinase C pathway, the advanced glycation end product formation pathway, and the hexosamine pathway.[2,3]

Other mechanisms include the anti-inflammatory effect of blocking activation of NF-κB, a pro-inflammatory transcription factor, and modulation of Vascular Endothelial Growth Factor Receptor 2 (VEGFR 2), which may benefit microvascular complications. Benfotiamine may also activate Protein Kinase B (PKB/Akt) to prevent hyperglycemia-induced apoptosis; inhibit activation of Mitogen-Activated Protein Kinases (MAPK) to diminish inflammation; and decrease activity of Glycogen Synthase Kinase-3β (GSK-3β), which modulates cell survival.[4]

Adverse Effects and Drug Interactions

There are no reports of major side effects, but those who are prone to allergies may experience skin rashes.[1]

Certain botanical supplements and some prescription medications may decrease thiamine activity. For instance, betel nuts (from the *Areca* palm tree), and metformin may decrease activity. Other supplements, such as horsetail plant (from the genus *Equisetum*), may cause thiamine deficiency. Some prescription drugs may decrease the body's natural thiamine levels, such as antibiotics, oral contraceptives, diuretics, some seizure medications, and chemotherapy drugs.[2]

Several studies have evaluated benfotiamine for neuropathy. Some studies are open label and others are randomized controlled trials. Due to less desirable study design, open-label studies will not be discussed here.

A 3-week randomized placebo-controlled trial reported improved neuropathy symptoms in 40 patients with type 1 or type 2 diabetes.[5] Half the group received two 50-mg benfotiamine tablets four times daily, and the other half received placebo. The neuropathy score evaluated polyneuropathy symptoms, vibration perception threshold, and the subjects' and physicians' assessment. The neuropathy score improved significantly ($P = 0.0287$). The authors also reported a significant decrease in pain ($P = 0.0414$).

A randomized double-blind placebo-controlled six-week study evaluated 133 subjects with type 1 or type 2 diabetes and distal polyneuropathy and compared two doses of benfotiamine (600 or 300 mg daily) to placebo.[6] The Neuropathy Symptom Score differed significantly between groups in the per protocol population ($P = 0.033$) but not in the intent to treat population ($P = 0.055$). There was no difference between the groups for the Total Symptom Score.

A randomized 12-week study in 24 patients with type 1 or type 2 diabetes comparing a benfotiamine plus vitamin B6 and B12 combination to placebo used higher benfotiamine doses (320 mg daily) for 2 weeks and then a lower dose (120 mg daily) for 10 weeks.[7] The benfotiamine group had improved vibration perception threshold scores in the metacarpal and metatarsal nerves, although the results were not significant. The benfotiamine group also had improved nerve conduction velocity in the peroneal nerve ($P = 0.006$) but not the median nerve.

Results are not always positive. A 24-month randomized double-blind placebo-controlled trial in 67 patients with type 1 diabetes found no benefit with 300 mg daily of benfotiamine for peripheral nerve function, which included peroneal nerve conduction velocity or other nerve conduction parameters.[8] However, the results of this study have been questioned by other researchers, secondary to what the persons providing the critique attributed to study design and definitions of abnormal nerve conduction velocity.[9]

A randomized double-blind crossover study investigated whether 900 mg daily of benfotiamine or placebo prevented postprandial endothelial dysfunction in 31 subjects with type 2 diabetes.[10] This study evaluated endothelial dysfunction by measuring flow-mediated dilatation. There was no difference between patients treated with benfotiamine and placebo. However, a subgroup of patients with the greatest endothelial dysfunction showed improvement with benfotiamine.

Summary

Benfotiamine is a fat-soluble thiamine pro-drug that has been evaluated in studies lasting 2 years.[8] Although highly studied for neuropathy, benfotiamine has also been studied for retinopathy in animal research.[3] In nephropathy, early research reported improvement in urinary albumin excretion with high-dose thiamine (not benfotiamine).[11] A later study evaluated 900 mg daily of benfotiamine or placebo in 82 subjects who had increased urinary albumin excretion (despite treatment with renin angiotensin aldosterone system inhibitors). Although urinary albumin excretion decreased, the change was not significant. Furthermore, kidney injury molecule (KIM-1), a marker of tubular damage, did not decrease.[12] Another study in subjects with nephropathy supplemented with benfotiamine also failed to find a decrease in urinary- or plasma-advanced glycation end products or markers of endothelial dysfunction and inflammation.[13]

There are numerous studies with varying results, and study design is not always optimal. At this time, results are more promising for neuropathy than nephropathy. The dose studied in diabetes is 300–600 mg a day, administered in divided doses.[1] Benfotiamine is also manufactured in combination with other B vitamins, as well as α-lipoic acid. Overall, benfotiamine is a promising agent and thus far has been safe.

References

1. Natural Medicines (Natural Medicines Database search engine). Available from https://naturalmedicines.therapeuticresearch.com. Accessed May 9, 2019
2. Head KA. Benfotiamine. *Altern Med Rev* 2006;11:238–242
3. Hammes H-P, Du X, Edelstein D, Taguchi T, Matsumura T, Ju Q, et al. Benfotiamine blocks three major pathways of hyperglycemic damage and prevents experimental diabetic retinopathy. *Nature Med* 2003;9:294–299
4. Raj V, Ojha S, Howarth FC, Belur PD, Subramanya SB. Therapeutic potential of benfotiamine and its molecular targets. *Eur Rev Med Pharmacol Sci* 2018;22:3261–3273
5. Haupt E, Ledermann H, Kopcke W. Benfotiamine in the treatment of diabetic polyneuropathy – a three-week randomized, controlled pilot study (BEDIP Study). *Int J Clin Pharmacol Ther* 2005;43:71–77
6. Stracke H, Gaus W, Achenbach U, Federlin K, Bretzel RG. Benfotiamine in diabetic polyneuropathy (BENDIP): results of a randomised, double-blind, placebo-controlled clinical study. *Exp Clin Endocrinol Diabetes* 2008;116:600–605
7. Stracke H. A benfotiamine-vitamin B combination in treatment of diabetic polyneuropathy. *Exp Clin Endocrinol Diabetes* 1996;104:311–316

8. Fraser DA, Diep LM, Hovden IA, et al. The effects of long-term oral benfotiamine supplementation on peripheral nerve function and inflammatory markers in patients with type 1 diabetes: a 24-month, double-blind, randomized, placebo-controlled trial. *Diabetes Care* 2012;35:1095–1097

9. Ziegler D, Tesfaye S, Kempler P: Comment on: Fraser et al. The effects of long-term long-term oral benfotiamine supplementation on peripheral nerve function and inflammatory markers in patients with type 1 diabetes: a 24-month, double-blind, randomized, placebo-controlled trial. *Diabetes Care* 2012;35:1095–1097

10. Stirban A, Pop A, Tschoepe D. A randomized, double-blind, crossover, placebo-controlled trial of 6 weeks benfotiamine treatment on postprandial vascular function and variables of autonomic nerve function in Type 2 diabetes. *Diabet Med* 2013;30:1204–1208

11. Rabbani N, Alam SS, Riaz S, et al: High-dose thiamine therapy for patients with type 2 diabetes and microalbuminuria: a randomized, double-blind placebo-controlled study. *Diabetologia* 2009;52:208–212

12. Alkhalaf A, Klooster A, van Oeveren W, et al: A double-blind, randomized, placebo-controlled clinical trial on benfotiamine treatment in patients with diabetic nephropathy. *Diabetes Care* 2010;33:1598–1601

13. Alkhalaf A, Kleefstra N, Groenier KH, et al. Effect of benfotiamine on advanced glycation endproducts and markers of endothelial dysfunction and inflammation in diabetic nephropathy. *PLoS One* 2012;7:e40427

COENZYME Q10

Coenzyme Q10 (CoQ10) is a lipid-soluble vitamin-like substance and is highly concentrated in the heart, liver, kidneys, and pancreas, as well as cell membranes.[1] It is thought to be deficient in many clinical conditions, including diabetes. Since the body manufactures adequate amounts of CoQ10, it is not considered a vitamin. Dietary sources include meats and fish as well as oils and nuts. Human CoQ10 levels decline with age, certain cardiac diseases, and different neurologic disorders, including diabetes-related neuropathy and Parkinson's Disease. CoQ10 is a popular supplement to treat cardiovascular diseases such as heart failure, hypertension, hyperlipidemia, and diabetes. It is widely used to offset the body's decreased CoQ10 levels secondary to statin use that may provoke myopathy. Smoking also depletes CoQ10 levels.[1]

Chemical Constituents and Mechanism of Action

CoQ10 is composed of a benzoquinone nucleus and a polyisoprenoid tail.[2] There are 10 Units in the isoprenoid tail, hence the number "10" as part of its name.[1] The benzoquinone nucleus is mostly derived from the amino acid tyrosine, and the isoprene tail is derived from the mevalonate pathway in cholesterol synthesis. CoQ10 may exist as the fully-oxidized (ubiquinone) or reduced (ubiquinol) forms, or as an intermediate. CoQ10 supplement bioequivalence may vary widely, and the manufacturing process is expensive. Microbial fermentation using various yeast and bacteria is used in the manufacturing process.[2]

The primary biochemical activity is as a cofactor in the electron transport chain involved in mitochondrial ATP production. CoQ10 may function as a direct membrane stabilizer, secondary to phospholipid-protein interactions. It serves as an antioxidant and free-radical scavenger. Oxygen-derived free radicals may inactivate endothelium-derived relaxing factor, which may result in arteriolar constriction. Ischemic tissues also may have oxygen-derived free radicals, and CoQ10 may be protective in tissues where these free radicals may exert damage.[1,3] In diabetes, it is theorized that there may be suboptimal CoQ10 activity in β-cells; by increasing activity of glycerol-3-phosphate dehydrogenase and improving ATP production, CoQ10 may improve glucose-stimulated insulin secretion.[4] In diabetes, it may improve endothelial dysfunction.[5]

In heart failure, CoQ10 may be important, since decreased mitochondrial CoQ10 may impair myocardial ATP production. Moreover, the failing myocardium may have difficulty dealing with increasing reactive oxygen species.[2] For hypertension, CoQ10 may work by producing vasodilatation via a direct effect on the endothelium and vascular smooth muscle, thus decreasing peripheral resistance.[6] In the past, there has been contradictory information as to whether CoQ10 may benefit statin-associated myopathy symptoms (SAMS). The possible mechanism of these symptoms is mitochondrial dysfunction secondary to decreased intramuscular and circulating CoQ10 levels.[7]

Adverse Effects and Drug Interactions

Adverse effects that may occur with CoQ10 are usually mild and include GI upset, anorexia, headache, and dizziness.[1] Overall, CoQ10 does not have any safety concerns, and even long-term administration for six years did not result in any adverse effects.[8]

There are several potential drug or disease interactions. The most concerning potential drug interaction is with warfarin, since CoQ10 is a vitamin K structural analog and thus may attenuate its anticoagulant effect and decrease the International Normalized Ratio (INR). As a result, a thromboembolic event may inadvertently occur. However, the effect on INR has not occurred consistently.[1] Statins, red yeast rice, and ω-3 fatty acids may decrease endogenous levels of CoQ10. Decrease in endogenous CoQ10 by statins has been theorized to be one possible mechanism responsible for statin-related myopathy.[9] Studies using low-dose atorvastatin and higher doses did indeed find CoQ10 depletion.[10,11] Other medications, including antihypertensives, diabetes medications, and amitriptyline (a tricyclic antidepressant) may also decrease CoQ10 levels.[1]

A potentially-beneficial drug interaction has occurred with doxorubicin, since CoQ10 supplementation may diminish doxorubicin-mediated cardiotoxicity by thwarting inhibition of CoQ10 enzymes.[12] However, a subsequent problematic issue is that, due to antioxidant properties, CoQ10 may diminish the cancer fighting benefits of doxorubicin.[1]

In heart failure, a disease interaction that is concerning is that patients on statins may have lower CoQ10 levels, which may possibly result in adverse outcomes.[2] In persons with diabetes, decreased CoQ10 concentrations have been reported.[13]

Clinical Studies

For over 40 years, CoQ10 has been evaluated extensively for different medical conditions.[2] CoQ10 has been studied for cardiovascular disease, including heart failure (HF) and hypertension as well as for hyperlipidemia, diabetes, and statin associated muscle symptoms. There is a plethora of studies; only a select few will be discussed here.

For primary prevention of cardiovascular disease, a Cochrane review determined that there are few studies that allow for an adequate evaluation to support its use.[14] For secondary prevention, there are several trials with small numbers of subjects and with limited follow up that show differing benefit. Most of these secondary prevention trials have evaluated CoQ10 administration after acute myocardial infarction (MI).

One trial of 144 patients post MI found that cardiac deaths and nonfatal MI had decreased at one year.[15] Thus, overall cardiac events, including cardiac mortality and nonfatal MI, was 24.6% in the CoQ10 group and 45% in the comparison group ($P < 0.02$). However, an issue with study design in this trial was that the active and control capsules were not identical, and subjects were instructed not to compare their pills with others in the study.[15]

A 2013 meta-analysis of 13 randomized controlled trials of CoQ10 for HF in 395 subjects showed improved ejection fraction of 3.67% and a slight improvement in New York Heart Association (NYHA) functional class.[16] However, the analysis included few studies, and many of these were older evaluations in which subjects were not taking agents that are now commonly used to treat HF, such as ACE inhibitors and beta blockers. Most of the trials showing Left Ventricular Ejection Fraction (LVEF) improvement were published earlier than 1993.

An important HF trial was the QSYMBIO study.[17] This two-year study was a randomized double-blind placebo-controlled trial that evaluated subjects with moderate to severe HF where 202 subjects took CoQ10 100 mg three times daily, and 218 took placebo. The study included mostly subjects with (NYHA) Class III disease and reduced ejection fraction. The study was a two-phase evaluation. The first assessment was done at 16 weeks and the second at 106 weeks. The primary outcomes for the first 16-week phase were NYHA functional class, a 6-minute walk test, and echocardiography, as well as measurement of N-terminal pro-B-type natriuretic peptide (NT-proBNP). The primary outcome for the second phase was a composite of major adverse cardiovascular events (MACE), consisting of unplanned hospitalization secondary to worsening HF, cardiovascular death, mechanical assist implantation, or urgent cardiac transplantation. There were no criteria for LVEF, but 93% of subjects had reduced ejection fraction with a LVEF < 40%. At week 16, there were no differences between the CoQ10 and placebo groups on LVEF, 6-minute walk distance, NYHA class, or plasma concentration of NT-proBNP. At the end of the second phase, MACE had occurred in 15% of the subjects on CoQ10 and 26% on placebo. Thus, the number needed to treat to prevent one major cardiovascular event was nine. The Hazard Ratio (HR) for CoQ10 compared to placebo was 0.5 and was significant at $P = 0.003$. In addition, there were more subjects with improved NYHA functional class in the CoQ10 group than subjects on placebo (58% vs. 45%, $P = 0.028$). Cardiovascular deaths were lower in the CoQ10 group than on placebo (9% vs. 16%, with a 43% relative reduction; $P = 0.039$). All-cause mortality was also lower in the CoQ10 group (10% vs. 18%, with a 42% relative reduction, $P = 0.036$). Although adverse events were lower on CoQ10 than placebo, the difference was not significant ($P = 0.110$). A limitation of this study was the relatively low number of subjects enrolled over a period of 8 years; enrollment was lower than the targeted number of 550 subjects and was closed prematurely due to slow recruitment. Other limitations include protocol changes in endpoints from the time of trial registration to publication as well as changes in CoQ10 dose; also of note is that the study was funded by the dietary supplement industry. Furthermore, since so many subjects had NYHA Class III function and reduced ejection fraction, results may not be easily extrapolated to all subjects with HF.

CoQ10 supplementation has also been frequently evaluated for hypertension. One trial evaluated blood pressure in subjects with hyperlipidemia and myocardial infarction who did not have diabetes.[18] This 12-week trial evaluated 200 mg of CoQ10 daily or placebo in 52 subjects. Systolic pressure declined from 143 to 131 mm Hg in the CoQ10 group and from 134 to 131 mm Hg in the placebo group ($P < 0.0001$ for CoQ10 versus placebo). The decrease in diastolic pressure was greater for the placebo than for CoQ10 group and was statistically significant. Thus, diastolic pressure declined from 90 to 82 mm Hg in the CoQ10 group and from 100 to 83 mm Hg in the placebo group ($P < 0.001$ in favor of placebo). The authors noted that a possible reason for the outcome was that the baseline blood pressures were markedly different in the two groups.

A 2012 randomized, double-blind crossover study evaluated 100 mg twice daily of CoQ10 versus placebo in 30 subjects with metabolic syndrome and used 24-hour ambulatory blood pressure and clinic based monitoring.[19] CoQ10 did not affect blood pressure or heart rate versus placebo in 24-hour ambulatory measurements. However, supplementation resulted in a lower daytime diastolic pressure compared to placebo.

Although several hypertension trials have assessed CoQ10 supplementation, the number of trials that may be included in a Cochrane evaluation are limited due to strict study design requirements. Thus, a 2016 Cochrane Evaluation of CoQ10 evaluated only two double-blind randomized placebo-controlled parallel or crossover trials with a duration of at least 3 weeks.[20] The primary outcome was to determine the impact of CoQ10 on systolic and diastolic blood pressure. The two trials of 50 subjects were included in the pooled analysis; a third study was excluded because of high risk of bias. One of the two included studies was the 2012 trial discussed previously (by Young et al) that incorporated 24-hour ambulatory blood pressure monitoring.[19] In the Cochrane analysis, systolic blood pressure declined nonsignificantly by 3.7 mm Hg and diastolic pressure also declined nonsignificantly by 2 mm Hg ($P = 0.16$ for both). The Cochrane evaluation concluded that CoQ10 does not have an effect on blood pressure.

Results for lipids have been varied. A 2014 study by Mosheni, et. al. evaluated lipid parameters.[18] There was a significant decrease from baseline in both the CoQ10 and placebo groups for total and LDL cholesterol. There was a 47-mg/dL (1.22 mmol/L) decrease for CoQ10 and 28-mg/dL (0.74 mmol/L) decrease for placebo for total cholesterol. For LDL cholesterol, the decrease was 30 mg/dL (0.76 mmol/L) for both CoQ10 and placebo. However, the difference between groups was not significant (P = 0.231 and P = 0.56 for total and LDL cholesterol, respectively). On the other hand, HDL cholesterol increased significantly from baseline only in the CoQ10 group (11.5 mg/dL [0.29 mmol/L] for CoQ10 and no change in placebo). The difference was significant for CoQ10 versus placebo (P < 0.001). Triglycerides did not decrease significantly in either group. Thus, the only significant change in lipids in this study was an increase in HDL cholesterol for CoQ10 versus placebo.

Some studies have evaluated both lipid and glycemic parameters using CoQ10. A 12-week lipid study by Aljawad evaluated patients with hyperlipidemia and type 2 diabetes.[21] In this study, 41 subjects were treated with daily doses of 150 mg of Coenzyme Q10, 20 mg of atorvastatin, or placebo while maintained on an oral sulfonylurea. At 12 weeks, total and LDL cholesterol as well as triglycerides had decreased significantly from baseline in the CoQ10 and atorvastatin groups (P < 0.001 for total and LDL cholesterol for both CoQ10 and atorvastatin; P < 0.05 for triglycerides for both CoQ10 and atorvastatin). This study did not assess differences between CoQ10 and atorvastatin. These lipid parameters did not change significantly in the placebo group. In the CoQ10 group, HDL cholesterol increased 11 mg/dL (0.28 mmol/L) from baseline (P < 0.05), and in the placebo group the increase was more modest (2 mg/dL [0.05 mmol/L]). HDL did not change in the atorvastatin group. Thus, increased HDL cholesterol was the lipid parameter that did change significantly in favor of CoQ10 (P < 0.001 for CoQ10 versus placebo). Another facet of this study was to evaluate fasting glucose and A1C at 12 weeks. Fasting glucose decreased significantly in the CoQ10 group, from 202 mg/dL (11.2 mmol/L) to 154 mg/dL (8.6 mmol/L), and remained the same in the placebo group. Fasting glucose difference was significant for CoQ10 compared to placebo (P < 0.05). In the atorvastatin group, fasting glucose increased. A1C decreased significantly in the CoQ10 group (7.8% to 6.4%; P < 0.001 versus baseline) and remained the same in the placebo group. The A1C difference was significant for CoQ10 compared to placebo (P < 0.05).

A 12-week randomized double-blind placebo-controlled trial in 50 subjects with type 2 diabetes evaluated the impact of daily doses of 150 mg of CoQ10 or placebo on lipids and glycemic parameters.[22] In this study, there were unusual changes in lipids. Total cholesterol increased in the CoQ10 group while the placebo group had a decrease. The difference was significant for placebo versus CoQ10 (P = 0.02). This result was mirrored for LDL cholesterol changes (an increase in the CoQ10 group and a decrease in the placebo group) and the difference was significant for placebo versus CoQ10 (P < 0.001). Triglycerides did decrease significantly from baseline in the CoQ10 group by 24 mg/dL (0.27 mmol/L; P = 0.004) but there was no difference compared to placebo. Thus, in this study, the only lipid parameter that decreased significantly was a significant decrease from baseline in triglycerides in the CoQ10 group. However, fasting glucose decreased significantly by 15.5 mg/dL (0.86 mmol/L) on CoQ10 and increased by 19.9 mg/dL (1.1 mmol/L) on placebo *(P = 0.02 for CoQ10 versus placebo)*. Similarly, there was a 0.4% decrease in A1C for CoQ10 and a 0.23% increase for placebo *(P = 0.01 for CoQ10 versus placebo)*.

A 2018 pooled analysis of 14 studies evaluated the impact of CoQ10 on metabolic biomarkers in 693 overweight and obese subjects with type 2 diabetes.[23] Daily doses of CoQ10 ranged from 100–400 mg for a follow up duration of 8–24 weeks. Each parameter was presented as a weighted mean difference (WMD) between CoQ10 and the control groups using a random-effects model. In 12 studies of fasting glucose, the WMD for CoQ10 decreased significantly by 10.6 mg/dL (0.59 mmol/L; *P* = 0.01). The WMD for A1C for CoQ10 was a significant decrease of 0.28% *(P* = 0.03) for 13 studies. The only lipid parameter that decreased significantly was triglycerides, with a WMD of 15 mg/dL (0.17 mmol/L; *P* = 0.02) in eight studies. Changes in other lipid parameters were not significant. Furthermore, changes in systolic and diastolic pressure were also not significant. A subgroup analysis based on CoQ10 daily doses lower than 200 mg also showed significant decreases in fasting glucose *(P* = 0.0006), A1C *(P* = 0.005), and triglycerides *(P* = 0.02). This subgroup analysis also showed a significant decrease in Homeostatic Model Assessment of Insulin Resistance (HOMA-IR) and fasting insulin *(P* = 0.0001 and *P* = 0.01, respectively), which were not significant in the overall pooled analysis. A post-hoc subgroup analysis also showed that supplementation with CoQ10 for less than 12 weeks also significantly decreased fasting glucose, A1C, and triglycerides *(P* = 0.01, *P* = 0.02, and *P* = 0.04, respectively). One strength of this evaluation was using the Grading of Recommendations Assessment, Development, and Evaluation (GRADE) approach to rate the quality of evidence that identified high-quality evidence for triglycerides and systolic blood pressure, moderate quality for fasting glucose and A1C, and low quality for diastolic blood pressure. Another strength was performing subgroup analyses. An important strength was evaluating safety that showed that there were no CoQ10-related adverse effects. Limitations include heterogeneity in reported outcomes that reflects study variability.

CoQ10 has often been used in combination with other supplements. In a study in elderly Swedish subjects, CoQ10 in combination with selenium administered for 4 years resulted in decreased cardiovascular mortality.[24] The effect persisted for eight years following the end of the study. The rationale for the study was that European selenium intake is low and CoQ10 levels decrease with age. However, the benefit was lower in those that had higher selenium levels. Thus, it is difficult to determine the impact of CoQ10 and separate it from the benefit provided by selenium.

A clinical controversy has been whether CoQ10 supplementation will improve statin-associated muscle symptoms (SAMS). Evidence has not consistently shown whether CoQ10 helps attenuate SAMS. Some studies have shown benefit, while others have not.[1] Results may vary, according to differences in product bioavailability and absorption. An important issue is the subjective nature of patient reports of muscle symptoms. A 2018 meta-analysis evaluating impact of CoQ10 on SAMS has included newer trials.[25] Twelve studies evaluated 575 subjects (294 on CoQ10 and 281 on placebo) that used daily doses of 100–600 mg of CoQ10 or placebo in studies that ranged from 30 days to 3 months. Nine randomized controlled trials evaluated the effect of CoQ10 on SAMS. Pooled weighted mean difference (WMD) using a fixed-effect model evaluated whether CoQ10 benefitted SAMS compared to placebo. Different components of SAMS were evaluated and showed a significant decrease in WMD for CoQ10 versus placebo. For muscle pain, the WMD was -1.60 $(P < 0.001)$ and for muscle weakness WMD was -2.28 $(P = 0.006)$. For muscle cramps, the WMD was -1.78, and for muscle tiredness the WMD was -1.75 $(P < 0.001$ for both). To confirm the effects, a random-effects model was also used and showed that WMD was -1.46 for muscle pain $(P < 0.001)$ and -2.54 for muscle weakness $(P = 0.006)$. In 10 trials, there was no decrease in plasma creatine kinase subsequent to CoQ10 supplementation, using a fixed-effect or random-effect model $(P = 0.23$ and $P = 0.85$, respectively). A limitation of this analysis was the low number of available randomized controlled trials, small numbers of subjects in the studies, heterogeneity due to characteristics of subjects, and dose and duration of CoQ10 supplementation.

Summary

CoQ10 is a popular supplement used by persons with and without diabetes. An important issue is that CoQ10 supplement bioequivalence may vary widely, and the manufacturing process is expensive.[2] A concern with CoQ10 use is in persons who take the anticoagulant warfarin, since CoQ10 has a structure similar to vitamin K and may result in breakthrough thromboembolism.[1] Most adverse effects are benign and include gastrointestinal upset, headache, and dizziness. In pregnancy, CoQ10 has been used after the 20th week of gestation. However, it is best to err on the side of caution, so it should probably not be used during pregnancy or lactation. There are no studies in lactation. CoQ10 has been used for a variety of disorders, and evidence is greater for some than others. For instance, for neurological disorders and diabetes-related neuropathy, there is less evidence.[1] Although blood pressure may decrease significantly, endpoint values are still higher than advocated for persons with diabetes. There is conflicting information on the effect of CoQ10 in lipid lowering, although in some individuals there is benefit. In diabetes, CoQ10 supplementation has shown improved effects on fasting glucose and

A1C, although endpoint values are higher than target goals. However, an important reason it is used in diabetes is because it improves endothelial dysfunction.[5]

In heart failure, the QSYMBIO study was a landmark trial that reported a 43% decrease in MACE and cardiovascular death, and a 42% decrease in all-cause mortality.[17] The impact of CoQ10 on mitigating SAMS is inconsistent. However, a 2018 meta-analysis reported positive results on amelioration of certain symptoms.[25] Thus, a trial for patients experiencing SAMS may be warranted. However, some sources have stated that if benefit occurs it will be seen within 30 days; 30 days may be an appropriate timeframe to evaluate whether benefit may occur.[1] Doses vary depending on the disease state. For hypertension and other cardiovascular diseases, a commonly used daily dose is 200–300 mg although higher doses have been used. There is no fixed dose for diabetes and doses used have ranged from 100–400 mg daily.[1] CoQ10 has been used safely long term.[8,25] CoQ10 is a highly studied and apparently safe supplement that has been used long term without serious adverse effects. Further studies will help determine its place in treatment.

References

1. Natural Medicines (Natural Medicines Database search engine). Available from https://naturalmedicines.therapeuticresearch.com. Accessed May 9, 2019

2. Ayer A, Macdonald P, Stocker R. Coq10 function and role in heart failure and ischemic heart disease. *Annu Rev Nutr* 2015;35:175–213

3. Bonakdar RA, Guarneri E: Coenzyme Q10. Am Fam Physician 2005;72:1065–1070.

4. McCarty MF. Can correction of sub-optimal coenzyme Q status improve beta-cell function in type II diabetics? *Med Hypotheses* 1999;52:397–400

5. Hamilton SJ, Chew GT, Watts GF. Coenzyme Q10 improves endothelial dysfunction in statin-treated type 2 diabetic patients. *Diabetes Care* 2009;32:810–812

6. Pepe S, Marasco SF, Haas SJ, et al. Coenzyme Q10 in cardiovascular disease. *Mitochondrion* 2007;7 Suppl:S154–S167

7. Stroes ES, Thompson PD, Corsini A, et al. Statin-associated muscle symptoms: impact on statin therapy – European Atherosclerosis Society Consensus Panel Statement on Assessment, Aetiology and Management. *Eur Heart J* 2015;36:1012–1022

8. Langsjoen P, Langsjoen P, Folkers K: Long-term efficacy and safety of coenzyme Q10 therapy for idiopathic dilated cardiomyopathy. *Am J Cardiol* 1990;65:521–523

9. Lamperti C, Naini AB, Lucchini V, et al.: Muscle coenzyme Q10 level in statin-related myopathy. *Arch Neurol* 2005;62:1709–1712

10. Mabuchi H, Higashikata T, Kawashiri M, et al. Reduction of serum ubiquinol-10 and ubiquinone-10 levels by atorvastatin in hypercholesterolemic patients. *J Atheroscler Thromb* 2005;12:111–119

11. Rundek T, Naini A, Sacco R, et al. Atorvastatin decreases the coenzyme Q10 level in the blood of patients at risk for cardiovascular disease and stroke. *Arch Neurol* 2004;61:889–892

12. Iarussi D, Auricchio U, Agretto A, et al. Protective effect of coenzyme Q10 on anthracycline cardiotoxicity: control study in children with acute lymphoblastic leukemia and non-Hodgkin's lymphoma. *Molec Aspects Med* 1994;15 (Suppl.):207–212

13. Miyake Y, Shouzu A, Nishikawa M, et al.: Effect of treatment with 3-hydroxy-3-methylglutaryl coenzyme A reductase inhibitors on serum coenzyme Q10 in diabetic patients. *Arzneimittelforschung* 1999;49:324–329

14. Flowers N, Hartley L, Todkill D, Stranges S, Rees K. Co-enzyme Q10 supplementation for the primary prevention of cardiovascular disease. *Cochrane Database Syst Rev* 2014;12:CD010405

15. Singh RB, Neki NS, Kartikey K, et al. Effect of coenzyme Q10 on risk of atherosclerosis in patients with recent myocardial infarction. *Mol Cell Biochem* 2003;246:75–82

16. Fotino AD, Thompson-Paul AM, Bazzano LA. Effect of coenzyme Q10 supplementation on heart failure: a meta-analysis. *Am J Clin Nutr* 2013;97:268–275

17. Mortensen SA, Rosenfeldt F, Kumar A, et al. The effect of Coenzyme Q10 on morbidity and mortality in chronic heart failure. Results from Q-SYMBIO: A randomized double-blind trial. *J Am Coll Cardiol HF* 2014;2:641–649

18. Mosheni M, Vafa MR, Hajimiresmail SJ, et al. Effects of coenzyme Q10 supplementation on serum lipoproteins, plasma fibrinogen, and blood pressure in patients with hyperlipidemia and myocardial infarction. *Iran Red Crescent Med J* 2014;16:e16433

19. Young JM, Florkowski CM, Molyneux SL, et al. A randomized, double-blind, placebo-controlled crossover study of coenzyme Q10 therapy in hypertensive patients with the metabolic syndrome. *Am J Hypertens* 2012;25:261–270

20. Ho MJ, Li ECK, Wright JM. Blood pressure lowering efficacy of coenzyme Q10 for primary hypertension. *Cochrane Database Syst Rev* 2016;3:CD007435

21. Aljawad FH, Hashim HM, Jasim GA, et al. Effects of atorvastatin and coenzyme Q10 on glycemic control and lipid profile in type 2 diabetic patients. *Int J Pharm Sci Rev Res* 2015;34:183–186

22. Zahedi H, Eghtesadi S, Seifirad S, et al. Effects of CoQ10 supplementation on lipid profiles and glycemic control in patients with type 2 diabetes: a randomized, double-blind, placebo-controlled trial. *J Diabetes Metab Disord* 2013;13:81

23. Huang H, Chi H, Liao D, Zou Y. Effects of coenzyme Q10 on cardiovascular and metabolic biomarkers in overweight and obese patients with type 2 diabetes mellitus: a pooled analysis. *Diabetes Metab Syndr Obes* 2018;11:875–886

24. Alehagen U, Asaeth J, Alexander J, Johansson P. Still reduced-cardiovascular mortality 12 years after supplementation with seleniuim and coenzyme Q10 for four years: A validation of previous 10-year follow-up results of a prospective randomized double-blind placebo-controlled trial in elderly. *PLoS One* 2018;13:e1093120. Available from https://doi.org/10.1371/journal.pone.0193120https://doi.org/10.1371/journal.pone.0193120. Accessed September 25, 2019

25. Qu H, Guo M, Chai H, et al. Effects of coenzyme Q10 on statin-induced myopathy: an updated meta-analysis of randomized controlled trials. *J Am Heart Assoc* 2018;7:e009835. Doi: 10.1161/JAHA.118.009835

FISH OIL (ω-3 Fatty Acids)

ω-3 fatty acids are essential fats mostly derived from marine sources and include eicosapentanoic acid (EPA) and docosahexanoic acid (DHA).[1] Fish oil and plant-based products are the primary sources of ω-3 fatty acids. The main use of ω-3 fatty acids is to lower lipids. Plant products with ω-3 fatty acids include flaxseed-derived α-linolenic acid, algal-derived eicosapentanoic acid (EPA), docosahexanoic acid (DHA), or a combination of these.[2] Oils from salmon, lake trout, mackerel, sturgeon, herring, tuna, and sardines are rich sources of EPA and DHA. Fish oil is the main type used for cardiovascular disease protection and treatment of hypertriglyceridemia, as well as for a variety of other medical problems, such as arthritis, dry eye syndrome, and psychiatric disorders.[1] The terms "ω-3 fatty acids" or "fish oil" will be used interchangeably to describe the same product in this monograph.

Chemical Constituents and Mechanism of Action

ω-3 fatty acids are characterized by a structure that has several carbon atoms and several double bonds. The structure contains a double bond at the third carbon atom from the methyl end of the fatty acid chain, hence the name n-3 or ω-3.[3] EPA and DHA are the main constituents. The activities of ω-3 fatty acids are complex and encompass a variety of multimodal effects. The major mechanisms of action include anti-inflammatory and antithrombotic effects, regulation of transcription factors, plaque and membrane stabilization, modulation of cardiac ion channels, and other physiologic effects.

ω-3 fatty acids inhibit inflammation by the following mechanisms: decreasing tumor necrosis factor-α (TNF-α); inhibiting activation of nuclear factor-κ light chain enhancer of activated β-cells (NF-κB); inhibiting different interleukins such as IL-6 and IL-1β; downregulating signaling molecules such as mitogen-activated protein kinases; decreasing monocyte infiltration and thus decreasing adhesion molecules such as vascular cell adhesion molecule-1 (VCAM-1), E-selectin, and other intercellular adhesion molecules associated with inflammation; and modulating transcription factors such as peroxisome proliferator-activated receptors (PPARα) to help regulate other inflammatory mediators.[3]

ω-3 fatty acids also exhibit antithrombotic effects by inhibiting prothrombotic and vasoconstrictive mediator production (thromboxane A2 and thromboxane B2) and by promoting production of thromboxane A3 (which does not produce thrombotic effects) in the arachidonic acid pathway.

ω-3 fatty acids may promote vasodilation by promoting prostacyclin synthesis. They may also have anti-arrhythmic properties, possibly through cardiac cell membrane stabilization by regulating calcium channels and suppressing intracellular calcium activity.[3]

ω-3 fatty acids have unique lipid-lowering activities that diminish lipogenesis and triglyceride production.[4] They not only decrease intestinal cholesterol absorption, but also decrease lipogenesis by inhibiting gene transcription for sterol regulatory element binding protein (SREBP) 1-c. Triglyceride production is decreased by suppressing activity of SREBP-1 and inhibiting hepatic diacyl-glycerol acyl transferase (the major enzyme involved in triglyceride production). Modulation of PPARα may also help regulate fasting triglyceride levels.[3] They may increase triglyceride clearance by upregulating lipoprotein lipase. They also promote intracellular degradation of apolipoprotein B, and thus interfere with very low density lipoprotein (VLDL) secretion.[4]

Adverse Effects and Drug Interactions

Adverse effects of ω-3 fatty acids include a "fishy after-taste" and eructation, halitosis, heartburn, nausea, and loose stools. A different concern is that persons allergic to fish may also react to ω-3 fatty acids, but this has not been definitively established. Certain fish, such as shark, mackerel, and swordfish, may contain high levels of mercury, and fish from polluted waters may contain unacceptable levels of PCBs (polychlorinated biphenyls).[1] Doses higher than 3 g per day may excessively inhibit platelet aggregation and lead to bleeding. In the past, it was thought that at higher doses glucose increased, but in a trial using 4 g daily of prescription ω-3 fatty acids, there was no increase in glucose.[5] There has also been some concern that LDL concentrations may increase with higher doses, although the LDL particles may not be the atherogenic type.

ω-3 fatty acids may have additive effects with antihypertensives, hypoglycemics, anticoagulants, and statins. A beneficial drug interaction is that ω-3 fatty acids decrease the hypertensive effects of cyclosporine. Oral contraceptives may interfere with the triglyceride-lowering effects of ω-3 fatty acids.[1]

Clinical Studies

Numerous studies have assessed ω-3 fatty acids for cardiovascular disease; only a few will be discussed here. In 1999, the famous Gissi (Gruppo Italiano per lo Studio della Sopravvivenza nell'Infarto miocardico) study evaluated ω-3 fatty acids (fish oil) for secondary prevention in 11,324 persons with a history of myocardial infarction (MI).[6] Patients were randomized to a 1-g daily dose of fish oil, vitamin E, a fish oil/vitamin E combination, or placebo. In the two-way analysis comparing fish oil with placebo, there was a 10% decrease in the primary endpoint of death, nonfatal MI, or nonfatal stroke for the fish oil group (P = .048). Risk of cardiovascular death decreased significantly by 17% in the two-way analysis.

In 2012, different analyses established doubt as to whether ω-3 fatty acids provided cardiovascular benefit since there were no decreases in adverse cardiovascular outcomes. In the ORIGIN (Outcome Reduction with Initial Glargine Intervention) trial, 12,536 subjects with type 2 diabetes or at risk for diabetes took approximately 1 g daily (840 mg/day of EPA plus DHA) of fish oil for 6 years.[7] Death from cardiovascular cause, the primary outcome, did not significantly decrease. A 2012 systematic review and meta-analysis of 20 randomized trials of 68,680 subjects (with coronary heart disease or at high risk for cardiovascular disease) evaluated the impact of mean daily doses of 1,000 or 1,510 mg (EPA plus DHA) for a duration of 1–6 years on cardiovascular events.[8] There was no difference between fish oil and comparators on all-cause mortality, cardiac death, myocardial infarction, sudden death, or stroke. One explanation is that subjects may have been on heart-protective medications such as statins, antihypertensives, and antiplatelets.

A 2018 meta-analysis from the ω-3 Treatment Trialists' Collaboration evaluated the impact of ω-3 fatty acid supplements on cardiovascular disease in 10 trials of 77,917 subjects.[9] The individuals were at high risk for cardiovascular events, and 37% had diabetes. The analysis evaluated eight double-blind randomized placebo-controlled trials and two open-label studies of subjects taking EPA (226–1,800 mg/day) or DHA (0–1,700 mg/day) for 1–6.2 years. There were no significant associations with rate ratios (RR) for several endpoints. These included coronary heart disease events (RR 0.96; 95% CI 0.90 to 1.01; $P = 0.12$), coronary heart disease death (RR 0.93; 99% CI 0.83 to 1.03; $P = 0.05$, considered nonsignificant), nonfatal MI (RR 0.97; 99% CI 0.87 to 1.08; $P = 0.40$), major vascular events (RR 0.97; 95% CI 0.93 to 1.01; $P = 0.10$), stroke (RR 1.03; 95% CI 0.93 to 1.13; $P = 0.56$), or revascularization events (RR 0.99; 95% CI 0.94 to 1.04; $P = 0.61$). Thus, the investigators concluded there was no impact on fatal or nonfatal coronary heart disease events or major vascular events.

The ASCEND (A Study of Cardiovascular Events in Diabetes) study was done in 15,480 subjects with diabetes who did not have cardiovascular disease and evaluated the impact of 1 g (460 mg EPA and 380 mg DHA) daily of ω-3 fatty acids or placebo (olive oil) for 7.4 years.[10] The primary endpoint was a first serious vascular event (a composite of nonfatal MI, stroke, transient ischemic attack, or vascular death) and occurred in 8.9% in the fish oil group and 9.2% in the placebo group ($P = 0.55$). The composite endpoint of any serious vascular event or revascularization occurred in 11.4% of the ω-3 fatty acids group and 11.5% of the placebo group and was not significant. Thus, this trial showed that in persons with diabetes without cardiovascular disease, ω-3 fatty acid supplementation did not decrease serious vascular events.

Another trial, the VITAL (vitamin D and ω-3 Trial) study, was done in 25,871 subjects without a prior history of cardiovascular disease and evaluated the impact of 1 g daily (460 mg of EPA and 380 mg of DHA) of marine ω-3 fatty acids or placebo on major cardiovascular events for a median follow up of 5.3 years.[11] The subjects were men ≥ 50 years and women ≥ 55 years with no prior history of cardio-vascular disease. The primary endpoint was a composite of MI, stroke, or death from cardiovascular causes and occurred in 386 subjects on ω-3 fatty acids and 419 on placebo (HR 0.92; 95% CI of 0.80 to 1.06; $P = 0.24$). There was also no significant decrease in the expanded composite end point of cardiovascular events, total MI, total stroke, or death from cardiovascular causes. This primary prevention trial only presented the results of ω-3 fatty acid supplementation and reported that ω-3 fatty acid supplements did not decrease cardiovascular events.

Previous trials have mostly used lower doses of ω-3 fatty acids. A landmark trial that used icosapent ethyl, a purified EPA ethyl ester, was the REDUCE-IT (Reduction of Cardiovascular Events with Icosapent Ethyl-Intervention Trial) study.[5] This product was not a supplement, but rather a prescription drug that contains only EPA. The study was a randomized double-blind placebo-controlled trial in 8,179 subjects. In this trial, 70.7% of subjects had pre-existing cardiovascular disease and thus were part of a secondary prevention group, while 29.3% of subjects enrolled were primary prevention. The latter group had diabetes and at least one additional risk factor. Patients took 2 g twice daily of icosapent ethyl or a mineral oil placebo for a median of 4.9 years. Subjects were on statins and had fasting triglycerides of 135–499 mg/dL (1.52 to 5.63 mmol/L) and LDL cholesterol of 41–100 mg/dL (1.06 to 2.59 mmol/L). A composite of cardiovascular death, nonfatal MI (including silent MI), nonfatal stroke, coronary revascularization, or unstable angina in a time to event analysis comprised the primary endpoint. A composite of cardiovascular death, nonfatal MI, or nonfatal stroke in a time-to-event analysis comprised the major secondary endpoint. In the icosapent ethyl group, there was a 25% reduction in the primary endpoint with a hazard ratio of 0.75; 95% CI of 0.68 to 0.83 ($P < 0.001$). This endpoint occurred in 17.2% of subjects on icosapent ethyl and in 22% on placebo. The secondary endpoint occurred in 11.2% on icosapent ethyl and in 14.8% on placebo (hazard ratio of 0.74, 95% CI of 0.65 to 0.83; $P < 0.001$). An important outcome was a significant decrease in fatal/nonfatal stroke in the icosapent ethyl group ($P = 0.01$). Notable adverse events were a significantly higher percentage of patients on icosapent ethyl than on placebo that were hospitalized for atrial fibrillation or flutter (3.1% versus 2.1%; $P = 0.004$). Serious bleeding events occurred in 2.7% of subjects on icosapent ethyl and in 2.1% on placebo, but the difference was not statistically significant ($P = 0.06$).

A 2019 meta-analysis updated the 2018 meta-analysis of 10 trials by Aung et al,[9] by adding the ASCEND,[10] VITAL,[11] and REDUCE-IT[5] study results to evaluate impact of ω-3 fatty acids on cardiovascular disease.[12] This meta-analysis included 13 trials with 127,477 subjects. Approximately 40% of subjects had diabetes, and 73% used lipid-lowering medications. The daily dose of ω-3 fatty acids ranged from 376–4,000 mg. Multiple endpoints were evaluated: MI (fatal/nonfatal); coronary heart disease (CHD) death; total CHD (MI, CHD death; or coronary revascularization), stroke (fatal/nonfatal), cardiovascular disease (CVD) death; total CVD (nonfatal MI, nonfatal stroke, CVD death, or hospitalization due to cardiovascular cause); and major vascular events (nonfatal MI, nonfatal stroke, any revascularization, or CVD death). The authors analyzed the data with and without inclusion of REDUCE-IT to determine whether results would vary, since REDUCE-IT it used a much higher ω-3 fatty acid dose than the other studies. Pooled rate ratios (RR) and 95% confidence intervals were used for statistical analysis. With or without REDUCE-IT, MI risk was lower (RR 0.88; $P < 0.001$; RR of 0.92; $P = 0.02$, respectively) and total CHD was lower (RR 0.93; $P < 0.001$; RR 0.95; $P = 0.008$, respectively). Total CVD risk was lower with or without REDUCE-IT (RR 0.95; $P < 0.001$; RR 0.97; $P = 0.015$, respectively), and CVD death risk was also lower with or without REDUCE-IT (RR 0.92; $P = 0.003$; RR 0.93; $P = 0.013$, respectively). When considered as a separate outcome, REDUCE-IT had a lower risk of fatal/nonfatal stroke (RR 0.73; $P = 0.017$). Overall, results of the meta-analysis did not show that stroke risk was decreased with or without inclusion of REDUCE-IT (RR 1.02; $P = 0.569$; RR 1.05; $P = 0.183$, respectively). Risk of major vascular events was also lower when REDUCE-IT was included (RR 0.95; $P < 0.001$), but was not lower if it was excluded (RR 0.97; $P = 0.058$). Thus, overall results showed that taking ω-3 fatty acids significantly lowered risk for several cardiovascular outcomes, even when excluding the REDUCE-IT study results. Moreover, the risk lowering was linearly associated with dose.

The STRENGTH trial (Statin Residual Risk Reduction with Epanova in High Cardiovascular Risk Patients with Hypertriglyceridemia) was intended to evaluate a daily dose of 4 g of ω-3-carboxylic acids plus statins in 13,086 high-risk subjects with high triglycerides.[13] It was hoped this trial could shed additional light on the role of high-dose ω-3 fatty acids in cardiovascular risk reduction in subjects with high triglycerides. However, this trial was discontinued in January 2020 by the manufacturer, Astra Zeneca, due to low likelihood of benefit.

Summary

ω-3 fatty acids (Fish oil) are highly-used supplements containing EPA and DHA with antithrombotic, anti-inflammatory, and cardiac cell membrane stabilization effects. In the past, some studies reported the benefit of ω-3 fatty acid consumption on glucose lowering. However, a 2019 meta-analysis of randomized controlled trials determined that higher intake compared to lower intake was not associated with developing diabetes or had any impact on glycemic parameters such as A1C or plasma glucose levels.[14]

Although early studies supported the therapeutic benefit of ω-3 fatty acids for cardiovascular disease prevention, recent studies do not. The early studies perhaps lacked the power to detect a benefit and also did not report baseline dietary fish intake. More recent studies include a 2018 meta-analysis[9] of 78,000 subjects as well as the ASCEND[10] and VITAL[11] studies. In the landmark REDUCE-IT study, there was a number needed to treat (NNT) of only 21 to prevent the primary endpoint, a composite of cardiovascular death, nonfatal MI, nonfatal stroke, coronary revascularization, or unstable angina.[5] A NNT of 28 prevented the secondary endpoint, a composite of cardiovascular death, nonfatal MI, or nonfatal stroke. It is unknown whether earlier trials lacked the benefit seen in REDUCE-IT because lower doses of ω-3 fatty acids or lower ratios of EPA to DHA were used. A 2019 meta-analysis that includes the ASCEND, VITAL, and REDUCE-IT studies has confirmed that ω-3 fatty acids lower risk for several cardiovascular outcomes, such as MI, total CHD, CHD death, total CVD, and CVD death.[12] Importantly, lowered risk was linearly correlated with the dose.

Per review of earlier randomized controlled trials, the 2017 American Heart Association (AHA) Scientific Advisory evaluated the impact of ω-3 fatty acid supplements on cardiovascular event prevention.[15] The advisory stated that in persons with established coronary heart disease (CHD), ω-3 fatty acid supplements are reasonable primarily due to their safety, even if there is only a modest reduction in CHD mortality. The advisory did recommend treatment for persons with heart failure without preserved left ventricular function to reduce hospitalizations and mortality. The advisory statement did not recommend supplements for CHD prevention for persons with diabetes or prediabetes. Treatment was not recommended to prevent stroke in persons at high cardiovascular risk and with recurrent atrial fibrillation. The 2017 AHA advisory did not include information from subsequent important trials, such as the ASCEND, VITAL, and REDUCE-IT studies.

However, the 2019 AHA Scientific Advisory of ω-3 fatty acids did include the ASCEND, VITAL, and REDUCE-IT results.[4] The advisory provided an overview of the evidence for high dose (4 g daily) prescription ω-3 fatty acids either as EPA only or EPA plus DHA as a safe and effective option to lower triglycerides either alone or concomitantly with other lipid lowering medications. The advisory also stressed that supplements are not FDA approved and differ from prescription ω-3 fatty acids.

Clinicians and consumers may be confused by the difference between supplements and other w-3 fatty acid prescription products. Approved prescription products include Lovaza® (GlaxoSmithKline) and Omtryg® (Trygg Pharma, Inc.). Both contain EPA and DHA (465 mg and 375 mg, respectively) per capsule. Icosapent ethyl (Vascepa® by Amarin) contains 960 mg of EPA per capsule. Another product that is approved but not commercially clinically available is Epanova® (Astra-Zeneca), which contains w-3 carboxylic acid as ≥ 850 mg of polyunsaturated fatty acids, including EPA, DHA, and other w-3 fatty acids. This product was being studied in the recently discontinued STRENGTH trial.[13]

In supplements, the most common EPA and DHA contents are 180 mg and 120 mg, respectively.[1] Thus, patients may need to take as many as 12 capsules daily to obtain the amount equivalent to prescription products. However, supplements **are not interchangeable** with prescription ω-3 fatty acid products. An important caveat is that REDUCE-IT study results cannot be applied to nonprescription ω-3 fatty acid supplements, since icosapent ethyl (Vascepa®) is a different product, and supplements may not produce the same effect.

Some tips to reduce gastrointestinal side effects include freezing the capsules and taking the product with food. A theoretical concern has been that persons with a fish allergy may react to ω-3 fatty acids, but this has not occurred. Nevertheless, the FDA urges caution in those with fish allergies. Some sources have stated that dietary or exogenous sources of ω-3 fatty acids are not beneficial for primary or secondary coronary heart disease prevention.[16] However, the AHA also recommends eating one to two servings weekly of non-fried fish as an alternative to less healthy protein consumption.[17] Overall, ω-3 fatty acids are not effective in primary prevention of coronary heart disease, including persons with diabetes who do not have cardiovascular risk. However, many persons with diabetes have elevated triglycerides, and ω-3 fatty acids may be beneficial. The American Diabetes Association clinical practice recommendations have been revised to include the REDUCE-IT trial results. The recommendations state that, in persons with diabetes and atherosclerotic cardiovascular disease or other cardiovascular risk factors who are on a statin and have controlled LDL cholesterol but have elevated triglycerides (135–499 mg/dL [1.52 to 5.64 mmol/L]), the addition of icosapent ethyl capsules may be considered to reduce cardiovascular risk.[18]

In December 2019, the FDA officially approved icosapent ethyl to decrease risk of cardiovascular events, based on REDUCE-IT trial results.[19] The approval applies to two groups of individuals with triglycerides of 150 mg/dL (1.69 mmol/L) or greater: one group includes those with diabetes and at least two other CVD risk factors on maximum tolerated statin doses; the other group is those with established cardiovascular disease. Critics of the REDUCE-IT trial have noted that the mineral oil placebo may have interacted with statins to reduce their benefit since the placebo group had a 10% increase in LDL cholesterol, thus possibly conferring an undue advantage to the icosapent ethyl group. Another caveat posed by critics was the increased risk of bleeding and atrial fibrillation (AF) in the icosapent ethyl group. However, bleeding was primarily found in subjects on anti-thrombotics, and increased AF was particularly noted in subjects who had AF at baseline. FDA panelists stated these adverse events did not negate the cardiovascular benefit. Moreover, the dreaded consequence of AF is stroke, and there was a significant decrease in stroke in the icosapent ethyl group in the REDUCE-IT trial.[5,19]

Overall, ω-3 fatty acids are safe and are used for a variety of medical conditions. There is a plethora of emerging information evaluating the impact on cardiovascular disease that should help guide clinicians and patients as to the most optimal dose and dosage form.

References

1. Natural Medicines (Natural Medicines Database search engine). Available from https://naturalmedicines.therapeuticresearch.com. Accessed May 9, 2019

2. Leslie MA, Cohen DJA, Liddle DM, Robinson LE, Ma DWL. A review of the effect of omega-3 polyunsaturated fatty acids on blood triacylglycerol levels in normolipidemic and borderline hyperlipidemic individuals. *Lipids Health Dis* 2015;14:53

3. Adkins Y, Kelley DS. Mechanisms underlying the cardioprotective effects of omega-3 polyunsaturated fatty acids. *J Nutr Biochem* 2010;21:781–792

4. Skulas-Ray A, Wilson PWF, Harris WS, et al. Omega-3 fatty acids for the management of hypertriglyceridemia: a science advisory from the American Heart Association. *Circulation* 2019;140:e673–e691.

5. Bhatt DL, Steg PG, Miller M, et al. for the REDUCE-IT Investigators. Cardiovascular risk reduction with icosapent ethyl for hypertriglyceridemia. *N Engl J Med* 2019;380:11–22

6. GISSI-Prevencione Investigators (Gruppo Italiano per lo Studio della Sopravvivenza nell'Infarto miocardico). Dietary supplementation with n-3 polyunsaturated fatty acids and vitamin E after myocardial infarction: results of the GISSI-Prevenzione trial. *Lancet* 1999;354:447–455

7. Origin Trial Investigators: Bosch J, Gerstein HC, Dagaenais GR, et al. n-3 fatty acids and cardiovascular outcomes in patients with dysglycemia. *N Engl J Med* 2012;367:309–318

8. Rizos EC, Ntzani EE, Bika E, Kostapanos MS, Elisaf MS. Association between omega-3 fatty acid supplementation and risk of major cardiovascular disease events: a systematic review and meta-analysis. *JAMA* 2012;308:1024–33

9. Aung T, Halsey J, Kromhout D, et al. for the Omega-3 Treatment Trialists' Collaboration. Associations of omega-3 fatty acid supplement use with cardiovascular disease risks – meta-analysis of 10 trials involving 77917 individuals. *JAMA Cardiology* 2018;3:225–234

10. Bowman L, Mafham M, Wallendszus K, et al. for the ASCEND Study Collaborative Group. Effects of n-3 fatty acid supplements in diabetes mellitus. *N Engl J Med* 2018;379:1540–1550

11. Manson JE, Cook NR, Lee IM, et al. for the VITAL Research Group. Marine n-3 fatty acids and prevention of cardiovascular disease and cancer. *N Engl J Med* 2019;380:23–32

12. Hu Y, Hu FB, Manson JE. Marine omega-3 supplementation and cardio-vascular disease: an updated meta-analysis of 13 randomized controlled trials involving 127,477 participants. *J Am Heart Assoc* 2019;8:e013543

13. Nicholls SJ, Lincoff AM, Bash D, et al. Assessment of omega-3 carboxylic acids in statin-treated patients with high levels of triglycerides and low levels of high-density lipoprotein cholesterol: Rationale and design of the STRENGTH trial. *Clin Cardiol* 2018;41:1281–1288

14. Brown TJ, Brainard J, Song F, et al. Omega-3, omega-6, and total dietary polyunsaturated fat for prevention and treatment of type 2 diabetes mel-litus: systematic review and meta-analysis of randomized controlled trials. *BMJ* 2019;Aug 21;366:l4697. doi: 10.1136/bmj.l4697

15. Siscovick DS, Barringer TA, Fretts AM, et al. Omega-3 polyunsaturated fatty acid (fish oil) supplementation and the prevention of clinical cardio-vascular disease: a science advisory from the American Heart Association. *Circulation* 2017;135:e867–e884

16. Abdelhamid AS, Brown TJ, Brainard JS, et al. Omega-3 fatty acids for the primary and secondary prevention of cardiovascular disease. *Cochrane Database Syst Rev* 2018,11:CD003177

17. Rimm EB, Appel LJ, Chiuve SE, et al. Seafood long-chain n-3 polyunsatu-rated fatty acids and cardiovascular disease: a science advisory from the American Heart Association. *Circulation* 2018;138:e35–e47

18. American Diabetes Association. 10. Cardiovascular disease and risk man-agement: Standards of Medical Care in Diabetes—2021. *Diabetes Care* 2021;44(Suppl. 1):S125-S150.

19. U.S. Food & Drug Administration. FDA approves use of drug to reduce risk of cardiovascular events in certain adult patient groups. Available from https://www.fda.gov/news-events/press-announcements/fda-approves-use-drug-reduce-risk-cardiovascular-events-certain-adult-patient-groups. Accessed December 18, 2019

GARCINIA (*Garcinia cambogia*)

Garcinia is a tree found in evergreen forests of India and Southeast Asia. It has shiny green leaves and produces a small pumpkin-shaped fruit that is reddish-yellow and about 1.5 inches in diameter.[1,2] The fruit rind is used for weight loss but is also used to treat constipation, hemorrhoids, intestinal parasites, edema, and menstrual disorders.[2] Garcinia is also used as a seasoning and for other culinary purposes.

Chemical Constituents and Mechanism of Action

The main chemical constituent is hydroxycitric acid (HCA).[1,2] It has a variety of actions including inhibition of adenosine triphosphate citrate lyase, ultimately resulting in lower acetyl-Coenzyme A (acetyl-CoA) levels. Acetyl-CoA is an enzyme necessary for fatty acid synthesis and lipogenesis. Additionally, there is decreased conversion of acetyl-CoA to malonyl-CoA. Overall, there is increased lipid oxidation, decreased fatty acid production, and decreased lipogenesis, and food intake may decrease. Garcinia may increase hepatic glycogen synthesis and subsequently influence glucoreceptors to increase satiety.[1] Garcinia may also decrease glucose. Additionally, HCA causes a 20% serotonin reuptake in brain tissue, which may enhance the feeling of well-being.[1,2]

Adverse Effects and Drug Interactions

The most common adverse effects are gastrointestinal upset (nausea, flatulence, and diarrhea), headache, and even pancreatitis.[1] There are some reports of increased blood pressure and one case of acute necrotizing eosinophilic myocarditis. Garcinia may also affect platelet aggregation.[2] The most concerning toxicity relates to the several serious reports of hepatotoxicity, including the need for liver transplantation.[1,3] Adverse impact on mood, including mania, has also been reported.

Since garcinia may lower glucose, it may result in additive hypoglycemia in combination with secretagogues. Additive hepatotoxicity with hepatotoxins (acetaminophen, kava, comfrey) may be possible. Serotonin syndrome in combination with a serotonergic antidepressant has also been reported.[1]

Clinical Studies

Several studies have evaluated the impact of garcinia on weight loss, and only a few will be discussed here. An early 12-week randomized controlled trial in 135 subjects compared 1,500 mg/day of HCA (1,000 mg three times daily of the extract) to placebo.[4] Sixty-six subjects were assigned to garcinia and 69 to placebo, and both groups were encouraged to follow a 1,200-calorie/day diet. The mean weight loss was 7 lb (3.2 kg) in the garcinia group and 9 lb (4.1 kg) in the placebo group, and there was no statistically significant difference between the two groups $(P = 0.14)$.

A 2011 systematic review and meta-analysis evaluated 12 randomized double-blind placebo-controlled trials comparing garcinia to placebo in 706 subjects.[5] However, only nine trials were appropriate to provide data for statistical pooling. Thus, in 459 subjects, the overall weight loss was 0.88 kg (1.9 lb). The difference was considered statistically significant $(P = 0.05)$. Per sensitivity analysis, however, the results were not significant; the authors noted that if three studies with small sample sizes were excluded from the analysis, the results would not be significant. There was significant heterogeneity in the trials. For instance, garcinia doses varied widely and there were varying amounts of study duration time—some trials lasted 2 weeks, some 8 weeks, and others 12 weeks.

Two other relevant studies assessed garcinia's impact on lipids as well as weight loss. In one 10-week randomized controlled trial in 86 persons, 2 g daily of garcinia was compared to 2 g daily of Glycine max (soybeans) and 2 g daily of placebo.[6] Subjects on garcinia gained 0.65 kg (1.4 lbs), the subjects on soybeans decreased weight by 0.18 kg (0.4 lbs), and subjects on placebo gained 0.68 kg (1.5 lbs). The results were not significant comparing garcinia to soybeans or placebo. Additionally, the garcinia group increased body fat by 0.67%, the soybean group decreased fat by 0.16%, and the placebo group had an increase of 1.4%. The results were significant for garcinia and soybeans versus placebo $(P < 0.05)$. There was no change in body mass index (BMI) in the three groups. Total cholesterol increased in all groups. Although triglycerides decreased in all groups, there were no significant changes between groups. The HDL cholesterol increased in both treatment groups, and the difference was significant only for the soybean group compared to placebo $(P < 0.05)$. A notable issue with this study is that a statistical power analysis was not calculated.

Another 60-day randomized double-blind study in 43 obese women compared 800 mg of garcinia three times daily to placebo and evaluated lipids as well as weight loss.[7] Before the start of the study, subjects were asked to decrease their daily caloric intake by 500 calories. In the garcinia group, BMI increased 0.17 kg/m^2, and in the placebo group, BMI decreased 0.24 kg/m^2, although the authors stated the difference was not significant. Body fat mass decreased by 0.12% in the garcinia group and increased by 0.21% in the placebo group; this difference was not statistically significant. Triglycerides decreased from 132.3 mg/dL (1.5 mmol/L) at baseline to 109.5 mg/dL (1.24 mmol/L) in the garcinia group $(P = 0.0002)$ and increased from 121.85 (1.38 mmol/L) to 127.1 mg/dL (1.44 mmol/L) in the placebo group (P value not stated). Overall, triglycerides decreased significantly in the garcinia group (23 mg/dL; [0.26 mmol/L) compared to placebo (increase of 4.5 mg/dL [0.05 mmol/L]; $P = 0.04$). Some issues with this study were the small number of participants and that *P* values were not reported for BMI and fat mass comparisons.

Summary

Garcinia is a supplement commonly used for weight loss. Since some persons with diabetes may struggle with weight management, they may turn to weight loss supplements such as garcinia. Garcinia has shown varying efficacy for weight loss; this may relate to doses or concentrations used as well as differences in study duration. Although an early study showed a 3-kg weight loss, the placebo group lost 4 kg.[4] However, this may have been associated with caloric restriction since a 1,200-calorie/day plan was encouraged. A meta-analysis showed marginal statistical significance, although a decrease in weight of only 0.88 kg (1.5 lb) is not clinically significant.[5] Studies evaluating weight and lipid parameters have shown that weight is not significantly impacted, although perhaps some lipids may improve slightly.

Garcinia has been combined with other supplements, such as glucomannan. In one study, the combination produced 16% weight loss, decreased total cholesterol by 13%, and decreased triglycerides by 15%. However, some subjects with certain genetic polymorphisms had diminished benefit.[8] A clinical controversy is that it would be difficult to determine whether garcinia or glucomannan was responsible for the impact on weight and lipids.

Doses of garcinia for weight loss have varied and are mostly 2 g daily, 800 mg three times daily, or up to 1,550 mg three times daily, administered 30 minutes before meals.[1] Although garcinia is a very popular supplement, there are worrisome adverse effects, such as hepatotoxicity and pancreatitis. Due to platelet aggregation effects and possible effects on glucose, it should be discontinued 2 weeks before surgery. Garcinia should not be combined with serotonergic drugs, such as dextromethorphan or tramadol or selective serotonin reuptake inhibitor (SSRI) antidepressants, such as fluoxetine (Prozac®), due to concern for serotonin syndrome. Another dangerous combination may be with hepatotoxic drugs or supplements (such as acetaminophen or isoniazid, or kava or comfrey). Thus, garcinia use is not warranted. Persons with diabetes should be counseled that weight loss achieved is suboptimal, and, most importantly, it is not a safe supplement.

References

1. Natural Medicines (Natural Medicines Database search engine). Available from https://naturalmedicines.therapeuticresearch.com. Accessed May 9, 2019

2. Haber SL, Awwad O, Phillips A, Park AE, Pham TM. Garcinia cambogia for weight loss. *Am J Health-Syst Pharm* 2018;75:17–22

3. Kothadia JP, Kaminski M, Samant H, Olivera-Martinez M. Hepatotoxicity associated with use of the weight loss supplement Garcinia cambogia: a case report and review of the literature. *Case Reports Hepatol* 2018;12:2018:6483605. doi: 10.1155/2018/6483605

4. Heymsfield SB, Allison DB, Vasselli JR, et al. Garcinia cambogia (hydroxy-citric acid) as a potential antiobesity agent. *JAMA* 1998;208:1596–1600

5. Onakpoya I, Hung SK, Perry R, Wider B, Ernst E. The use of Garcinia extract (hydroxycitric acid) as a weight loss supplement: a systematic review and meta-analysis of randomized clinical trials. *J Obes* 2011;2011:509038

6. Kim J-E, Jeon S-M, Park KH, et al. Does Glycine max leaves or Garcinia cambogia promote weight-loss or lower plasma cholesterol in overweight individuals: a randomized control trial. *Nutrition J* 2011;10:94

7. Vasques CAR, Schneider R, Klein-Junior LC, et al. Hypolipemic effect of Garcinia cambogia in obese women. *Phytother Res* 2014;28:887–891

8. Maia-Landim A, Ramirez JM, Lancho C, Poblador MS, Lancho JL. Long-term effects of Garcinia cambogia/Glucomannan on weight loss in people with obesity, PLIN4, FTO and Trp64Arg polymorphisms. *BMC Complement Altern Med* 2018;18:26

GARLIC (*Allium sativum*)

Garlic is a member of the lily family that has been used in cooking for thousands of years.[1] Garlic is used for hyperlipidemia, hypertension, cancer prevention, and antibacterial activity.[1,2] More recently, evidence has supported its use for diabetes.[3] Highly valued in ancient Egypt and ancient Chinese medicine, garlic has a rich history of thousands of years of medicinal use.[2]

Chemical Constituents and Mechanism of Action

Garlic contains the sulfur-based chemical constituent alliin, which must be converted to the active form, allicin, by the enzyme alliinase. This reaction occurs when the garlic bulb is chewed or crushed. Active constituents include allicin as well as ajoene, which is formed by the acid-catalyzed reaction of two allicin molecules. However, there are other important organosulfur compounds, such as S-allyl-L-cysteine, S-allyllmercaptocysteine, diallyldisulfide, and dimethyltrisulfide.[2] The primary active ingredient in aqueous garlic extract and raw garlic is allicin. Aged garlic extract is an important garlic product; its key component is S-allylcysteine.[4] Commercial garlic products may contain alliin, but not allicin or ajoene. Conversion to allicin requires alliinase, which is unstable in stomach acids. Dried garlic preparations may be effective only if the product is enteric coated to prevent gastric acid breakdown and permit release in the small intestine. Fresh garlic, however, is effective.[1]

Antihypertensive properties are related to the modulation of endothelium relaxing and constricting factors.[5] On the one hand, garlic stimulates production of the vasorelaxants nitric oxide and hydrogen sulfide. On the other hand, garlic also decreases production of the vasoconstrictors endothelin 1 and angiotensin II.[5,6] For hyperlipidemia, garlic decreases the activity of enzymes involved in cholesterol synthesis, such as hepatic glucose-6-phosphate dehydrogenase, as well as others that catalyze fatty acid synthesis, such as fatty acid synthetase. It also inhibits HMG-CoA reductase and suppresses LDL oxidation.[1,7] Aged garlic extract may contribute to lipid-lowering activity.[4] Ajoene has antiplatelet activity and interferes with thromboxane synthesis.[1] In diabetes, garlic may increase endogenous insulin production, increase insulin sensitivity, enhance pancreatic β-cell regeneration, inhibit carbohydrate absorption, and improve oxidative stress.[3]

Adverse Effects and Drug Interactions

Overall garlic is relatively safe and has been used for several years in clinical studies. Common side effects of garlic include breath odor, mouth and gastrointestinal burning or irritation, heartburn, flatulence, allergic reactions, and, rarely, topical lesions and burns. There are case reports of spontaneous spinal epidural hematoma, retrobulbar hemorrhage, and postoperative bleeding associated with garlic use. Use in pregnancy may be safe, although not in lactation.[1]

Bleeding may occur if a patient takes antiplatelet agents such as warfarin or aspirin or CAM supplements with antiplatelet activity such as ginkgo, ginger, feverfew, or others. Garlic may induce CYP 3A4 isoenzyme activity, thus decreasing the effects of drugs that are metabolized through this pathway. Decreased efficacy of cyclosporine, protease inhibitors in antiretroviral treatment, calcium-channel blockers, certain statins, certain non-nucleoside reverse transcriptase inhibitors, certain anticonvulsants, certain macrolides, and others. A major interaction is that it decreases levels of the important antibiotic, isoniazid, by 65%. Garlic oil may also inhibit CYP 2E1 activity and result in increased concentrations of ethanol, acetaminophen, and other products. Combining with antihypertensives or diabetes medications may result in additive effects such as hypotension and hypoglycemia, respectively.[1]

Clinical Studies

Numerous studies have evaluated the impact of garlic on dyslipidemia, blood pressure, and diabetes, but only a few will be presented here. A 2016 meta-analysis evaluated 20 trials in 970 subjects.[5] Studies in the analysis ranged from 2–24 weeks in duration, and the majority included garlic powder supplements. Other preparations included aged garlic extract, garlic oil, and an egg yolk-enriched garlic powder. The mean decrease in systolic blood pressure (SBP) was 5.1 mm Hg ($P < 0.001$), whereas the mean decrease in diastolic blood pressure (DBP) was 2.5 mm Hg ($P < 0.002$). Subgroup analysis of studies that included hypertensive subjects found that mean SBP and DBP decreases were 8.7 mm Hg and 6.1 mm Hg, respectively ($P < 0.001$ for both). This meta-analysis depicts the problematic issues of including normotensive as well as hypertensive individuals in different studies and using various preparations.

A different systematic review and meta-analysis evaluated seven randomized controlled trials in 391 subjects, ranging from 8–12 weeks.[6] This analysis included studies that used six different garlic preparations—aged garlic extract, dried garlic homogenate, processed garlic capsule, time-released garlic powder tablet, regular garlic pills, and garlic powder. The primary outcome measure was a composite of mortality and cardiovascular events, including coronary heart disease, MI, heart failure, and stroke. Secondary outcomes were SBP and DBP at treatment end. The authors stated that primary outcome measures were not reported in all trials and thus could not make conclusions about mortality or cardiovascular events, but they did report secondary outcomes. Three trials of 125 subjects were used for the meta-analysis statistical evaluation. Systolic pressure decreased significantly by 6.7 mm Hg ($P = 0.02$), and DBP also decreased significantly by 4.8 mm Hg ($P < 0.00001$). The main strength of this study was including only studies with hypertensive subjects, but a limitation was the inability to assess the primary outcome as well as the heterogeneity of different products used.

A 2013 meta-analysis of 39 trials in 2,298 subjects evaluated the impact of garlic on lipids.[7] Trials lasting anywhere from 2–52 weeks used garlic powder, garlic oil, aged garlic extract, or raw garlic. In 29 studies, total cholesterol was ≥ 200 mg/dL (5.2 mmol/L) and in eight studies, it was < 200 mg/dL (5.2 mmol/L). In trials where cholesterol was ≥ 200 mg/dL (5.2 mmol/L) and lasted longer than two months, total cholesterol decreased 17 mg/dL (0.44 mmol/L) compared to placebo ($P < 0.0001$). The LDL cholesterol decreased by 9 mg/dL (0.23 mmol/L; $P = 0.0004$) in trials where the baseline LDL cholesterol was > 130 mg/dL (3.4 mmol/L) and lasted longer than 2 months. Triglycerides did not decrease significantly ($P = 0.22$), whereas HDL cholesterol improved slightly (1.5 mg/dL [0.04 mmol/L]) but significantly ($P = 0.02$). For total cholesterol lowering, aged garlic extract was more effective than garlic powder or garlic oil. Garlic powder reduced LDL cholesterol more effectively, and garlic oil was more effective for increasing HDL cholesterol. However, the authors noted that conclusions regarding the impact of different garlic types should be cautiously interpreted.

Although animal data has indicated that garlic improves glucose, studies demonstrating benefit in humans have emerged only relatively recently.[1] In one small study, 300 mg three times daily of garlic powder was combined with metformin 500 mg twice daily for 24 weeks and compared to the same dose of metformin plus placebo.[8] In the garlic plus metformin group, fasting glucose decreased from 128 to 125 mg/dL (7.1 to 6.9 mmol/L, respectively). In the metformin-plus-placebo group, fasting glucose decreased from 113 to 110 mg/dL (6.3 to 6.1 mmol/L, respectively). The decrease was significantly greater for the garlic-plus-metformin group compared to metformin only ($P < 0.005$). Moreover, decreases in total and LDL cholesterol, triglycerides, and increases in HDL cholesterol were all significant compared to the metformin-only group ($P < 0.005$ for all).

A 2015 meta-analysis of seven randomized controlled trials in 513 subjects evaluated the effect of garlic on glycemic parameters.[3] The study duration ranged from 4–24 weeks and studies were heterogeneous, since two trials included healthy subjects. Per Jadad scores ≥ 4, only two studies were of high quality, and five studies were of low quality. The studies included garlic powder, garlic oil, or aged garlic extract, compared to control. A total of 390 subjects had elevated baseline fasting glucose. The standardized mean difference decrease in fasting glucose was 1.67 mg/dL (0.09 mmol/L) and was significant ($P = 0.004$). The greatest benefit was in studies where treatment lasted at least 12 weeks and for garlic powder or aged garlic extract formulations. Only one study reported a decrease in postprandial glucose, which was significant, compared to control ($P < 0.01$). Two studies reported A1C outcomes—one showed garlic decreased A1C significantly compared to control ($P < 0.005$) and the other did not show a difference between garlic and control ($P > 0.05$). Thus, the pooled analysis was underpowered and did not provide any conclusions regarding postprandial glucose or A1C.

Summary

Garlic is a popular product that may be used by persons with diabetes for hypertension, hyperlipidemia, or to manage glucose. It contains the sulfur-based chemical constituent alliin, which must be converted to the active form, allicin, by the enzyme alliinase. Active constituents include allicin and ajoene as well as other important organosulfur compounds, such as S-allyl-L-cysteine. Commercial preparations of garlic usually contain alliin, not allicin or ajoene.[2,4] Enteric-coated products are recommended to prevent gastric acid breakdown of allinase and thus permit release of the active forms in the small intestine.[1]

Animal studies have suggested that garlic may decrease glucose and increase insulin sensitivity.[9] Human studies are emerging, and primarily demonstrate a significant lowering of fasting glucose, but thus far have not significantly impacted postprandial glucose or A1C.[3,8] One potential benefit for diabetes complications is that garlic may inhibit formation of advanced glycation end products that contribute to microvascular disease.[10] For hyperlipidemia, garlic extracts of 600–1,200 mg per day in divided doses have been used, and doses for hypertension range from 300–1,500 mg. For diabetes, 600–1,500 mg daily has been used. Garlic is sometimes combined with other products such as fish oil or B vitamins. Fresh garlic may be effective but the exact amount is unknown.[1] The most appropriate doses and forms are unknown.

Garlic demonstrates an important controversy regarding supplements—numerous product types and dosage forms are used, subjects with normal baseline parameters are sometimes included in clinical studies, and varying results are reported. Nevertheless, garlic is highly used, and it is estimated that up to half of patients with hypertension may take garlic in various forms. A Cochrane Review that assessed the impact of garlic in hypertensive patients reported that garlic decreases blood pressure, but there is insufficient evidence to determine the effect on reducing cardiovascular morbidity and mortality.[11] It is important that clinicians instruct individuals that antiplatelet activity is a serious potential problem and that they may experience bleeding reactions, especially if using drugs or CAM therapies with antiplatelet properties. There are also numerous potentially serious interactions, particularly with antiretroviral treatments.[1] As a food, garlic is safe; however, when used as a supplement, close monitoring is advised, due to the potential for bleeding and drug interactions. Clinicians should remind patients to discontinue garlic supplements 2 weeks before surgery. Although garlic may lower blood pressure, lipids, and glucose, the impact is not as potent as conventional medications to treat these disorders.

References

1. Natural Medicines (Natural Medicines Database search engine). Available from https://naturalmedicines.therapeuticresearch.com. Accessed May 9, 2019

2. Ali M, Thomson M, Afzal M. Garlic and onions: their effect on eicosanoid metabolism and its clinical relevance. Prostaglandins, Leukot and Essent Fatty Acids 2000;62:55–73

3. Hou Li-Q, Liu Y-H, Zhang Y-Y. Garlic intake lowers fasting blood glucose: meta-analysis of randomized controlled trials. *Asia Pac J Clin Nutr* 2015;24:575–582

4. Zhu Y, Anand R, Geng X, Ding Y. A mini review: garlic extract and vascular diseases. *Neurol Res* 2018;40:421–425

5. Ried K. Garlic lowers blood pressure in hypertensive individuals, regulates serum cholesterol, and stimulates immunity: an updated meta-analysis and review. *J Nutr* 2016;146 (Suppl):389S–396S

6. Xiong XJ, Wang PQ, Li SJ, et al. Garlic for hypertension: a systematic review and meta-analysis of randomized controlled trials. *Phytomedicine* 2015;22:352–361

7. Ried K, Toben C, Fakler P. Effect of garlic on serum lipids: an updated meta-analysis. *Nutr Rev* 2013;71:282–299

8. Ashraf R, Khan RA, Ashraf I. Garlic (Allium sativum) supplementation with standard antidiabetic agent provides better diabetic control in type 2 diabetes patients. *Pak J Pharm Sci* 2011;24:565–570

9. Augusti KT, Sheela CG. Antiperoxide effect of S-allyl cysteine sulfoxide, an insulin secretagogue, in diabetic rats. *Experientia* 1996;52:115–120

10. Ahmad MS, Ahmed N. Antiglycation properties of aged garlic extract: possible role in prevention of diabetic complications. *J Nutr* 2006;136:796S–799S

11. Stabler SN, Tejani AM, Huynh F, Fowkes C. Garlic for the prevention of cardiovascular morbidity and mortality in hypertensive patients. *Cochrane Database Syst Rev* 2012;8:CD007653

GINKGO (*Gingko biloba L.*)

Gingko biloba, also known as the maidenhair tree or ginkgo, has unique bi-lobed, fan-shaped leaves. Ginkgo has a unique history. It is one of the world's oldest living tree species, dating back over 200 million years. It was introduced to Europe and North America in the 1700s. The ginkgo tree lives a long time—possibly as long as 1,000 years.[1] Extracts from dried leaves of younger trees are used in complementary therapies.[2] Gingko biloba is one of the most commonly used supplements worldwide.

Ginkgo is used to treat Alzheimer's Disease, multi-infarct dementia, cerebral insufficiency, peripheral arterial disease, antidepressant-induced sexual dysfunction, chilblains (hand and foot swelling from cold exposure), vertigo and tinnitus, altitude sickness, and asthma. Ginkgo has been used for glaucoma and macular degeneration.[3] In diabetes, gingko biloba may be useful for peripheral circulatory problems (such as intermittent claudication) and retinopathy. Persons with diabetes often may have dementia or Alzheimer's disease, and thus there is interest in using ginkgo to treat or prevent these conditions. Although ginkgo may improve some symptoms of cognitive impairment, it does not reduce the risk of developing dementia or Alzheimer's disease, and does not alter disease progression.[1]

Chemical Constituents and Mechanism of Action

Active ingredients include flavonoids (ginkgo flavone glycosides) and terpenoids (ginkgolides and bilobalides).[1,2] The flavone glycosides include quercetin, kaempferol, and isorhamnetin. These are thought to have antioxidant activity and inhibit platelet aggregation. The ginkgolides, one of the chemical constituents of terpenoids, are thought to improve circulation and inhibit platelet-activating factor. The bilobalides, the other constituents of the terpenoids, are thought to have neuroprotective properties.[1] Ginkgo may help visual problems such as glaucoma and macular degeneration by increasing ocular blood flow.[3] For diabetes, ginkgo may increase insulin secretion. Clinical studies have used products containing 24% flavone glycosides and 6% terpene lactones.[1]

Adverse Effects and Drug Interactions

Overall ginkgo has been used for several years in clinical studies. Reported side effects have included various maladies. In a few patients, gastrointestinal upset may occur. Transient headache for the first two-three days has been a common complaint. Exposure to the fruit pulp may result in cross-allergic reactions with members of the *Rhus* species (poison ivy). Eating the seed may result in seizures, due to the ginkgotoxin content.[1] Providers should note that concomitant use of ginkgo with drugs that lower seizure threshold should be avoided.

Some of the most worrisome adverse effects have been bleeding reactions, including subdural hematoma, subarachnoid hemorrhage, hyphema (bleeding from the margin of the iris), and retrobulbar hemorrhage. A review of case reports concluded that there may be a causal association of increased bleeding with ginkgo use, and further study is warranted.[4]

The main drug interaction is the potential for additive antiplatelet activity when combined with antiplatelet drugs, such as warfarin and aspirin, or Cox-2 inhibitors such as celecoxib, or with botanical products that also have antiplatelet activity, such as ginger, garlic, and feverfew. A large database evaluation has suggested that warfarin and ginkgo co-administration may result in increased risk of bleeding events. A case report indicated that concomitant use with trazodone (an antidepressant) resulted in coma in a patient with dementia. Moreover, a 17% decrease in alprazolam (an anxiolytic benzodiazepine) serum concentrations with concomitant ginkgo use has been reported.[1] Hypomania due to a combination of ginkgo with melatonin, St. John's wort, and fluoxetine (Prozac®) has also been reported.

Emerging evidence has shown that ginkgo may mildly or moderately inhibit metabolism of drugs that are metabolized by various CYP 450 isoenzymes, including CYP 2D6, 1A2, and 2C9. However, there are varying reports on the degree of enzyme inhibition, depending on in vitro or in vivo evaluation, and the clinical significance has not yet been determined. Clinicians should therefore monitor the effects of certain medications and look for slightly increased blood levels with some antipsychotics and some cardiac medications (metabolized through CYP 2D6), caffeine and some dementia medications (metabolized through CYP 1A2), and warfarin (metabolized through CYP 2C9). In addition, certain sulfonylureas are metabolized through 2C9, including glipizide and glyburide, so a theoretical potentiation of these drugs may occur. Ginkgo has been reported to induce metabolism of CYP 2C19. Since the anticonvulsant phenytoin (Dilantin®) is metabolized by CYP 2C19, decreased serum concentrations of phenytoin (and thus resultant seizures) may occur. A case report of fatal seizures attributed to a drug interaction between ginkgo biloba and two anticonvulsants illustrates this point.[5] Effects on CYP 3A4 are variable, with some reports that indicate that ginkgo inhibits metabolism (and thus the affected drug may have increased serum concentrations) and others that indicate induction (and thus the affected drug may have decreased serum concentrations). Some examples of drugs metabolized through CYP3A4 are cyclosporine, some statins, and some calcium channel blockers.[1]

Clinical Studies

The effect of 120 mg/day ginkgo for 3 months has been evaluated in three different studies that evaluated insulin secretion. In individuals with normal glucose, there was an increase in pancreatic insulin and C-peptide response measured as area under the curve during a 75-g OGTT.[6] In individuals with diet-controlled type 2 diabetes, there was no effect on insulin area under the curve with ginkgo. In the same study, however, in gingko administration in type 2 diabetes patients on secretagogues (with β-cell exhaustion), glucose loading resulted in increased insulin and C-peptide levels, although glucose levels did not decrease.[7] The third report was a crossover comparison of ginkgo or placebo for 3 months in subjects with normal glucose tolerance, impaired glucose tolerance, and type 2 diabetes. Subjects underwent a two-step euglycemic insulin clamp after taking ginkgo or placebo. There was no difference in glucose metabolic rates at low or high insulin infusion rates. Thus, there was no indication of insulin resistance in the three populations.[8]

A randomized double-blind placebo-controlled trial evaluated the impact of ginkgo added to metformin or placebo in 60 subjects with type 2 diabetes.[9] In this 90-day study, subjects took daily doses of 120 mg of ginkgo or placebo plus metformin (1,360 or 1,240 mg/day, respectively). In the ginkgo group, A1C decreased significantly from 8.6% to 7.7% ($P < 0.001$ versus baseline) and in the placebo group, A1C decreased nonsignificantly from 8.8% to 8.4% ($P > 0.05$). Fasting glucose also decreased significantly from 194 mg/dL (10.8 mmol/L) to 155 mg/dL (8.6 mmol/L) in the ginkgo group ($P < 0.001$ versus baseline), and in the placebo group fasting glucose decreased from 174 mg/dL (9.7 mmol/L) to 167 mg/dL (9.3 mmol/L; $P = 0.53$), but the change was not significant. BMI also decreased significantly in the ginkgo group ($P < 0.001$) and did not change in the placebo group. Although this study involved only a few subjects, it is notable in that it is the first time ginkgo has been shown to improve glycemic parameters in a human study.

Patients with diabetes may have peripheral arterial disease and calf pain while walking, classified as intermittent claudication. Studies have evaluated ginkgo in intermittent claudication and found that ginkgo may increase pain-free walking distance.[1] A 2013 Cochrane Review evaluated 14 trials of ginkgo versus placebo in 739 subjects.[10] Eleven trials of 477 subjects compared ginkgo with placebo to assess absolute claudication distance. The researchers reported that subjects were able to increase walking distance by 64.5 meters (212 ft.) on a flat treadmill, although the improvement was not significant.

Persons with diabetes may develop microvascular complications such as retinopathy. A 3-month open-label study was conducted in 25 patients with type 2 diabetes and retinopathy.[11] The study evaluated 240 mg/day of the ginkgo biloba extract EGb 761. Retinal capillary blood flow increased significantly, by 0.44 mm/sec, in the ginkgo group ($P < 0.05$). Blood viscosity decreased at high, medium, and low shear rates (a measure of red blood cell strength). The results were −0.44 ($P < 0.05$), −0.52 ($P < 0.05$), and −2.88 ($P < 0.01$), respectively. Oxygen transport efficiency increased significantly at all shear rates ($P < 0.05$). Erythrocyte rigidity decreased only at shear rates of 150 and 5 per second (−0.02 at both rates,

$P < 0.05$). Erythrocyte malondialdehyde levels (a product of lipid peroxidation) also decreased (-0.92×10^{10} nmol/cell; $P < 0.05$), indicating that oxidative stress decreased. Overall, ginkgo use results in improved retinal capillary circulation without increasing blood glucose.

Other ocular disorders that persons with diabetes may experience are glaucoma and age-related macular degeneration. Vasculature dysfunction is associated with glaucoma. One small randomized crossover study used placebo or 120 mg daily of ginkgo in an antioxidant dietary supplement in 45 subjects with open angle glaucoma.[12] The antioxidant supplement showed improved ocular blood flow. Compared to placebo, the ginkgo group had several blood flow improvements. These included increased superior and inferior temporal retinal capillary mean blood flow, improved blood velocities in the retrobulbar blood vessels (peak systolic and/or end diastolic blood velocities), decreased vascular resistance in the nasal short posterior ciliary and central retinal arteries, and increased ratio of active to nonactive retinal capillaries.

A 2013 Cochrane Review evaluated ginkgo for macular degeneration in two 6-month trials of 119 subjects.[13] One trial compared ginkgo to placebo, and the other trial evaluated two different doses of ginkgo. Both studies showed some benefit, but the author stated they were unable to pool the results for evaluation. The author stated that although it is widely used in China and some European countries, research has not provided evidence that ginkgo may be helpful for age-related macular degeneration.

Summary

Ginkgo biloba is a very popular product used for a variety of disease states. An issue that has emerged in product quality is the occasional addition of rutin or quercetin to improve the quality of substandard ginkgo. Because of historical use of ginkgo for dementia or peripheral vascular disease, persons with diabetes may decide to take it. Other likely reasons for use include ophthalmic disorders such as glaucoma, macular degeneration, or retinopathy. The theorized mechanism of action involves improved blood flow. Accordingly, patients should be counseled about the potential for bleeding and hemorrhage if combined with drugs or CAM supplements with antiplatelet effects. Thus, patients should be counseled to discontinue ginkgo 2 weeks before surgery. Persons with seizure disorders should not take ginkgo. Doses of gingko biloba are variable: 120–240 mg/day for dementia, 120–160 mg/day for peripheral vascular disease, and 240 mg/day for retinopathy.[1] Gingko biloba is best administered in divided doses, usually twice or three times daily. Administration for 6–8 weeks is required to determine the benefit. Although ginkgo biloba may benefit retinopathy and other ocular disorders, its role in consistently lowering blood glucose in diabetes is unknown. However, one study reported that combined administration with metformin resulted in a significant improvement in glycemic parameters.[9] Since ginkgo may affect insulin secretion, close monitoring of blood glucose and A1C is warranted. Caution with concomitant medications is warranted due to varying and complex drug interactions. Overall, the benefit of ginkgo in diabetes is still being investigated and is not well established.

References

1. Natural Medicines (Natural Medicines Database search engine). Available from https://naturalmedicines.therapeuticresearch.com. Accessed May 9, 2019
2. Singh B, Kaur P, Singh GRD, Ahuja PS. Biology and chemistry of Ginkgo biloba. *Fitoterapia* 2008;79:401–418
3. Kang JM, Lin S. Ginkgo biloba and its potential role in glaucoma. *Curr Opin Ophthalmol* 2018;29:116–120
4. Bent S, Goldberg H, Padula A, Avins AL: Spontaneous bleeding associated with ginkgo biloba: a case report and systematic review of the literature. *J Gen Intern Med* 2005;20:657–661
5. Kupiec T, Raj V. Fatal seizures due to potential herb-drug interactions with Ginkgo biloba. *J Anal Toxicol* 2005;29:755–758
6. Kudolo GB. The effect of 3-month ingestion of ginkgo biloba extract on pancreatic beta-cell function in response to glucose loading in normal glucose tolerant individuals. *J Clin Pharmacol* 2000;40:647–654
7. Kudolo GB. The effect of 3-month ingestion of gingko biloba extract (EGb 761) on pancreatic beta-cell function in response to glucose loading in individuals with non-insulin-dependent diabetes mellitus. *J Clin Pharmacol* 2001;41:600–611
8. Kudolo GB, Wang W, Elrod R, et al. Short-term ingestion of ginkgo biloba extract does not alter whole body insulin sensitivity in non-diabetic, pre-diabetic or type 2 diabetic subjects: a randomized double-blind placebo-controlled crossover study. *Clin Nutr* 2006;25:123–134
9. Aziz TA, Hussain SA, Mahwi TO, et al. The efficacy and safety of Ginkgo biloba extract as an adjuvant in type 2 diabetes mellitus patients ineffectively managed with metformin: a double-blind, randomized, placebo-controlled trial. *Drug Des Devel Ther* 2018;12:735–742
10. Nicolai SPA, Kruidenier LM, Bendermacher BLW, et al. Ginkgo biloba for intermittent claudication. *Cochrane Database Syst Rev* 2013;6:CD006888
11. Huang SY, Jeng C, Kao SC, et al.: Improved haemorrheological properties by ginkgo biloba extract (EGb 761) in type 2 diabetes mellitus complicated with retinopathy. *Clin Nutr* 2004;23:615–621

12. Harris A, Gross J, Moore N, et al. The effects of antioxidants on ocular blood flow in patients with glaucoma. *Acta Ophthalmol* 2018;96:e237–e241
13. Evans JR. Ginkgo biloba extract for age-related macular degeneration. *Cochrane Database Syst Rev* 2013;1:CD001775

GLUCOMANNAN (*Amorphophallus konjac K. Koch*)

Glucomannan is derived from the root of the konjac plant and is known as konjac or konjac mannan.[1] The plant grows in Asia and Africa. In Asia, it has been popular as a medicinal agent and food for thousands of years. Glucomannan is extracted from tubers and is a traditional food in the form of noodles, jelly, tofu, and other culinary products.[2] Glucomannan has been used for constipation, obesity, hyperlipidemia, acne, and diabetes.[1]

Chemical Constituents and Mechanism of Action

Glucomannan is a highly viscous hydrocolloidal dietary fiber polysaccharide comprised of D glucose and D mannose, linked by β-1,4 glycosidic bonds.[2] It is derived from konjac flour and treated with ethanol washings to remove impurities. It absorbs high liquid volumes and turns into mucilage by increasing its volume. It binds food and forms a nondigestible mixture that is not assimilated and absorbed.

Glucomannan has multimodal mechanisms of action. It may promote weight loss by fecal energy loss, prolonging gastric emptying and thus promoting satiety.[1,3] Another potential mechanism of weight loss is increased chewing time.[1] This agent is very high in soluble fiber and may delay glucose absorption and decrease cholesterol absorption. It may inhibit cholesterol absorption in the jejunum, inhibit bile acid absorption in the ileum, and possibly reduce stimulation of hydroxy-3-methyl-glutaryl CoA reductase (HMG-CoA-reductase).[2] Another possible lipid-lowering mechanism is decreased hepatic synthesis of cholesterol and increased fecal sterol excretion. Prebiotic effects may occur due to production of short-chain fatty acids. Effects on lowering blood glucose may be related to increased viscosity and subsequent slowed rate of food absorption in the small intestine.[2] Glucomannan is one of the most highly viscous fibers, which facilitates postprandial glucose reduction.[4] Additionally, glucomannan may bind to ingested polysaccharides and block carbohydrate hydrolyzing enzymes, thus resulting in postprandial glucose lowering.[5]

Adverse Effects and Drug Interactions

The most dangerous adverse effect is esophageal, throat (choking), or intestinal obstruction due to fluid absorption and swelling.[2] It may cause stomach upset, including flatulence, loose stools, and diarrhea.

Drug interactions may include binding of oil-soluble vitamins such as A, D, E, and K. It may also bind other medications if taken at the same time and thus decrease their absorption. Also, there may be additive effects with glucose-lowering agents as well as with antihyperlipidemics.[1]

There are various studies of glucomannan; only a few will be presented here. A 2008 systematic review and meta-analysis of 14 randomized controlled trials of glucomannan in various dosage forms in 531 subjects found a significant weighted mean difference decrease in weight of 1.7 lb (0.79 kg; $P < 0.05$).[6] This analysis included trials ranging from three to 16 weeks and used daily doses of 1.2 to 15.1 g. All of the trials had a placebo control group, except for three studies that used diet as control. The authors stated that results were considered significant at a P level < 0.05. The authors reported a significant weighted mean difference decrease in total cholesterol of 19.3 mg/dL (0.5 mmol/L), LDL decrease of 16 mg/dL (0.41 mmol/L), and triglyceride decrease of 11.1 mg/dL (0.125 mmol/L). Fasting glucose also decreased significantly by 7.4 mg/dL (0.41 mmol/L). There were no changes in HDL cholesterol, systolic, or diastolic blood pressure. The authors stated that a limitation of the study was the inclusion of crossover as well as parallel trials. Crossover trials may contribute to bias and have diminished internal validity.

A 2014 systematic review and meta-analysis of nine randomized placebo-controlled trials evaluated glucomannan for obesity.[3] In the meta-analysis, eight trials using daily doses of 1,000–3,870 mg and lasting 3–12 weeks in 301 subjects were included in the statistical evaluation. In the glucomannan group, there was a non-significant mean difference in weight loss versus placebo of only 0.22 kg (0.48 lb, 95% CI of −0.62 to 0.19; $P = 0.3$). Two trials were analyzed for mean difference in Body Mass Index (BMI). There was a decrease that was not significant of −0.42 kg/m^2 (95% CI of −2.27 to 1.43). The authors reported that some of the included studies reported significant reductions in lipids, but did not provide details. Adverse effects reported included abdominal discomfort, meteorism, diarrhea, and constipation. The authors stated that most of the included trials had flawed methodology reporting, including omission of details regarding randomization or blinding. Overall, there was no significant decrease in weight or BMI, compared to placebo.

A 2017 systematic review and meta-analysis of randomized controlled trials evaluated the effect of glucomannan on lipids.[7] This analysis evaluated 12 studies in 370 subjects using a median daily dose of 3 g (with a range of 2.5–15.1 g) and with a duration of 3–12 weeks. Significant mean difference decreases were reported for LDL cholesterol (13.5 mg/dL [-0.35 mmol/L]; $P < 0.00001$) and non-HDL cholesterol decrease of 12.4 mg/dL (-0.32 mmol/L; $P < 0.00001$). There was no impact on apolipoprotein B ($P = 0.22$). The authors did not report impact on other lipid parameters.

Summary

Glucomannan is a polysaccharide that has been used for weight loss, hyperlipidemia, and hyperglycemia. As of January 2020, glucomannan is on the list of nondigestible carbohydrates that are considered dietary fiber, and this may be stated in the Supplement Facts label.[1] Trials have shown conflicting results on weight loss, but more consistently show lower lipids, and show small decreases in glycemic parameters, including postprandial glucose lowering.[1,5] Glucomannan has been used in combination with other supplements, such as American ginseng.[8] There is no problem with its use as a food, but as a supplement in tablet form, it has caused esophageal obstruction. This may be averted if used in powder or capsule form. It may cause gastrointestinal upset and may have additive effects with diabetes and lipid-lowering medications. It should not be taken at the same time as oil-soluble vitamins (A,D,E, and K) or other medications. Patients should be counseled to take other medications 1 hour before or 4 hours after glucomannan administration. The dose used has been variable. For obesity, daily doses range from 1,000–3,870 mg. For lipids, the daily dose has ranged from 1.2–15.1 g. However, there are also newer supplements with various doses used, and often in combination with other ingredients, such as *Garcinia cambogia*.[1] Glucomannan use warrants caution, particularly in elderly individuals who may have trouble swallowing and may be vulnerable to suffocation or esophageal obstruction.

References

1. Natural Medicines (Natural Medicines Database search engine). Available from https://naturalmedicines.therapeuticresearch.com. Accessed May 9, 2019
2. Devaraj RD, Reddy CK, Xu B. Health-promoting effects of konjac glucomannan and its practical applications: a critical review. *Int J Biol Macromol* 2019;126:273–281
3. Onakpoya I, Posadzki P, Ernst E. The efficacy of glucomannan supplementation in overweight and obesity: a systematic review and meta-analysis of randomized clinical trials. *J Am Coll Nutr* 2014;33:70–78
4. Vuksan V, Sievenpiper JL, Xu Z, et al. Konjac-mannan and American ginsing: emerging alternative therapies for type 2 diabetes mellitus. *J Am Coll Nutr* 2001 Oct;20(5 Suppl):370S–380S; discussion 381S–383S
5. Trask LE, Kasid N, Homa K, Chaidarun S. Safety and efficacy of the nonsystemic chewable complex carbohydrate dietary supplement PAZ320 on postprandial glycemia when added to oral agents or insulin in patients with type 2 diabetes mellitus. *Endocr Pract* 2013;19:627–632

6. Sood N, Baker WL, Coleman CJ. Effect of glucomannan on plasma lipids and glucose concentrations, body weight, and blood pressure: a systematic review and meta-analysis. *Am J Clin Nutr* 2008;88:1167–1173

7. Ho HVT, Jovanovski E, Zurbau A, et al. A systematic review and meta-analysis of randomized controlled trials of the effect of konjac glucomannan, a viscous soluble fiber, on LDL cholesterol and the new lipid targets non-HDL cholesterol and apolipoprotein B. *Am J Clin Nutr* 2017;105:1239–1247

8. Jenkins AL, Morgan LM, Bishop J, et al. Co-administration of a konjac-based fibre blend and American ginseng (Panax quinquefolius L.) on glycemic control and serum lipids in type 2 diabetes: a randomized, controlled, crossover clinical trial. *Eur J Nut* 2018;57:2217–2225

HIBISCUS (*Hibiscus sabdariffa L.*)

Hibiscus is a shrub that bears brightly colored flowers and is grown in Africa, India, Asia, the Americas, and the West Indies. In Egypt, flower parts are used to make a drink called "karkade." Various plant parts are used to prepare sauces, jams, and soups. The seeds are used for their oil and in different foods, and the leaves are used for culinary purposes.[1] The flower and calyx are used to make a tea to treat hypertension or hyperlipidemia. This product is known by a variety of names, including "hibiscus tea," "roselle," "agua de Jamaica," "sour tea," and others.[2]

Chemical Constituents and Mechanism of Action

Hibiscus contains several active constituents, including organic acids (malic, hibiscus, or citric acid), anthocyanins, polyphenols, and flavonoids (gossypetine, hibiscetin, and various glycosides), which are all found in the flower.[3]

Anthocyanins, including delphinidin-3-sambubioside and cyanidin-3-sambubioside may exert the antihypertensive effects through angiotensin converting enzyme inhibition, diuretic effects, and vasorelaxation.[2,4] Potential lipid-lowering effects may be due to inhibition of LDL-C oxidation by anthocyanins and polyphenols.[5] Moreover, anthocyanins and polyphenols may also contribute to weight loss by inhibiting intracellular lipid accumulation and decreasing adipose tissue inflammation.[6] There is evidence that hibiscus may lower glucose.[7] The mechanism of action for glucose lowering is possible α-glucosidase inhibition activity.[4]

Adverse Effects and Drug Interactions

The main side effects include gastrointestinal upset, including constipation and abdominal distention. Rarely, dysuria, headache, tremor, and tinnitus have also been reported.[1] There is conflicting information regarding some potential adverse effects. Per murine data, prolonged use may cause hepatotoxicity.[8] Conversely, also per murine research, hibiscus has been reported to provide hepatic benefit in diabetes-induced liver damage.[9] Hibiscus should not be used during pregnancy due to possible abortifacient properties. Although hibiscus is rumored to promote lactation, per animal research, in large quantities it may decrease water and food intake during lactation, and thus should possibly not be used by nursing mothers.[1]

The most serious drug interaction is with chloroquine, the anti-malarial drug, since hibiscus may decrease its bioavailability and thus efficacy.[1,10] It has also increased the clearance, thus decreasing efficacy, of the statin simvastatin. With antihypertensives there may be hypotension, and with diabetes medications there may be hypoglycemia due to additive effects.[1]

Hibiscus flowers and tea sachets steeped in water have shown blood-pressure-lowering effects. In comparison with angiotensin converting enzyme inhibitors (ACE Is), hibiscus was as effective as captopril but less effective than lisinopril in lowering blood pressure.[11,12] Compared to hydrochlorothiazide, hibiscus was more effective in lowering blood pressure in Nigerian subjects with newly-diagnosed hypertension.[13]

In a 4-week comparison of hibiscus versus black tea, 53 persons with hypertension and type 2 diabetes experienced a significant decrease in systolic blood pressure (SBP).[14] Both groups drank the tea twice daily. In the hibiscus group, SBP decreased significantly from 134.4 mm Hg to 112.7 mm Hg, while the black tea group had an increase in SBP of 118.6 mm Hg to 127.3 mm Hg ($P < 0.001$ for hibiscus versus black tea). The diastolic blood pressure (DBP) decreased slightly in the hibiscus group, from 81.6 mm Hg to 80.5 mm Hg, while DBP increased in the black tea group from 76.7 mm Hg to 80 mm Hg (P value for hibiscus versus black tea was not significant at $P = 0.8$).

A 2010 Cochrane review attempted to review evidence from randomized controlled trials that compared hibiscus to placebo or no treatment.[15] After an extensive search, the authors were unable to find appropriate studies to review. They stated that evidence favoring use of hibiscus for hypertension is inconclusive and recommended that rigorous trials be conducted. Another 2010 systematic review evaluated four clinical trials in 390 subjects.[16] Two trials compared hibiscus to ACE inhibitors, and two compared it to black tea. The authors stated that the studies were short term and of poor quality. Issues included randomization, blinding, and details regarding the preparations. The authors concluded that evidence is limited to support hibiscus use for hypertension.

A 2015 systematic review and meta-analysis of randomized controlled trials evaluated the effect of hibiscus versus control on hypertension.[17] This review of five studies with seven treatment arms excluded trials that compared hibiscus to prescription medications and included 225 subjects who drank hibiscus tea or took hibiscus extract and 165 subjects on control (black or green tea, diet treatment, or placebo). The studies ranged in duration from 15 days–6 weeks. Hibiscus products included daily doses of 3.75 mg–2 spoonfuls (or 100 mg) of aqueous extract. The evaluation included one trial in healthy individuals and other trials in persons with metabolic syndrome or diabetes. Pooled estimates of the effect of hibiscus included a weighted mean difference (WMD) that showed a significant decrease in systolic blood pressure of 7.6 mm Hg ($P < 0.00001$) and a significant decrease in diastolic blood pressure of 3.5 mm Hg ($P < 0.0001$) for hibiscus versus control. However, the quality of the studies was not optimal. The sample sizes were small and diverse, and some healthy individuals were included. There was also heterogeneity in products included in the control groups. Nevertheless, the analysis provided some evidence for potential benefit, and the authors reiterated the need for well-designed and large scale trials.

Lipid lowering has been shown in some individual studies. In a 4-week study of 53 subjects with type 2 diabetes that had been evaluated for hypertension,[14] a separate publication evaluated impact of hibiscus on lipids.[18] LDL cholesterol decreased from 137.5 mg/dL (3.6 mmol/L) to 128.5 mg/dL (3.3 mmol/L) in the hibiscus group, while the comparison group had an increase in LDL from 124.9 mg/dL (3.2 mmol/L) to 130.1 mg/dL (3.4 mmol/L; $P = 0.003$ for hibiscus vs. black tea). There was a significant increase from baseline in HDL cholesterol in the hibiscus group ($P = 0.002$). Otherwise, other lipid parameters improved, but differences between the groups were not significant.

A 2013 systematic review and meta-analysis of randomized controlled trials did not support the benefit of hibiscus for lipids.[19] The authors of this analysis evaluated six studies in 474 subjects ranging in duration from 15 to 90 days. The control groups were heterogeneous and included placebo, diet, black tea, or pravastatin. When hibiscus was compared to pravastatin, the statin group showed benefit, although hibiscus did not. The authors noted that the quality of evidence in the individual studies was suboptimal and suggested future trials be done with improved rigor in study design and larger sample sizes.

Hibiscus may potentially have some beneficial effect on weight loss. A two-month study in 54 overweight and obese subjects evaluated the impact of a combination product containing hibiscus and lemon verbena extracts compared to placebo.[6] After 2 months, subjects on the combination extract lost 7.7 lb (3.5 kg) and those on placebo lost 4.6 lb (2.1 kg). Results were significant for the supplement combination versus placebo ($P < 0.05$). The authors reported that subjects who took the extract had decreased hunger and weight as well as a significant 6% decrease in heart rate and decreased systolic and diastolic blood pressure. An interesting finding was a statistically significant increase in GLP-1, a satiety hormone, in the supplement combination versus placebo. In the supplement group, GLP-1 increased from 5.22 pg/mL to 6.82 pg/mL and decreased in the placebo group from 5.66 pg/mL to 4.23 pg/mL ($P < 0.05$). However, it was unknown whether these effects were due to the impact of hibiscus, the lemon verbena extract, or the combination. Thus, although there may be some benefit, evidence is limited.

Summary

Hibiscus contains anthocyanins and polyphenols that may contribute to blood pressure and lipid lowering. It is used as a tea, and there are no standardized doses, although extracts are now being used. What has been described in the literature is a process to steep the flowers in boiling water.[5] Overall, reported benefits are mainly for mild hypertension in trials that are small in number of patients, of short duration, and have sub-optimal study design. Other reviews have not reported benefit, although a more recent meta-analysis reported benefit.[15-17] Although studied for lipid lowering, strong evidence of benefit has not been shown.[19] Impact on weight loss has been reported with a combination supplement product.[6] Evidence for glucose lowering is emerging.[7] The most important caution is that persons taking chloroquine for malaria should not use hibiscus due to increased clearance and thus possible suboptimal malaria treatment.[1,10] Moreover, patients on simvastatin may experience subtherapeutic effects in lipid-lowering, since hibiscus may increase its clearance.[1] Clinicians are advised to closely monitor lipid laboratory values if patients are taking a statin concomitantly. Conflicting adverse effects have been reported in animal studies—hepatotoxicity with prolonged use and conversely hepatic benefit.[8,9] In short-term human studies, hepatotoxicity has not been reported, but clinicians should err on the side of caution and monitor liver enzymes. Pregnant and lactating women should not use hibiscus.[1] Hispanic patients often report "agua de Jamaica" is a commonly used beverage and they may not recognize the term "hibiscus." Patients may report they are consuming "teas" that will benefit diabetes or its comorbidities, so clinicians should inquire about the product name in order to provide the most appropriate individualized patient information. Overall, hibiscus used for hypertension, hyperlipidemia, hyperglycemia, and weight loss. However, the quality of studies is not sufficiently optimal to recommend its use.

References

1. Natural Medicines (Natural Medicines Database search engine). Available from https://naturalmedicines.therapeuticresearch.com. Accessed May 9, 2019

2. McKay DL, Chen CYO, Saltzman E, Blumberg J. Hibiscus Sabdariffa L. tea (Tisane) lowers blood pressure in prehypertensive and mildly hypertensive adults. *J Nutr* 2010;140:298–303

3. Riaz G, Chopra R. A review on phytochemistry and therapeutic uses of Hibiscus sabdariffa L. *Biomed Pharmacother* 2018;102:575–586

4. Da-Costa-Rocha I, Bonnlaender B, Sievers H, Pischel I, Heinrich M. Hibiscus sabdariffa L. – a phytochemical and pharmacological review. *Food Chem* 2014;165:424–443

5. Hopkins AL, Lamm MG, Funk JL, Ritenbaugh C. Hibiscus sabdariffa L, in the treatment of hypertension and hyperlipidemia: A comprehensive review of animal and human studies. *Fitoterapia* 2013;85:84–94

6. Boix-Castejon M, Herranz-Lopez M, Perez Gago A, et al. Hibiscus and lemon verbena polyphenols modulate appetite-related biomarkers in overweight subjects: a randomized controlled trial. *Food Funct* 2018;9:3173–3184

7. Gurrola-Díaz CM, García-López PM, Sánchez-Enríquez S, et al. Effects of Hibiscus sabdariffa extract powder and preventive treatment (diet) on the lipid profiles of patients with metabolic syndrome. *Phytomedicine* 2010;17:500–505

8. Akindahunsi AA, Olaleye MT. Toxicological investigation of aqueous-methanolic extract of the calyces of Hibiscus sabdariffa L. *J Ethnopharmacol* 2003;89:161–164

9. Adeyemi DO, Ukwenya VO, Obuotor EM, Adewole SO. Anti-hepatotoxic activities of Hibiscus sabdariffa L. in animal model of streptozotocin diabetes-induced liver damage. *BMC Complement Altern Med* 2014;14:277. doi: 10.1186/1472-6882-14-277

10. Mahmoud BM, Ali HM, Homeida MM, Bennett JL. Significant reduction in cholorquine bioavailability following coadministration with the Sudanese beverages aradaib, karkadi and lemon. Antimicrob Chemother 1994;33:1005–1009

11. Herrera-Arellano A, Flores-Romero S, Chavez-Soto MA, and Tortoriello J. Effectiveness and tolerability of a standardized extract from Hibiscus sabdariffa in patients with mild to moderate hypertension: a controlled and randomized clinical trial. *Phytomedicine* 2004;11(5):375–382

12. Herrera-Arellano A, Miranda-Sanchez J, Avila-Castro P, et al. Clinical effects produced by a standardized herbal medicinal product of Hibiscus sabdariffa on patients with hypertension. A randomized, double-blind, lisinopril-controlled clinical trial. *Planta Med* 2007;73:6-12

13. Nwachukwu DC, Aneke E, Nwachukwu NZ, et al. Effect of Hibiscus sabdariffa on blood pressure and electrolyte profile of mild to moderate hypertensive Nigerians: a comparative study with hydrochlorothiazide. *Niger J Clin Pract* 2015;18:762–770

14. Mozaffari-Khosravi H, Jalali-Khanabadi BA, Afkhami-Ardekani M, et al. The effects of sour tea (Hibiscus sabdariffa on hypertension in patients with type II diabetes. *J Hum Hypertens* 2009;23:48–54

15. Ngamjarus C, Pattanittum P, Somboonporn C. Roselle for hypertension in adults. *Cochrane Database of Sys Rev* 2010, Issue 1. Art. No.: CD007894. doi: 10.1002/14651858.CD007894.pub2

16. Wahabi HA, Alansary LA, Al-Sabban AH, Glasziuo P. The effectiveness of Hibiscus sabdariffa in the treatment of hypertension: a systematic review. Phytomedicine 2010;17:83–86

17. Serban C, Sahebkar A, Ursoniu S, Andrica F, Banach M. Effect of sour tea (Hibiscus sabdariffa L.) on arterial hypertension: a systematic review and meta-analysis of randomized controlled trials. *J Hypertension* 2015;33:1119–1127

18. Mozaffari-Khosravi H, Jalali-Khanabadi BA, Afkhami-Ardekani M, Fatehi F. Effects of sour tea (Hibiscus sabdariffa) on lipid profile and lipo-proteins in patients with type II diabetes. *J Alt Compl Med* 2009;15:899–903

19. Aziz J, Wong SY, Chong NJ. Effects of Hibiscus sabdariffa L. on serum lipids: a systematic review and meta-analysis. *J Ethnopharmacol* 2013;150:442–450

PINE BARK EXTRACT (*Pinus pinaster Ait*)

Pine bark extract is a unique product obtained from French maritime pine bark, although the tree grows in Mediterranean countries.[1] It is widely available as Pycnogenol®, a standardized extract obtained from pines grown in southwestern France.[2] Pine bark extract has been used for numerous conditions, including chronic venous insufficiency, asthma, inflammatory states such as arthritis, and is also used for ergogenic effects and to slow aging.[1] It has been evaluated for lowering blood pressure and lipids. In diabetes, it has been used for microvascular disease, including retinopathy, as well as reduction of blood glucose. In recent years, it has been evaluated for metabolic syndrome (including elevated glucose, blood pressure, lipids, and weight issues) due to several properties that may help persons with this condition.[3]

Chemical Constituents and Mechanism of Action

Pycnogenol is standardized to $70 \pm 5\%$ procyanidins. It also contains catechin, taxifolin, and phenolic acids.[3] The phenolic components are derived from benzoic and cinnamic acids and include gallic, caffeic, and ferulic, as well as other acids.[1,2]

Pine bark extract is thought to work as an antioxidant that potently scavenges free radicals. It also has anti-inflammatory properties. It enhances endothelial production of nitric oxide from L-arginine via the enzyme nitric oxide synthase. Nitric oxide mediated vasodilation improves blood flow, and thus may improve perfusion in the peripheral circulation, the retina, and the kidneys. Enhanced endothelial function and vasodilation may be responsible for decreasing blood pressure in hypertensive individuals.[3] Pine bark extract also has anti-thrombotic effects, slight inhibition of angiotensin-converting enzyme, and some spasmolytic activity. It protects against ultraviolet radiation-induced oxidative stress.[1,2] Pine bark extract also inhibits α-glucosidase and therefore may be of benefit in persons with diabetes.[3] It mitigates LDL oxidation, which may decrease lipids. A unique activity is that pine bark extract may boost the immune system and enhance natural killer cell activity.[1]

Adverse Effects and Drug Interactions

Most adverse effects of pine bark extract are benign and transient. The most common is gastrointestinal upset, but diarrhea, headache, and rash have been reported.[1,3] An overview of 104 studies in 8,134 subjects that took pine bark extract reported that the global rate of adverse effects was 1.66%. The commonly reported gastric upset did not occur when taken with meals.[4] Blood chemistries have shown no changes in liver or renal function.[5]

Possible drug interactions include additive lowering of blood glucose with some diabetes medications and supplements that lower glucose (such as chromium or gymnema sylvestre). Possible bleeding may occur when combined with antiplatelet agents, such as clopidogrel or warfarin, or supplements that may result in bleeding, such as ginkgo. Since pine bark extract may have immunostimulant effects, it may antagonize the effects of immunosuppressants such as corticosteroids, cyclosporine, or tacrolimus.[1] The same line of reasoning would also apply in suggesting avoidance by people who have autoimmune diseases such as lupus or multiple sclerosis.

Clinical Studies

Pine bark extract, primarily in the form of Pycnogenol®, has been studied for a variety of uses. Only a few studies will be discussed here. Five major studies evaluated its use for retinopathy in 1,289 patients, but these were mainly published in languages other than English.[6] One study published in English was a randomized, double-blind study of 20 subjects with diabetes.[5] Subjects took placebo or 50 mg three times daily of Pycnogenol® for two months. This was followed by an open-label phase in which another 20 people were treated with the same dose of Pycnogenol® for two months. For visual acuity determined through a Snellen test, values improved nonsignificantly in the right eye (from 7.57 at baseline to 8.0, $P > 0.05$) and significantly in the left eye (8.1 to 8.67, $P < 0.01$). An ocular exam of retinal damage showed improvement in both the right and left eyes. Mean scores declined from 1.6 at baseline to 1.33 at the end in the right eye ($P < 0.01$) and 1.57 to 1.43 in the left eye ($P < 0.05$). Visual field scores remained unchanged in both the placebo and Pycnogenol® groups. The researchers provided a subjective judgment that 53% of the Pycnogenol® group had "good to very good" efficacy and 47% had "moderate" efficacy.

Forty-six subjects with diabetes and moderate macular edema participated in a randomized control study where approximately half the group received daily doses of 150 mg Pycnogenol®; the other half received placebo.[7] Retinal edema scores decreased significantly in subjects treated with Pycnogenol compared to placebo in both mild and moderate edema groups ($P < 0.05$). After three months, Doppler flow velocity measurements showed a significant increase from 34 to 44 cm/seconds in the Pycnogenol™ group compared to a slight effect in the control group ($P < 0.05$). Per Snellen test, the visual acuity improved from a baseline of 14/20 to 17/20 in the Pycnogenol group, whereas the control group did not have any improvement ($P < 0.05$).

For diabetes, researchers conducted a randomized double-blind placebo-controlled multicenter study in 77 subjects with type 2 diabetes.[8] Of 77 subjects, 43 were randomized to placebo, and 34 took 100 mg/day of Pycnogenol® in addition to conventional diabetes medications for 12 weeks. The Pycnogenol® group had lower glucose and A1C. Results were reported for median but not mean values. After 12 weeks, the median plasma glucose level decline was 36 mg/dL (2.0 mmoL/L) from a baseline of 218.5 mg/dL (12.1 mmoL/L; $P < 0.01$). The researchers stated that A1C had a greater decrease in the Pycnogenol® group, but did not report actual values. They stated the median decrease was 0.32% after one month ($P < 0.01$) and 0.69% after three months (P not significant).

Studies have also evaluated pine bark for hypertension. One randomized double-blind placebo-controlled study evaluated 125 mg daily of Pycnogenol® in 23 subjects compared to 22 subjects on control.[9] All subjects had diabetes and hypertension and were taking an angiotensin converting enzyme inhibitor (ACE inhibitor). Based on blood pressure measurements taken every 2 weeks, the researchers left the dose of the ACE inhibitor unchanged, decreased the dose by half, or reinstated the pre-intervention dose until a stable blood pressure was obtained. After 12 weeks, 58.3% of the subjects in the Pycnogenol® group achieved their blood pressure target, versus only 20.8% of subjects in the control group with a 50% ACE inhibitor dose decrease. Moreover, at 12 weeks, fasting glucose decreased significantly by 23.7 mg/dL (1.32 mmol/L) and 5.7 mg/dL (0.32 mmol/L) in the Pycnogenol® and control groups, respectively ($P < 0.0001$). A1C decreased 0.8% in the Pycnogenol® group, but only 0.1% in the control group ($P < 0.001$). LDL cholesterol decreases were also greater in the Pycnogenol® group at 12 weeks ($P < 0.001$).

A different study evaluated Pycnogenol® in hypertensive subjects taking the ACE inhibitor ramipril.[10] One group of 29 subjects took 150 mg daily of Pycnogenol® plus 10 mg of ramipril, and 26 took only the ramipril for 6 months. The primary intent was to evaluate urinary albumin excretion (UAE), which decreased from 91 to 39 mg/day in the combination treatment group and from 87 to 64 mg/day in the ramipril monotherapy control group ($P = 0.0021$ for the combination group versus control). Systolic blood pressure (SBP) decreased from 188 to 119 mm Hg in the combination group and from 186 to 123 mm Hg in the control group. Diastolic blood pressure (DBP) significantly decreased from 96 to 83 mm Hg in the combination group and from 96 to 88 mm Hg in the control group ($P < 0.05$ for Pycnogenol compared to control). Thus, the addition of Pycnogenol® to the ACE inhibitor resulted in lower blood pressure and UAE.

Although there are several individual studies that have shown significant decreases in blood pressure, a 2019 meta-analysis of studies with optimal study design (randomized double-blind placebo-controlled trials) did not find a significant decrease in systolic and diastolic blood pressure.[11] Seven trials evaluated Pycnogenol® in 323 subjects compared to 326 subjects on control, ranging in duration from 2 weeks–6 months. The effect sizes were stated as weighted mean differences (WMD) and 95% Confidence Intervals. For SBP, the WMD was −0.028 mm Hg,

(95% CI of −1.82 to 0.127, $P = 0.726$). For DBP, the WMD was −0.144 mm Hg (95% CI of −0.299 to 0.010; $P = 0.067$).

A 2014 meta-analysis of seven trials in 442 subjects evaluated the impact of Pycnogenol® on cholesterol.[12] Daily doses varied from 120–200 mg, and study duration ranged from 2–24 weeks. There was no significant impact on total cholesterol ($P = 0.83$), LDL cholesterol ($P = 0.54$), HDL cholesterol ($P = 0.86$), or triglycerides ($P = 0.55$). A 2019 meta-analysis of 14 studies in 1,065 subjects verified a lack of benefit on lipid parameters, with one exception.[13] There was an overall significant increase in HDL cholesterol of 3.27 mg/dL (0.085 mmol/L; $P = 0.038$) in 10 studies that evaluated this parameter. However, in this analysis, there was substantial heterogeneity, and some of the evaluated studies included subjects without hyperlipidemia. These two meta-analyses demonstrated that although individual studies may show a decrease in lipids, when grouped together, there was no significant impact.

Summary

Bark derived from maritime pine is primarily available as the extract form in Pycnogenol®. This product has been used widely for chronic venous insufficiency, inflammatory disorders, and retinopathy. Combination products of Pycnogenol® and other supplements such as those that contain other anthocyanidins (such as bilberry) have been used for ophthalmic health. Pycnogenol has even been used topically for diabetes-related foot ulcers.[1] It has a variety of actions that relate to antioxidant effects and dilation of the microcirculation. Pycnogenol® may provide benefit in persons with diabetes, although long-term studies are not available. There is emerging interest in evaluating the impact of Pycnogenol® in hypertension and hyperlipidemia. A potential benefit is that, in combination with antihypertensives, Pycnogenol® may allow for improved blood pressure while possibly using lower antihypertensive doses. Pycnogenol® also improves urinary albumin excretion (UAE). Adverse effects are mostly benign and include gastric upset and dizziness; however, gastric upset may be mitigated if taken with meals. Individuals with autoimmune diseases, such as lupus and multiple sclerosis, should not take Pycnogenol®. Although there are numerous studies evaluating its use, there are problems with study design and reporting results. Doses are variable, and a common daily dose for diabetes has been 100–200 mg. For hypertension, daily doses have ranged from 60–200 mg, and for hyperlipidemia, from 120–200 mg. For chronic venous insufficiency, the dose has been from 45–360 mg taken in three divided doses.[1] Pine bark has great appeal for many individuals, due to antioxidant, anti-inflammatory, and vasodilation effects, with only minimal adverse effects. However, there is a need for studies with better study design that report long-term results. Although it is likely a safe agent, and there is promising evidence supporting its use, there is not enough consistent information to recommend that patients with diabetes use pine bark extract.

References

1. Natural Medicines (Natural Medicines Database search engine). Available from https://naturalmedicines.therapeuticresearch.com. Accessed May 9, 2019
2. Rohdewald P. A review of the French maritime pine bark extract (Pycnogenol®), a herbal medication with a diverse clinical pharmacology. *Int J Clin Pharmacol Ther* 2002;40:158–168
3. Gulati OP. Pycnogenol® in metabolic syndrome and related disorders. *Phytother Res* 2015;29:949–968
4. Gulati OP. Pycnogenol® in chronic venous insufficiency and related venous disorders. *Phytother Res* 2014;28:348–362
5. Spadea L, Balestrazzi E. Treatment of vascular retinopathy with Pycnogenol®. *Phytother Res* 2001;15:219–223
6. Schonlau F, Rohdewald P. Pycnogenol® for diabetic retinopathy. *Int Ophthalmology* 2001;24:161–171
7. Steigerwalt R, Belcaro G, Cesarone MR, et al. Pycnogenol® improves microcirculation, retinal edema, and visual acuity in early diabetic retinopathy. *J Ocul Pharmacol Ther* 2009;25:537–540
8. Liu X, Wei J, Tan F, et al. Antidiabetic effect of Pycnogenol® French maritime pine bark extract in patients with diabetes type II. *Life Sci* 2004;75:2505–2513
9. Zibadi S, Rohdewald PJ, Park D, Watson RR. Reduction of cardiovascular risk factors in subjects with type 2 diabetes by Pycnogenol supplementation. *Nutr Res* 2008;28:315–320
10. Cesarone MR, Belcaro G, Stuard S, et al. Kidney flow and function in hypertension: protective effects of pycnogenol in hypertensive participants – a controlled study. *J Cardiovasc Pharmacol Ther* 2010;15:41–46
11. Fogacci F, Tocci G, Sahebkar A, et al. Effect of pycnogenol on blood pressure: findings from a PRISMA compliant systematic review and meta-analysis of randomized, double-blind, placebo-controlled, clinical studies. *Angiology* 2019; Nov 25:3319719889428. doi: 10.1177/0003319719889428
12. Sahebkar A. A systematic review and meta-analysis of the effects of Pycnogenol on plasma lipids. *J Cardiovasc Pharmacol Ther* 2014;19:244–255
13. Hadi A, Pourmasoumi M, Mohammadi H, Javaheri A, Rouhani MH. The impact of pycnogenol supplementation on plasma lipids in humans: a systematic review and meta-analysis of clinical trials. *Phytother Res* 2019;33:276–287

RED YEAST RICE (*Monascus Purpureus Went*)

Red yeast rice (RYR) is the product of white rice fermented with the yeast *Monascus purpureus*.[1] It is also known by several other names, including "XueZhiKang." Red yeast rice contains several compounds, called the monacolins. RYR was described in 800 AD in the Tang Dynasty. It is used in Asian folk medicine to treat diarrhea and indigestion.[2] RYR has also been used to make rice wine, and is used as a food preservative, flavor enhancer, and coloring agent for fish, meat, and vegetables. The red color is secondary to pigments produced by fermentation.[3] A highly prevalent use is to treat hyperlipidemia.[1,3]

Chemical Constituents and Mechanism of Action

RYR consists of different unsaturated fatty acids, polyketides, phytosterols, pigments (such as rubropunctamine and monascorubramine), and several monacolins.[3] The monacolins include compactin and monacolin M, L, J, X, and K.[4] Monacolin K, or mevinolin, has a chemical structure identical to lovastatin, a 3-hydroxy-3-methylglutaryl-coenzyme A (HMG-CoA) reductase inhibitor—a conventional lipid lowering statin. However, the pharmacokinetic profile and bioavailability of RYR may differ from lovastatin.[3] The mechanism of action of RYR is HMG-CoA reductase inhibitory activity to prevent cholesterol formation. Products may contain citrinin, a Monascus purpureus metabolite.[1,3,5]

Adverse Effects and Drug Interactions

RYR has several potential adverse effects and drug interactions. Citrinin is a nephrotoxin that may be inadvertently produced by Monascus purpureus in the fermentation process.[1,3,5] Red yeast rice may cause gastrointestinal upset, allergic reactions, and myalgias. RYR should not be used in pregnancy, due to the possibility of teratogenic effects, and should not be used in lactation due to unknown effects.[1] A caution to note is that various databases may differ in the number of adverse events that are recorded.[6]

RYR has been reported to increase liver function tests.[1] The Italian Surveillance System of Natural Health Products collected and evaluated adverse reports involving RYR from 2002 to 2015.[7] There were 55 reports, including 19 cases of myalgia and/or increase in creatine phosphokinase, 10 cases of liver injury, 12 cases of gastrointestinal upset, nine cutaneous reactions, one case of rhabdomyolysis, and other effects. Hospitalization was required in 27% of cases, due to serious reactions, and 71% of the reactions occurred in women. The report stated the most common daily dose of monacolin K was 3 mg.

A controversy is that some published reports state that adverse reports of RYR tend to be lower than for statins, whereas others report that adverse effects are comparable. A systematic review and meta-analysis of 53 randomized controlled trials ranging from 4 weeks–4.5 years evaluated safety of RYR in 4,437 subjects compared to 4,303 subjects on control (placebo and other agents).[4] The primary outcomes were musculoskeletal disorders and secondary outcomes were non-musculoskeletal as well as serious adverse events. Musculoskeletal events consisted of muscle weakness or stiffness, myalgias, body aches, back pain, or creatine kinase increase of four or greater times the upper limit of normal. Non musculoskeletal events consisted of gastrointestinal upset, urinary tract infections, pruritus, rash, and general discomfort. Serious adverse effects were defined as those that were life threatening or required urgent care or hospitalization. For the primary outcomes, RYR was not associated with an increased risk of musculoskeletal disorders (OR 0.94; 95% CI 0.53-1.65). There was no increased risk in certain sub-analyses that evaluated daily doses, treatment duration, comparator type, or whether subjects were statin intolerant. Moreover, the researchers found a reduced risk of non-musculoskeletal disorders (OR 0.59; 95% CI 0.5 to 0.69) and serious adverse events (OR 0.54; 95% CI 0.46 to 0.64), compared to control.

The International Lipid Expert Panel (ILEP) has evaluated the role of nutraceuticals, such as RYR, berberine, green tea, garlic, and others in statin-intolerant persons.[8] The panel stated that nutraceuticals as monotherapy or in combination with other nutraceuticals may be considered. The conclusion was that there are three situations where nutraceuticals may be considered: in persons with high or very high cardiovascular (CV) risk with complete statin intolerance who have not reached LDL targets with nonstatin treatment; in persons with high or very high CV risk with partial statin intolerance who have not reached LDL targets with tolerable statin and/or nonstatin treatment; and in persons with intermediate CV risk with high lipid levels and statin intolerance who have not reached LDL targets.

In another manuscript, a researcher that conducted many of the original lovastatin studies stated that his lipid research laboratory was commissioned by a Chinese manufacturer of RYR to perform a clinical trial in hyperlipidemic subjects, in hopes of obtaining FDA approval to sell the product as an over-the-counter (OTC) supplement.[9] However, the researcher stated that FDA had concerns about reproducibility of results with unregulated RYR supplements since they could become part of the OTC market. The researcher stated that the FDA thus denied approval of the product.

Another issue with RYR is that there may be considerable product variability. Researchers evaluated 28 different RYR products found at four major retailers in the United States.[10] The intent was to determine whether there were standard monacolin K concentrations in RYR products. In 26 brands, the quantity ranged from 0.09–5.48 mg per 1,200 mg of RYR—a range of more than 60 fold. Moreover, monacolin K was not detected in two products. The researchers noted that monacolin content was not stated on any of the brands, and only two products advised consumers to avoid its use if taking prescription statins.

As far as drug interactions are concerned, RYR may have additive cholesterol lowering with other antihyperlipidemic agents.[1] Grapefruit may increase RYR serum concentrations through CYP 450 3A4 inhibition. Increased RYR concentrations may lead to adverse effects. Other medications that may produce the same effect due to similar CYP 3A4 inhibition include certain macrolides, azole antifungals, protease inhibitors, and the antidepressant nefazodone.[1,3] On the other hand, St. John's wort and certain anticonvulsants (phenobarbital, carbamazepine, and phenytoin) may reduce serum RYR concentrations, because they induce CYP 3A4 isoenzymes. In combination with gemfibrozil there is a theoretical concern of rhabdomyolysis. With high-dose niacin there is also the theoretical potential for myopathy and liver toxicity. Concomitant use with thyroid supplements may result in thyroid function abnormalities. Red yeast rice use may also lower endogenous CoQ10 concentrations.[1]

Clinical Studies

The China Coronary Secondary Prevention Study evaluated 300 mg twice daily of Xuezhikang (XZK, a RYR product) or placebo in 4,870 subjects with previous myocardial infarction over a mean duration of treatment of 4.5 years.[11] Each capsule contained 2.5–3.2 mg of monacolin K, equivalent to a total daily dose of 10–12.8 mg of lovastatin. The primary endpoint was a major coronary event, including nonfatal MI and death from coronary heart disease. The primary endpoint occurred in 5.7% and 10.4% of subjects in the RYR and placebo groups, respectively, and was significantly lower in the RYR group ($P < 0.001$). Other outcomes included a significant decrease in cardiovascular and total mortality by 30 and 33%, respectively, and the need for coronary revascularization by one third. Moreover, the RYR also decreased lipid parameters. However, the study has not been replicated, and the results may not be transferable to other populations outside of China.

A 2015 systematic review and meta-analysis of trials found benefit for RYR use.[5] The 20 studies with a duration of 4–168 weeks involved 6,663 subjects comparing daily doses of 1,200–4,800 mg of RYR to other agents, including placebo, statins, and non-statin lipid lowering agents. The amount of monacolin K contained in the supplements ranged from 4.8–24 mg of monacolin K. The average daily dose of monacolin K was 10.8 mg. The pooled estimate determined that, compared to placebo, LDL decreased in the RYR group by 39.4 mg/dL (1.02 mmol/L; $P < 0.00001$). Compared to placebo, total cholesterol decreased 38.6 mg/dL (1 mmol/L; $P < 0.00001$). Also compared to placebo, HDL increased 2.7 mg/dL (0.07 mmol/L; $P = 0.001$), and triglycerides decreased 23 mg/dL (0.26 mmol/L; $P < 0.00001$). Compared to three different statins (lovastatin, pravastatin, and simvastatin), the effect on lowering LDL was not significant (1.16 mg/dL [0.03 mmol/l]; $P = 0.89$). Compared to non-statin active comparators, LDL decreased to a greater extent in the RYR group (20.1 mg/dL [0.52 mmol/l]; $P = 0.008$). Also compared to non-statin active comparator, HDL increased to a greater extent in the RYR group (3.1 mg/dL [0.08 mmol/L]; $P < 0.00001$). The authors noted that liver transaminases increased in seven RYR studies. In addition, muscle symptoms ranged from 0–24% in the RYR group versus 0–36% in the control groups. Another commonly reported adverse effect was gastrointestinal upset. Overall, this study demonstrated greater efficacy compared to placebo and non-statin active comparators, but no difference from the three statins evaluated in this study.

A 2016 systematic review of ten randomized controlled trials compared RYR with simvastatin in 905 Chinese subjects with hyperlipidemia.[12] The studies ranged from 4–12 weeks; daily doses of RYR ranged from 1.2–3.6 g/day, and simvastatin ranged from 10–20 mg. Overall, there was no significant difference between RYR and simvastatin lowering of total cholesterol ($P = 0.44$), LDL ($P = 0.10$), or triglycerides ($P = 0.57$), and no difference in HDL increase ($P = 0.33$). Adverse effects were similar in the RYR and simvastatin groups and included gastrointestinal upset, increased transaminases, and anorexia. Creatine phosphokinase elevations were reported only in the simvastatin groups. The authors noted that the trials lacked methodological rigor. The authors also stated they did not think there was justification to replace simvastatin with RYR. Moreover, since this was done in Chinese subjects, the results cannot be extrapolated to other populations.

Summary

Red yeast rice is a product used to treat hyperlipidemia and is often combined with other lipid-lowering ingredients such as berberine.[1] Indeed, a 2016 systematic review and meta-analysis of 14 trials evaluated the effects of a combination of RYR (3 mg monacolin), berberine (500 mg), policosanol (10 mg) and three other nutraceuticals in 1,670 subjects compared to 1,489 subjects on control.[13] The control group consisted mostly of placebo, although three studies used berberine or ezetimibe (a lipid lowering drug). Compared to control, significant decreases were reported in favor of the combination nutraceutical for total cholesterol (26.15 mg/dL [0.68 mmol/L]); LDL cholesterol (23.85 mg/dL [0.62 mmol/L]); and triglycerides (13.83 mg/dL [0.16 mmol/L]. HDL cholesterol increased significantly by 2.53 mg/dL (0.07 mmol/L). The P value was < 0.001 compared to control for all lipid parameters. Moreover, glucose decreased significantly by 2.6 mg/dL (0.14 mmol/L; $P = 0.01$) in 10 trials.

RYR is a controversial product in that some reports highlight its safety whereas others cite the potential dangers associated with its use. One potential problem is that commercial products do not typically list the monacolin content.[5] Studies show commercially available preparations may contain variable monacolin K or lack monacolin K content.[10] Commonly used daily doses range from 200–4,800 mg.[5]

The issue of RYR monacolin K content is controversial. Per Natural Medicines, the FDA considers that RYR supplements that contain a *significant* amount of monacolins are unapproved drugs.[1] Supplement manufacturers are not required to register products or dietary supplement ingredients with the FDA; thus, it may be difficult to determine whether any manufacturers have been inspected to evaluate RYR products. However, the Natural Products Association states that RYR manufacturers are being inspected, and some have been inspected according to 21 Code of Federal Regulations 111 (part of the Good Manufacturing Practices Rule).[14] In the past, the FDA has taken action against companies that sell products that contain more than trace amounts of monacolin K and has stated that these products should not be marketed as supplements.[15] However, it may be difficult for consumers to select appropriate products since the labels may only state the RYR amount, not whether there is any monacolin content. Moreover, considerable variability may exist in monacolin content in products sold over the counter.[16] In Germany, RYR products containing 5 mg or more of monacolin K are considered drugs.[1,6]

Although RYR may decrease lipids, individuals may experience side effects and drug interactions similar to statins. Many consider red yeast rice to be another statin, and it may have the same side effects as other statins. It may cause myalgias and has the potential to cause rhabdomyolysis. If not appropriately manufactured, RYR may contain an inadvertent nephrotoxin, citrinin.[1] There is only one study in Chinese patients that showed improved parameters for secondary prevention, but in American or other populations, primary and secondary prevention results are not available.[11] This is in contrast to statins, which have shown a role in both primary and secondary prevention. A population that merits extreme caution is young women of childbearing age since RYR may be teratogenic.[1] Consumers do not know whether products contain monacolins or citrinin. RYR should not be combined with statins. Due to differences in adverse events reported in different databases, clinicians should be diligent in searching adverse event reports.[6] Clinicians should also counsel persons that RYR use requires extreme caution, and they must closely monitor not only the efficacy, but side effects and drug interactions.

References

1. Natural Medicines (Natural Medicines Database search engine). Available from https://naturalmedicines.therapeuticresearch.com. Accessed May 9, 2019

2. Burke FM. Red yeast rice for the treatment of dyslipidemia. *Curr Atheroscler Rep* 2015; Apr;17(4):495. doi: 10.1007/s11883-015-0495-8

3. Cicero AFG, Fogacci F, Banach M. Red yeast rice for hypercholesterolemia. *Methodist Debakey Cardiovasc J* 2019;15:192–199

4. Fogacci F, Banach M, Mikhailidis DP, et al. Safety of red yeast rice supplementation: a systematic review and meta-analysis of randomized controlled trials. *Pharmacol Res* 2019;143:1–16

5. Gerards MC, Terlou RJ, Yu H, Koks CHW, Gerdes VEA. Traditional Chinese lipid-lowering red yeast rice results in significant LDL reduction but safety is uncertain—a systematic review and meta-analysis. Atherosclerosis 2015;240:415–423

6. Raschi E, Girardi A, Poluzzi E, et al. Adverse events to food supplements containing red yeast rice: comparative analysis of FAERS and CAERS reporting systems. *Drug Saf* 2018;41:745–752

7. Mazzanti G, Moro PA, Raschi E, Da Cas R, Menniti-Ippolito F. Adverse reactions to dietary supplements containing red yeast rice: assessment of cases from the Italian surveillance system. *Br J Clin Pharmacol* 2017;83:894–908

8. Banach M, Patti AM, Giglio RV, et al. The role of nutraceuticals in statin intolerant patients. *J Am Coll Cardiol* 2018;72:96–118

9. Dujovne CA. Red yeast rice preparations: are they suitable substitutions for statins? *Am J Med* 2017;130:1148–1150

10. Cohen PA, Avula B, Khan IA. Variability in strength of red yeast rice supplements purchased from mainstream retailers. *Eur J Prev Cardiol* 2017;24:1431–1434

11. Lu Z, Kou W, Du B, et al. Effect of Xuezhikang, an extract from red yeast Chinese rice, on coronary events in a Chinese population with previous myocardial infarction. *Am J Cardiol* 2008;101:1689–93

12. Ong YC, Aziz Z. Systematic review of red yeast rice compared with simvastatin in dyslipidaemia. *J Clin Pharm Ther* 2016;41:170–179

13. Pirro M, Mannarino MR, Bianconi V, et al. The effects of a nutraceutical combination on plasma lipids and glucose: a systematic review and meta-analysis of randomized controlled trials. *Pharmacol Res* 2016;110:76–88

14. FDA is regulating red yeast rice manufacturers, say ABC and NPA. Available from https://www.nutraingredients-usa.com/Article/2013/02/21/FDA-is-regulating-red-yeast-rice-manufacturers-say-ABC-NPA-as-scientists-question-safety-and-labels. Accessed January 18, 2020

15. Red yeast rice. NIH. National Center for Complementary and Integrative Health. Available from https://nccih.nih.gov/health/redyeastrice. Accessed January 18, 2020

16. Gordon RY, Cooperman T, Obermeyer W, et al. Marked variability of monacolin levels in commercial red yeast rice products: buyer beware!*Arch Intern Med* 2010;170:1722–1727

ST. JOHN'S WORT (*Hypericum perforatum L.*)

St John's wort is a perennial that grows throughout the United States, Canada, and Europe. The bright yellow flowers bloom in late June and constitute the primary ingredient used in the product. St John's wort (SJW) has been used for a variety of purposes, including antiviral and antibacterial effects, as well as to treat a variety of psychiatric disorders, such as depression and anxiety.[1] Many persons with diabetes have depression, and many clinicians consider this an important comorbidity that warrants evaluation.

Chemical Constituents and Mechanism of Action

St. John's wort contains different active chemical constituents, such as naphthodianthrones, flavonoids, phloroglucinols (including hyperforin), and essential oils. Hypericin was once thought to be the major active constituent with antidepressant activity; however, hyperforin and adhyperforin may be the most significant contributors to antidepressant effects.[1] Nevertheless, many trials have used the hypericin extract.

The mechanism of action is thought to be inhibition of reuptake of serotonin, norepinephrine, and dopamine. Other neurotransmitters that are also affected include gamma-aminobutyric acid (GABA) and glutamate.[1,2] Impact on serotonin reuptake inhibition may be the most significant factor involved in antidepressant activity.

Adverse Effects and Drug Interactions

Side effects of St. John's wort include phototoxicity, photosensitivity, sleep difficulties, gastrointestinal upset, anxiety, and withdrawal-like symptoms if discontinued abruptly. St. John's wort may also increase TSH (thyroid stimulating hormone) in laboratory analyses.[1] Overall, a systematic review indicated that St. John's wort is well tolerated, and adverse effects in surveillance studies evaluating 34,804 patients have ranged from 0% to 6%. This is a much lower rate than with conventional antidepressants.[3]

Through different effects on P-glycoprotein modulation with CYP 450 3A4 and 2C9 isoenzyme system induction, St. John's wort may decrease serum concentrations of several drugs that a patient with diabetes may be taking.[1,2] Hyperforin is the chemical constituent thought to be primarily responsible for the interactions. Hyperforin activates the pregnane x receptor, subsequently resulting in drug metabolism and transporter gene activation. Of note: if very low doses of hyperforin are used, the risk of drug interactions is minimized.[2] Examples of drugs where metabolism may be induced, and thus have decreased efficacy, include oral contraceptives, cyclosporine, warfarin, angiotensin-receptor blockers, certain statins, and digoxin. Other important drugs that may be induced and thus have decreased efficacy are protease inhibitors.[1,2] Moreover, SJW has been found to produce serotonin syndrome, and subsequent toxicity, when combined with serotonergic agents, due to high serotonin levels. Examples of serotonergic drugs include fluoxetine (Prozac®), sertraline (Zoloft®), and paroxetine (Paxil®). Additive sedation may also occur when combined with narcotics.[1]

Clinical Studies

Many published studies have evaluated SJW for depression, but only a few will be discussed here. SJW has been studied in comparisons to placebo as well as conventional antidepressants. The most recent Cochrane Review evaluating SJW for depression was published in 2008.[4] A total of 5,489 persons were assessed in 29 randomized controlled trials. In 18 trials SJW was compared to placebo, and in 19 trials, it was compared to conventional antidepressants, including tricyclic or tetracyclic antidepressants and selective serotonin reuptake inhibitors (SSRIs). Compared to placebo, the overall response rate (indicating a 50% decrease in Hamilton Depression Scale scores) for SJW was 1.48 (95% CI of 1.23 to 1.77), but the trials were quite heterogeneous. However, there were no differences in response between SJW and conventional antidepressants (RR 1.01; 95% CI of 0.93 to 1.09). A unique finding was that subjects on SJW were less likely than those on conventional antidepressants to drop out of studies due to adverse effects. Compared to tricyclic antidepressants, those on SJW were 76% less likely to discontinue treatment ($P < 0.0001$). Compared to SSRIs, those on SJW were 47% less likely to stop treatment ($P = 0.005$). The review found that trials performed in German-speaking countries tended to report results that are more favorable.

Results of a 2016 systematic review of 35 trials in 6,993 subjects were similar to results of the Cochrane Review.[5] In the 2016 systematic review, there were more treatment responders on SJW compared to placebo (RR 1.53; 95% CI of 1.19 to 1.97) and there was no difference in response compared to standard antidepressants (RR 1.01; 95% CI of 0.90 to 1.14). The authors noted that since trials were heterogeneous and did not evaluate impact on severe depression, the evidence for benefit is limited.

A 2017 meta-analysis evaluated the impact of SJW for depression compared to SSRIs.[6] The analysis included 27 trials in 3,808 subjects, and treatment duration ranged from 4–12 weeks. The pooled response rate showed no significant difference (or equal response) between SJW and SSRIs (RR 0.983; 95% CI of 0.924 to 1.042). The authors defined remission as a greater than 75% decrease in Hamilton Depression Scale scores. There was no difference in remission rates between subjects on SJW and SSRIs (RR 1.013; 95% CI of 0.892 to 1.134). Overall, there was no difference in standardized mean difference (SMD) Hamilton Depression Scale scores between subjects on SJW and SSRIs. (Pooled SMD –0.068; 95% CI of –0.127

to 0.021). One study favoring SJW over SSRIs evaluated the discontinuation rate due to adverse effects. The discontinuation rate was significantly lower among subjects taking SJW than those prescribed SSRIs (OR 0.587; 95% CI of 0.478 to 0.697).

Summary

St John's wort is a unique botanical product that has been used for centuries to treat depression, although studies show it may be useful only for mild to moderate depression. Long-term studies are not available. Two of the chemical constituents, hypericin and hyperforin, have been used as standardized extracts, but some researchers believe the constituents most likely to produce antidepressant effects are hyperforin, adhyperforin, and other related compounds.[1] These compounds modulate different neurotransmitters, including serotonin, norepinephrine, dopamine, GABA, and glutamate. The serotonergic effects may be the major antidepressant activity.

St John's wort use may have significant consequences because of the potential for serious drug interactions. SJW is a potent CYP450 enzyme inducer of important drugs that persons with diabetes may be taking, such as certain statins, calcium channel blockers, angiotensin receptor blockers, oral contraceptives, warfarin, and cyclosporine. It may also reduce serum concentrations of digoxin and interact adversely with serotonergic drugs (such as fluoxetine, sertraline, or paroxetine) or narcotics, subsequently resulting in toxicity. Doses used are 300–600 mg three times daily. Standardized extracts used in studies include 0.3% hypericin and the hyperforin-stabilized version of this extract.[1] Patients should always inform their healthcare providers if they are taking SJW, particularly because of the potential for serious drug interactions with medications they may be using. Patients should be informed that SJW might reduce serum concentrations of certain drugs to subtherapeutic levels. Conversely, patients should also be informed that abrupt discontinuation might result in dangerously increased serum concentrations of drugs that normally have lower concentrations during coadministration. St John's wort may not be considered a safe agent to use in diabetes because of the potential harm if it lowers serum concentrations of medications critical for diabetes management or its comorbidities. If a person is depressed, clinicians may wish to emphasize the important role of a traditional antidepressant and promote careful monitoring to obtain optimal and safe results.

References

1. Natural Medicines (Natural Medicines Database search engine). Available from https://naturalmedicines.therapeuticresearch.com. Accessed May 9, 2019

2. Chrubasik-Hausmann S, Viachojannis J, McLachlan AJ. Understanding drug interactions with St. John's wort (Hypericum perforatum L.): impact of hyperforin content. *J Pharm Pharmacol* 2019;71:129–138

3. Schulz V. Safety of St. John's wort extract compared to synthetic antidepressants. *Phytomedicine* 2006;13:199–204

4. Linde K, Berner MM, Kriston L. St John's wort for major depression. *Cochrane Database Syst Rev* 2008:CD000448

5. Apaydin EA, Maher AR, Shanman R, et al. A systematic review of St. John's wort for major depressive disorder. *Syst Rev* 2016;5:148

6. Ng QX, Venkatanarayanan N, Ho CYX. Clinical use of Hypericum perforatum (St. John's wort) in depression: a meta-analysis. *J Affect Disord* 2017;210:211–221

VITAMIN D

Vitamin D is a fat-soluble vitamin.[1] It is considered a hormone because the active form is produced in one part of the body (kidneys) but its effects are exerted throughout the body.[1-4] A highly-prevalent role of vitamin D has been in the prevention and treatment of osteoporosis. It is an important nutrient, and consumption may benefit many individuals, including those with diabetes. Vitamin D is synthesized in the human body but is also found in certain foods and as a dietary supplement. Two major forms include vitamin D2 and vitamin D3. Vitamin D2 is synthesized by plants, and vitamin D3 is produced in the skin as a result of exposure to ultraviolet B rays from sunlight. Examples of foods containing vitamin D include salmon, sardines, cod liver oil, egg yolks, and fortified foods such as milk and orange juice.[1-4] Vitamin D is involved in many metabolic processes and disease states, and it tends to be deficient in persons who live in northern latitudes, who have less exposure to sunshine, and those who are dark skinned.

Chemical Constituents and Mechanism of Action

Vitamin D supplements are available as ergocalciferol (vitamin D2) and cholecalciferol (vitamin D3).[1,4] Vitamin D2 is considered one third as potent as vitamin D3. Either form must undergo two hydroxylations for activation to 25-hydroxyvitamin D (25[OH] D), or calcidiol, and to 1,25-dihydroxyvitamin D (1,25[OH]2D), or calcitriol.[4] The active form is essential for calcium absorption in the digestive tract. The most appropriate indicator of vitamin D status is 25-hydroxyvitamin D, abbreviated as 25(OH)D. To meet most overall health needs, a serum concentration of at least 20 ng/mL (50 nmol/L) of 25(OH)D is considered appropriate. Lower concentrations are thought to indicate deficiency (< 12 ng/mL [<30 nmol/L]).[4]

Vitamin D has multimodal mechanisms of action. A main function is to regulate serum calcium and phosphorous concentrations, and it has an important role in regulating bone health and muscle strength.[4] In diabetes, low vitamin D levels are thought to be associated with impaired pancreatic β-cell function and insulin resistance.[5] It also increases calcium concentrations, which may improve insulin action. A few studies have shown there may be an association between vitamin D deficiency and statin associated muscle symptoms (SAMS), and in some cases vitamin D supplementation may help mitigate these symptoms.[6] However, there have been no randomized controlled studies to determine whether vitamin D supplementation definitively corrects SAMS.

Vitamin D is also thought to improve inflammation by interfering with cytokine generation and action. It may also downregulate activation of pro-inflammatory markers (nF-κB); thus, there has been interest in a potential role in cardiovascular health.[1,7]

Adverse Effects and Drug Interactions

Side effects may occur when toxic concentrations of 25-hydroxyvitamin D are reached (> 150 ng/mL [374.4 nmol/L]); these manifest as nausea, vomiting, poor appetite, weight loss, weakness, and constipation. Hypercalcemia is possible, due to increased calcium absorption, and may result in confusion, tinnitus, ataxia, arrhythmias, and deposition of calcium phosphate in soft tissues.[1] A three-year randomized study in 311 healthy persons without osteoporosis evaluated administration of daily doses of 400 IU, 4,000 IU, or 10,000 IU of vitamin D. The study found that bone loss occurred in the two highest-dose groups compared to 400 IU, but the highest dose resulted in much lower bone mineral density.[8] Thus, taking very high daily doses of vitamin D may result in bone loss. The National Academy of Medicine (formerly Institute of Medicine) has stated that the safe upper limit of daily vitamin D is 4,000 IU.[9]

Drug interactions with vitamin D mostly involve depletion by certain medications. Certain anticonvulsants (such as phenobarbital or phenytoin), antibiotics (such as rifampin), and certain HIV medications may decrease vitamin D concentrations. Steroids impair calcium absorption and vitamin D metabolism. Orlistat and cholestyramine may impair vitamin D absorption. Arrhythmias may occur if taken with digoxin, due to hypercalcemia. Finally, hypermagnesemia may occur if taken with magnesium-containing antacids.[1]

Clinical Studies

There is a large body of published information evaluating the role of vitamin D in different disease states, such as osteoporosis.[2] Vitamin D deficiency is associated with muscle weakness and with certain cancers such as pancreatic, colon, prostate, ovarian, and breast cancer, as well as Hodgkin's lymphoma. Supplementation may benefit certain autoimmune diseases, such as multiple sclerosis, because it acts as an important immunomodulator. Although many studies have been published, only a few will be presented here.

Observational studies have suggested a connection between vitamin D and diabetes. For instance, a 2008 systematic review and meta-analysis evaluated the impact of vitamin D supplementation in infants and later risk of type 1 diabetes.[10] Five observational studies found that vitamin D supplementation during early childhood was associated with a significant 29% decreased risk of type 1 diabetes (OR 0.71; 95% CI of 0.60 to 0.84). Observational data has also associated a correlation between low serum 25-hydroxyvitamin D levels and type 2 diabetes.[11]

Other trials have evaluated the outcomes of vitamin D supplementation in subjects with diabetes. One 48-week randomized double-blind placebo-controlled study evaluated daily administration of 4,000 IU of vitamin D3 in 127 subjects with well-controlled type 2 diabetes (baseline A1C of 6.6%).[12] At baseline,

25-hydroxy vitamin D levels were considered adequate (26.6 ng/mL [66.4 nmol/L]), and the levels increased significantly in the supplemented group compared to placebo by 24 weeks ($P < 0.001$). Compared to placebo, A1C did not decrease significantly at 48 weeks in the vitamin D group ($P = 0.87$). There were no other significant changes in insulin sensitivity or insulin secretion rate. Vitamin D supplementation had no impact in persons with well-controlled type 2 diabetes subjects with adequate baseline 25-hydroxy vitamin D levels.

A 2017 systematic review and meta-analysis of 24 studies evaluated the impact of vitamin D supplementation in type 2 diabetes.[13] In a pooled analysis of information from 23 studies, A1C decreased significantly by 0.25% ($P = 0.01$). In 17 studies that analyzed impact on fasting glucose, there was no decrease with vitamin D supplementation ($P = 0.10$). However, per subgroup analysis, subjects with baseline vitamin D deficiency (25 hydroxy Vit D levels less than 20 ng/mL [50 nmol/L]) had a significant decline not only in A1C but also fasting glucose ($P = 0.009$ and $P = 0.007$, respectively, compared to control). A 2019 meta-analysis of 19 randomized controlled studies in subjects with type 2 diabetes showed that mean A1C decreased significantly ($P = 0.007$) in short-term studies (less than 6 months duration).[14] Thus, vitamin D supplementation in subjects with diabetes has shown varying results on glycemic parameters.

The D2d trial was a randomized double-blind placebo-controlled trial that evaluated the impact of a daily vitamin D3 dose of 4,000 IU on prevention of type 2 diabetes in 2,423 subjects with prediabetes.[15] There were 1,211 subjects on vitamin D3 and 1,212 on placebo, and the median follow up was 2.5 years. Subjects on vitamin D had a baseline 25(OH)D level of 27.7 ng/mL (69.1 nmol/L), and this increased to 54.3 ng/mL (135.5 nmol/L) at 24 months. The placebo group had a baseline level of 28.2 ng/mL (70.4 nmol/L) which essentially remained the same at 24 months (28.8 ng/mL [71.90 nmol/L]). At the end of the trial, 293 subjects (24.2%) in the vitamin D group had developed diabetes, compared to 323 (26.7%) in the placebo group, but the difference was not significant (HR 0.88 [95% CI 0.75 to 1.04]; $P = 0.12$). For adverse effects the researchers cited as being of interest, there were no differences between the vitamin D and placebo groups. These included nephrolithiasis, hypercalcemia, low estimated glomerular filtration rate, or a fasting urine calcium:creatinine ratio exceeding 0.375. In a post-hoc analysis of 4.3% of subjects with low baseline 25(OH)D levels (less than 12 ng/mL [30 nmol/L]), the hazard ratio in the vitamin D3 group was 0.38 (95% CI 0.18 to 0.80). This suggested that perhaps vitamin D may be of benefit in those subjects with prediabetes who have insufficient 25(OH)D levels. Trial strengths were inclusion of a large number of subjects, a diverse and appropriately-randomized study population, study design, and duration. However, the dose used was higher than what most persons will generally use, which could limit generalizability. The overall conclusion was that vitamin D supplementation does not prevent type 2 diabetes.

The VITAL DKD trial evaluated the impact of vitamin D and ω-3 fatty acid supplementation in subjects with type 2 diabetes who were at risk for development of kidney disease.[16] The study was a 5-year randomized clinical trial with a two-by-two factorial design in 1,312 subjects with type 2 diabetes. Subjects were randomized to receive vitamin D3 and ω-3 fatty acids, vitamin D3 and placebo, ω-3 fatty acids and placebo, or two placebos. Daily doses used were 2,000 IU of vitamin D3 and 1 g of ω-3 fatty acids. The primary outcome was the 5-year glomerular filtration rate (eGFR) change, estimated from serum creatinine and cystatin C. The mean baseline eGFR was 85.8 mL/min/1.73m.[2] At endpoint (year 5), the mean change in eGFR was −12.3 (95% CI of −13.4 to −11.2) mL/min/1.73m^2 for vitamin D3 compared to −13.1 (95% CI of −14.2 to −11.9) mL/min/1.73m^2 for placebo. The difference was 0.9 (95% CI of −0.7 to 2.5) mL/min/1.73m^2 and was not significant. For ω-3 fatty acids, the mean change in eGFR was −12.2 (95% CI of −13.3 to −11.1) mL/min/1.73m^2 compared to −13.1 (95% CI of −14.2 to −12.0) mL/min/1.73m^2 for placebo. The difference was 0.9 (95% CI of −0.7 to 2.6) mL/min/1.73m^2. Thus, neither vitamin D3 nor ω-3 fatty acids had an impact on decreasing kidney disease in at-risk subjects with type 2 diabetes. The authors noted there was no interaction between the assigned treatments ($P = 0.42$). Notable adverse outcomes were kidney stones in 32 subjects on vitamin D and 26 on placebo, and gastrointestinal bleeding in 28 on ω-3 fatty acids and 17 on placebo. The authors noted that—in subgroup analyses of subjects with lower vitamin D levels (< 30 ng/mL [75 nmol/L]), lower eGFR levels (< 60 mL/min/1.73m^2) or albumin/creatinine > 30 mg/g or normal baseline BMI—results favored vitamin D supplementation, but they were not statistically significant. Study strengths were the large sample size and long study duration. A limitation was limited power to assess effects among subgroups that may benefit from study interventions. The overall conclusion was that vitamin D3 or ω-3 fatty acid supplements do not preserve renal function in subjects with type 2 diabetes.

There has been interest in the possible benefit of vitamin D on cardiovascular outcomes. However, a 2019 meta-analysis of 21 randomized clinical trials found that vitamin D supplementation did not decrease major adverse cardiovascular events ($P = 0.85$).[17] There were 41,669 subjects that received vitamin D and 41,622 that received placebo. There was also no significant reduction in secondary outcomes, including myocardial infarction ($P = 0.92$), stroke ($P = 0.16$) cardiovascular mortality ($P = 0.68$), or all-cause mortality ($P = 0.23$).

The VITAL (Vitamin D and ω-3 Trial) study was a two-by-two factorial design trial done in 25,871 subjects that evaluated the impact of daily doses of vitamin D at 2,000 IU or 1 g daily of marine ω-3 fatty acids or placebo on cancer and cardiovascular disease (CVD) prevention.[18] There was no impact on CVD prevention, since 396 subjects in the vitamin D group and 409 in the placebo group experienced a major cardiovascular event (HR 0.97; 95% CI 0.85 to 1.12; $P = 0.69$). Vitamin D supplementation also did not prevent cancer.

The Vital-HF was an ancillary study of the VITAL trial that evaluated the impact of a daily dose of 2,000 IU of vitamin D3 and 1 g daily of ω-3 fatty acids compared to placebo on the incidence of hospitalization for heart failure in a multi-ethnic sample of 25,871 subjects.[19] The researchers found that first hospitalization for heart failure occurred in 240 subjects on vitamin D and 259 on placebo (HR 0.93; 95% CI of 0.78 to 1.11; $P = 0.41$). In the ω-3 fatty acids group, 244 subjects were hospitalized compared to 255 on placebo (HR 0.96; 95% CI of 0.80 to 1.14; $P = 0.61$). In a secondary analysis, recurrent heart failure hospitalization did not differ between the vitamin D and placebo groups (HR 0.94; 95% CI of 0.81 to 1.09; $P = 0.44$). However, the reduction in recurrent hospitalizations was significantly decreased by 14% in the ω-3 fatty acids group compared to placebo (HR 0.86; 95% CI of 0.74 to 0.998; $P = 0.048$). Overall, the authors concluded that vitamin D and ω-3 fatty acids did not reduce first heart failure hospitalizations. Moreover, although vitamin D did not reduce recurrent heart failure hospitalizations, the authors stated that the benefit of ω-3 fatty acids on this outcome requires confirmation.

Summary

Vitamin D is an important nutrient necessary for different body functions as well as bone and muscle health. Most supplements that individuals use contain vitamin D3 (cholecalciferol), although vitamin D2 (ergocalciferol, found in high doses—50,000 IU) is sometimes used. The appropriate measurement to assess vitamin D status is serum 25(OH)D. Osteoporosis is of concern, particularly in the elderly (including persons with diabetes), because of the possibility of falls and fractures. However, there are varying recommendations by different organizations regarding vitamin D intake with regard to bone health. For instance, the National Academy of Medicine recommends that adults up to age 70 should receive a recommended daily allowance of 600 IU of vitamin D, and 800 IU if older than 70 years of age.[9] The National Osteoporosis Foundation recommends vitamin D3 daily doses of 800–1,000 IU along with calcium to prevent osteoporosis in adults 50 years and older.[20] A systematic review and meta-analysis in community-dwelling elderly without osteoporosis did not support calcium or vitamin D supplementation for fracture prevention.[21] Accordingly, the US Preventive Services Task Force Recommendation Statement does not support routine vitamin D supplementation in individuals without known deficiency, prior fracture, or osteoporosis.[22]

In the past, observational studies showed an association between low vitamin D levels and development of diabetes. The D2d study provided evidence that supplementation does not prevent diabetes.[15] Additionally, vitamin D supplementation does not improve glycemic parameters in subjects with diabetes.[12-14] Trials have also provided evidence that supplementation does not reduce kidney disease, prevent adverse cardiovascular outcomes, or decrease heart failure hospitalizations.[16-19] Vitamin D is considered a relatively safe supplement, although kidney stones, hypercalcemia, and GI upset at high doses may occur.[1] Patients should be counseled that they should not take daily doses of vitamin D3 higher than 4,000 IU. They should also be told that if they are taking certain medications, such as certain anticonvulsants, cholestyramine, or orlistat, that these may decrease vitamin D serum concentrations. Although research is prolific, there are still many unknowns, such as the most optimal serum concentration and when routine screening should be done. In many cases, however, clinicians may wish to assess vitamin D levels and recommend supplementation, if necessary, to improve the overall health, particularly bone health, of individuals with diabetes.

References

1. Natural Medicines (Natural Medicines Database search engine). Available from https://naturalmedicines.therapeuticresearch.com. Accessed May 9, 2019
2. Pittas AG, Lau J, Hu FB, Dawson-Hughes B. The role of vitamin D and calcium in type 2 diabetes: a systematic review and meta-analysis. *J Clin Endocrinol Metab* 2007;92:2017–29
3. Holick MF. Vitamin D deficiency. *N Engl J Med* 2007;357:266–81
4. NIH Office of Dietary Supplements. Vitamin D. Fact sheet for health professionals. Available from http://ods.od.nih.gov/factsheets/VitaminD-HealthProfessional/?print=1. Accessed December 2, 2019
5. Kayaniyil S, Vieth R, Retnakaran R, et al. Association of vitamin D with insulin resistance and beta-cell dysfunction in subjects at risk for type 2 diabetes. *Diabetes Care* 2010;33:1379–1381
6. Lowe K, Kubra KT, He ZY, Carey K. Vitamin D supplementation to treat statin-associated muscle symptoms: a review. *Sr Care Pharm* 2019;34:253–257
7. Mozos I, Marginean O. Links between Vitamin D deficiency and cardiovascular diseases. *Biomed Res Int* 2015;2015:109275. doi: 10.1155/2015/109275. Epub 2015 Apr 27
8. Burt LA, Billington EQ, Rose MS, et al. Effect of high-dose Vitamin D supplementation on volumetric bone density and bone strength: a randomized clinical trial. *JAMA* 2019;322:736–745
9. Institute of Medicine. Dietary Reference Intakes for Calcium and Vitamin D. Washington, DC: National Academies Press: 2011

10. Zipitis CS, Akobeng AK. Vitamin D supplementation in early childhood and risk of type 1 diabetes: a systematic review and meta-analysis. *Arch Dis Child* 2008;93:512–517

11. Song Y, Wang L, Pittas AG, et al. Blood 25-hydroxy vitamin D levels and incident type 2 diabetes: a meta-analysis of prospective studies. *Diabetes Care* 2013;36:1422–1428

12. Angellotti E, D'Alessio D, Dawson-Hughes B, et al. Vitamin D supplementation in patients with type 2 diabetes: the vitamin D for established type 2 diabetes (DDM2) study. *J Endocr Soc* 2018;2:310–321

13. Wu C, Qiu S, Zhu X, Li L. Vitamin D supplementation and glycemic control in type 2 diabetes patients: a systematic review and meta-analysis. *Metabolism* 2017;73:67–76

14. Hu Z, Chen J, Sun X, Wang L, Wang A. Efficacy of vitamin D supplementation on glycemic control in type 2 diabetes patients. *Medicine* (Baltimore). 2019 Apr;98(14):e14970. doi: 10.1097/MD.0000000000014970

15. Pittas AG, Dawson-Hughes B, Sheehan P, et al. Vitamin D supplementation and prevention of type 2 diabetes. *N Engl J Med* 2019;381:520–530

16. de Boer IH, Zelnick LR, Ruzinski J, et al. Effect of vitamin D and omega-3 fatty acid supplementation on kidney function in patients with type 2 diabetes: a randomized clinical trial. *JAMA* 2019;322:1899–1909

17. Barbarawi M, Kheiri B, Zayed Y, et al. Vitamin D supplementation and cardiovascular disease risks in more than 83,000 individuals in 21 randomized clinical trials: a meta-analysis. *JAMA Cardiol* 2019;4:765–775

18. Manson JE, Cook NR, Lee IM, et al. Vitamin D supplements and prevention of cancer and cardiovascular disease. *N Engl J Med* 2019;380:33–44

19. Djousse L, Cook NR, Kim E, et al. Supplementation with vitamin D and/or omega-3 fatty acids and incidence of heart failure hospitalization: VITAL-heart failure. *Circulation* 2019; Nov 11. doi: 10.1161/CIRCULATIONAHA.119.044645.

20. Cosman F, de Beur SJ, LeBoff MS, et al. Clinician's Guide to Prevention and Treatment of Osteoporosis. *Osteoporos Int* 2014;25:2359–2381

21. Zhao JG, Zeng XT, Wang J, Liu L. Association between calcium or vitamin D supplementation and fracture incidence in community-dwelling older adults: a systematic review and meta-analysis. *JAMA* 2017;318:2466–2482

22. US Preventive Services Task Force Recommendation Statement. Vitamin D, calcium, or combined supplementation for the primary prevention of fractures in community-dwelling adults. *JAMA* 2018;319:1592–1599

Closing Comments and Advice for Clinicians

In this book, 38 different supplements for diabetes and related comorbidities have been highlighted. Some studies in this book have evaluated the impact of supplements on prediabetes. Hopefully, emerging research may address whether these products may decrease or delay diabetes onset. The reader should be apprised that there are literally thousands of available supplements on the market. Some examples of other popular plant products for diabetes or its comorbidities include soy (Glycine max), guarumo (Cecropia obtusifolia), caiapo (Ipomoea batatas), the common bean (Phaseolus vulgaris), guar gum (Cyamopsis tetragonolobus [L.] Taub), policosanol (Saccharum officinarum L.), guggul (Commiphora mukul), and ginger (Zingiber officinale). There are also non botanical products such as vanadium, nicotinamide, and selenium that are also used. The reader is encouraged to learn more about these and other products, including more specifics about product effectiveness and safety ratings, at the Natural Medicines website.[1]

An emerging trend in complementary health approaches is focused on hemp-based cannabidiol (CBD) supplements. The Agriculture Improvement Act of 2018, more commonly known as the "2018 Farm Bill," was enacted in December 2018; this act declassified hemp as a controlled substance, legalizing hemp cultivation.[2] Marijuana and hemp are two forms of the plant *Cannabis sativa*. Marijuana contains more than 15% of delta-9-tetrahydrocannabinol (THC), whereas hemp contains less than 0.3% of THC, per dry weight. CBD is a non-psychoactive component of *Cannabis sativa*, whereas THC is psychoactive. A complicated issue is that CBD is not allowed to be marketed for therapeutic purposes, because it is FDA approved as a prescription drug (Epidiolex®) for certain seizure disorders. However, CBD is sold without a prescription in various formulations—oils, sprays, balms, capsules, gummy bears, and vapes. CBD content must not exceed 0.3% of THC per dry weight.

CBD has been used as an anxiolytic, for pain, opioid withdrawal, smoking cessation, and diabetes. There are various theorized mechanism of action. Some mechanisms include inhibiting uptake and degradation of andanamide (an endo-cannabinoid neurotransmitter), increasing activity of 5-HT1A serotonin recep-tors, enhancing nuclear peroxisome proliferator-activated receptor γ (PPARγ) activity, and activation of transient receptor potential of vanilloid type 1 (TRPV1) and 2 (TRPV2) channels. Adverse effects include gastrointestinal upset, weight loss, and elevated liver enzymes. Moreover, CBD may inhibit several CYP 450 enzymes, resulting in increased concentrations of many drugs, such as some ben-zodiazepines, certain anticonvulsants, macrolide antibiotics, and anticoagulants.[1] A serious issue, however, has been that commercial CBD products have shown problems with product content. In one assessment of 84 products in the United States, only 26 were accurately labeled, and 21% contained THC.[3] Other assays have also shown measurable quantities of THC in European and vaping products.[1]

In diabetes, benefit may be related to anti-inflammatory activity and dimin-ished insulin resistance. A 13-week proof of concept study evaluated CBD and another plant cannabinoid, delta-9-tetrahydrocannabivarin (THVC), in subjects with type 2 diabetes.[4] This study reported that CBD did not improve glycemic or lipid parameters or inflammatory markers. However, the other cannabinoid, THCV, decreased fasting glucose and improved pancreatic β-cell function.

Supplement-related research has been prolific, and clinicians are advised to stay abreast of research in this area. NIH has a website that provides information on dietary supplement research.[5]

It is imperative for clinicians to inform their patients that supplement use is not advocated by the American Diabetes Association.[6,7] The ADA has issued a position statement on unproven therapies, and the Standards of Medical Care also emphasize that vitamins, antioxidants, herbal therapies, and other supplements, such as aloe vera, chromium, cinnamon, or curcumin are not recommended for elevated glucose. Nevertheless, it is important for clinicians to maintain an open, nonjudgmental dialogue with their patients to ask about supplements they may be taking and include them in their list of medications. Guiding individuals regarding supplements is an important aspect of clinical care. Persons with diabetes (PWD) should be encouraged to take all of their supplements, as well as prescription med-ications, to their provider visits.

PWD should be asked at each visit whether they have started or stopped taking any supplements. Individuals who take supplements should be congratulated for taking an active interest in their own health care. This provides an opportunity to make the point that supplements may not be benign, and using them could pos-sibly result in adverse effects and interactions with comorbid conditions, other medications, supplements, alcohol, or nutrients. Clinicians should advise PWD that a particularly vulnerable time is when they are about to have surgery—supple-ments should be discontinued 2 weeks prior.

PWD often take supplements because they believe they are natural. Clinicians should, however, remind them that supplements are not necessarily safer than conventional medications. Although the FDA does regulate supplements, the evaluation process is not as rigorous as for prescription medications.

Clincans need to teach PWD about third-party verification to ensure safety, such as that provided by the U.S. Pharmacopoeia, NSF International, or Consumer Lab. These certifications ensure that the ingredients stated on the label are actually contained in the product. However, although the product may have been appropriately scrutinized through verification processes, that does not guarantee efficacy or safety.

PWD should be encouraged to research a product before they start taking it, especially since some products may be very expensive and only provide minimal benefit. PWD should be reminded that they deserve to find and use quality products. PWD should be encouraged to read labels carefully and look for telephone numbers, addresses, and websites on the labels. If there is any doubt, PWD should be encouraged to contact manufacturers and ask questions. If a manufacturer is willing to provide published information rather than testimonials, that may indicate they are a more reliable company. PWD should be wary of products lacking a lot number or expiration date. When in doubt, recommend discarding the product 1 year from date of purchase. There is new information on the "Nutrition Facts Label" effective January 1, 2020.[8] Manufacturers that earn at least $10 million in annual sales are required to make these changes. Smaller manufacturers are not required to make the change until 2021. One specific change for supplements is that actual quantities must be clearly stated along with the percent daily value, such as for vitamin D or other nutrients. The intent is to assist consumers in making better-informed decisions.

Patients should be taught to scrutinize the dose provided and ask their provider, pharmacist, or diabetes care and education specialist to make sure it is the most appropriate dose for them. They should avoid products that do not include dosing instructions. Also, clinicians should teach patients about identifying the best possible product based on active ingredients. For instance, although a product lists an ingredient such as "turmeric" on the label, that does not mean it has been standardized to contain sufficient curcuminoids to provide benefit as shown in evidence-based studies. The Natural Medicines website is a good reference to consult in the Standardization and Formulation section of the product monograph in question.[1] The next step is to check the Pharmacokinetics section in the product monograph to determine which formulations provide the best bioavailability.

Another counseling point is to compare ingredients when making repeat purchases to verify that ingredients, amounts, and doses do not vary. It is best not to change brands. PWD should also be wary of purchasing different products that may duplicate the same ingredient and inadvertently result in overdoses or toxicity. PWD may be advised to save a few pills from a bottle should there be a need to perform a product assay in case of adverse effects.

Clinicans should remind PWD to be especially careful with supplement use in vulnerable populations, such as children, pregnant or lactating women, the elderly, and those with certain comorbidities such as cancer or Human Immunodeficiency Virus. Moreover, persons with several allergies (such as to different plant products) or on anticoagulants or blood thinners may also be vulnerable. Starting with single-ingredient rather than multiple-ingredient products is a safer way to initiate supplement use. Accordingly, if an adverse effect, such as hypoglycemia or changes in blood pressure or other untoward events occur, it is easier to determine the responsible ingredient. Along those lines, it would be advisable to initiate treatment with a small dose and titrate up to the recommended dose to evaluate whether the product impacts blood glucose or other parameters and to avoid dose-related adverse effects.

PWD should be advised to monitor glucose values frequently and to share any concerns with their health care team. It takes 3 months to see any impact on A1C, and if there is no benefit after that time, then it is a good idea to determine whether the supplement should be continued. Clinicians should advise record keeping to assess progress on glucose, blood pressure, lipids, weight, and other important aspects of diabetes care.

A critical clinician role is to empower PWD to determine what they hope to achieve in taking supplements. It is important for PWD to realize that supplements may improve certain outcomes but may not help achieve target goals for glucose, blood pressure, lipids, or weight. Reminding PWD that there are many scams and false claims made regarding supplements is another key role for clinicians. For instance, claims of a "miracle cure" or benefitting a wide variety of disease states should warrant further information and be considered as suspect statements. PWD should be taught in a caring and positive manner that supplements are not a substitute for conventional medications or for an unhealthy lifestyle.

In the past, some clinicians may have been reluctant to initiate a conversation about supplement use because they personally do not believe in their efficacy or because they lack confidence in their own knowledge of these products. Perhaps this book may help mitigate these concerns and may promote a positive patient-clinician relationship. It is crucial to emphasize that the products discussed in this book have not demonstrated ADA-recommended target goals for glucose, blood pressure, lipids, or weight.

Conclusions

Information and studies on supplements continue to be published at an exponentially increasing rate, and consumer use mirrors that increase. Some of the supplement types that are increasingly popular include protein drinks and powders, energy drinks, certain vitamins, and probiotics. The future portends continued research and an ever-evolving supplement market that will continue to be of importance and interest to clinicians and persons with diabetes.

References

1. Natural Medicines (Natural Medicines Database search engine). Available from https://naturalmedicines.therapeuticresearch.comhttps://natural-medicines.therapeuticresearch.com. Accessed January 29, 2020
2. FDA regulation of Cannabis and Cannabis-Derived Products, Including Cannabidiol (CBD). US Food & Drug Administration website. Available from www.fda.gov/news-events/public-health-focus/fda-regulation-cannabis-and-cannabis-derived-products-questions-and-answers#other cbdapproved. Accessed Jan 30, 2020
3. Bonn-Miller MO, Loflin MJE, Thomas BF, et al. Labeling accuracy of cannabidiol extracts sold online. *JAMA* 2017;318:1708–1709
4. Jadoon KA, Ratcliffe SH, Barrett DA, et al. Efficacy and safety of cannabidiol and tetrahydrocannabivarin on glycemic and lipid parameters in patients with type 2 diabetes: a randomized, double-blind, placebo-controlled, parallel group pilot study. *Diabetes Care* 2016;39:1777–1786
5. NIH Office of Dietary Supplements. Computer Access to Research on Dietary Supplements (CARDS) database. Available from https://ods.od.nih.gov/Research/CARDS_Database.aspx. Accessed January 29, 2020
6. American Diabetes Association. Unproven therapies (Position Statement). *Diabetes Care* 2003;26:S142
7. American Diabetes Association. 5. Facilitating behavior change and well-being to improve health outcomes: Standards of Medical Care in Diabetes—2020. *Diabetes Care* 2020;43(Suppl. 1):S48–S65
8. U.S. Food and Drug Administration. Changes to the Nutrition Facts Label. Available from https://www.fda.gov/food/food-labeling-nutrition/changes-nutrition-facts-label. Accessed January 29, 2020

CASE STUDY

EBM is a 62-year-old woman with diabetes, retinopathy, and peripheral neuropathy asking her clinician about using supplements to treat her diabetes and its comorbidities. She also has hypertension, hyperlipidemia, intermittent claudication, knee osteoarthritis, history of a deep-vein thrombosis (DVT) one month prior, depression, and has a BMI of 29 kg/m^2. EBM is taking metformin (Glucophage®), and injecting weekly dulaglutide (Trulicity®) and daily degludec (Tresiba®) for her diabetes. Additionally, she takes atorvastatin (Lipitor®) for hyperlipidemia, losartan (Cozaar®) for hypertension, acetaminophen (Tylenol®) for the osteoarthritis, warfarin (Coumadin®) for the DVT, and escitalopram (Lexapro®) for depression. EBM asks about taking berberine, turmeric, flaxseed, garcinia, and fish oil (ω-3 fatty acids) to supplement her current medications.

Questions for Discussion

1. Can these supplements help her diabetes?
2. What supplements may be useful for her diabetes-related comorbidities?
3. What potential drug interactions may occur if the patient takes these supplements?

The supplements EBM is asking about have been used to treat diabetes, cardiometabolic complications, and weight loss. Berberine is a much-studied supplement and may have some efficacy in lowering glucose, blood pressure, and lipids. However, it may interact with medications EBM is taking for these conditions. Thus, berberine use may result in hypoglycemia and hypotension. Since it may increase the effects of the statin EBM is taking, she may have additional lipid lowering but may experience myalgias due to increased statin effects. Additionally, it may interact with the warfarin and result in bleeding reactions. It may promote endogenous incretin effects, but EBM is already taking the GLP-1-analog, dulaglutide, and berberine may not provide any additional benefit. Thus, EBM should be told that it may not be advisable to take the berberine.

Turmeric is a product with anti-inflammatory and antioxidant activity. It has shown benefit for glucose and lipid lowering as well as benefit for osteoarthritis. The main concern is that since EBM is taking warfarin, she may experience bleeding with the turmeric. Flaxseed is a product that has shown benefit for lowering glucose, blood pressure, and lipids. As a food it may be an excellent source of fiber that may be of benefit to EBM. Garcinia is another supplement that has been used for weight loss. However, it has shown limited benefit and may cause serotonin toxicity when combined with the escitalopram. Fish oil supplements (ω-3 fatty acids) have now been shown to have limited efficacy in different disease states, so she should not take the supplement. However, EBM may benefit from the prescription product, icosapent ethyl (Vascepa®), a prescription ω-3-fatty acid, to diminish the possibility of major adverse cardiovascular events.

Other agents that may be useful for diabetes include cinnamon and milk thistle. For the retinopathy, bilberry and pine bark extract may be considered. For peripheral neuropathy, α-lipoic acid and benfotiamine may be helpful. For all of these agents, careful use would be advocated. For the intermittent claudication, ginkgo may help, but bleeding reactions may occur in combination with the warfarin. Garlic may help for hypertension and hyperlipidemia, and St. John's wort for depression. Garlic in food form is absolutely appropriate, but as a supplement tablet there may be issues with side effects and drug interactions. If St. John's wort is added, the combination with the antidepressant may result in serotonin syndrome. Additionally, St. John's wort may lower blood levels of EBM's antihypertensive and the statin. Thus, EBM may have a spike in blood pressure, and her cholesterol may increase. If St. John's wort is used and then stopped, the dose of the antihypertensive and the statin may have to be adjusted. Specifically, the doses of these medications (antihypertensive and statin) may have to initially be increased and then eventually decreased when St. John's wort is stopped.

If EBM decides to take any of the supplements mentioned, she should try only one at a time to determine the impact since doses of her other medications may need to be adjusted. The products should be obtained from a reputable manufacturer that uses appropriate third-party verification and is appropriately standardized. For instance, the turmeric should be appropriately standardized to reflect curcuminoid content that is used in evidence-based studies. The clinician may help guide EBM in seeking appropriate Standardization and Formulation information mentioned in the Natural Medicines website for each of the products in question.

Appendix
Tables 1 and 2

In the following tables, using information obtained from the Natural Medicines website, ratings are classified according to evidence from randomized controlled trials or meta-analyses, with consideration of the number of subjects, risk of bias, and positive or negative outcomes.[1] Sometimes a product may have several different ratings, depending on use. For instance, a product may be rated as "possibly effective for diabetes" and "insufficient reliable evidence to rate" for hyperlipidemia.

"Effective" – very high level of reliable clinical evidence supporting a specific use. The evidence is consistent with passing a review via a rigorous process, such as passing a Food and Drug Administration or Health Canada review and approval. Evidence is consistently positive and supported by two or more randomized clinical trials (RCTs) or meta-analysis, including several hundred to several thousand subjects. Evidence has a low risk of bias and high level of validity.

"Likely Effective" – high level of reliable clinical evidence to support positive outcomes for a specific use, from two or more RCTs or meta-analysis involving hundreds of subjects. Evidence has a low risk of bias and high level of validity.

"Possibly Effective" – some evidence to support a specific use, provided by one or more RCTs or meta-analysis, or two or more epidemiological or population based studies. Evidence has low to moderate risk of bias and moderate to high level of validity. Generally positive outcomes are reported that may outweigh contrary evidence.

"Possibly Ineffective" – some evidence showing ineffective results for a specific indication from one or more RCTs or meta-analysis or two or more epidemiological or population based studies. Trials have low-to-moderate bias and moderate to high validity level and positive evidence generally outweighs negative evidence.

"Likely Ineffective" – high level of reliable evidence showing ineffectiveness for a specific indication, from two or more RCTs or meta-analysis in hundreds of subjects. Trials have low risk of bias and high level of validity, and evidence shows negative evidence without significant contrary evidence. Use is discouraged.

"Ineffective" – highly reliable evidence that shows ineffectiveness for use for a specific indication, from two or more RCTs or meta-analysis involving several hundred to thousands of subjects. Use is discouraged.

"Insufficient Reliable Evidence to Rate" – There is insufficient reliable evidence to provide an effectiveness rating.

Table 1—Botanical and Nonbotanical Products Used to Lower Blood Glucose

Product & Natural Medicines Rating	Chemical Constituents	Mechanism of Action	Side Effects & Drug Interactions
Aloe vera *Diabetes, Obesity:* Possibly Effective *Hyperlipidemia, Prediabetes:* Not Rated by Natural Medicines	Various ingredients[1-39] • Aloe gel contains acemannan (polysaccharide similar to guar gum and glycoprotein) • Aloeresin A • Phenolic and saponin contents	Various mechanisms[1-39] *Diabetes:* • Fiber may delay or prevent glucose absorption • Aloeresin may inhibit α-glucosidases • Decrease insulin resistance by AMPK activation • Acemannan may decrease inflammation • Acemannan may promote benefit through gut microbiota via production of short chain fatty acids *Hyperlipidemia:* • Altered lipid metabolism • Decreased lipid absorption	*Side effects:*[1,4-6] • Abdominal pain, diarrhea • Acute hepatitis • Thyroid dysfunction • Possible carcinogenicity *Drug interactions:*[1,7] • Possible digoxin toxicity due to potential hypokalemia • Intraoperative blood loss in surgery patients where sevoflurane was used • Additive glucose lowering effects with sulfonylureas and insulin

Banaba	Various ingredients[1,3]	Various mechanisms[1,3-4]	Side effects:[1,5-7]	Drug interactions:[1,8]
Diabetes: Possibly Effective	• Corsolic acid	*Diabetes:*	• Lactic acidosis in renal impairment	• Possible hypotension if combined with antihypertensives
Prediabetes: Insufficient Reliable Evidence to Rate	• Ellagitannins: – Lagerstroemin – Flosin B – Reginin A	• Enhanced glucose transport • May stimulate glucose uptake • Insulin-like activity (increased tyrosine phosphorylation of insulin receptor β-subunit)	• In combination products: – Stomach upset – Dizziness, weakness – Diaphoresis – Palpitations – Tremor	• Additive glucose-lowering effects with sulfonylureas and insulin • OATP inhibition may decrease absorption of statins, sulfonylureas, some antihypertensives, fluoroquinolones

Note: Reference numbers correspond to the subject's references in the text

(Continued)

Table 1 *continued*

Product & Natural Medicines Rating	Chemical Constituents[1,3]	Mechanism of Action	Side Effects & Drug Interactions
Berberine	• Isoquinoline alkaloid[1,3]	Various mechanisms[1-5]	*Side effects:[1,2,6]*
Diabetes, Hypertension, Hyperlipidemia: Possibly Effective		*Diabetes:* • Enhanced glucose-stimulated insulin secretion • Increased insulin receptor expression • GLUT4 translocation • α-glucosidase inhibition • Enhanced AMPK • Increased GLP-1 activity • PPARγ receptor activation • Stimulates gut microbiota	• Abdominal upset, constipation, diarrhea • Headache • Muscle pain • May stimulate uterine contractions • Kernicterus
Obesity; Metabolic Syndrome, Non Alcoholic Fatty Liver Disease (NAFLD): Insufficient Reliable Evidence to Rate		*Hyperlipidemia:* • Decreased cholesterol absorption • Upregulates LDL receptors • PCSK9 inhibition	*Drug interactions:[1]* • Increased levels of drugs metabolized by CYP3A4 (cyclosporine, certain statins, and calcium channel blockers) • Increased levels of drugs metabolized by CYP2C9 (warfarin, losartan) • Increased levels of drugs metabolized by CYP2D6 (metoprolol, certain tricyclic antidepressants, tramadol)
Diabetic Nephropathy: Not Rated by Natural Medicines		*Hypertension:* • α-2 agonist activity • Blocks α adrenergic activity	• Additive glucose-lowering effects with sulfonylureas and insulin • Additive hypotension if combined with antihypertensives • Sedation if combined with CNS depressants
		Diabetic Nephropathy: • Inhibits aldose reductase	

Bilberry	Various ingredients[1-5]	Various mechanisms[1-5]	Side effects:[1-5]
Chronic venous insufficiency: Possibly Effective	• Anthocyanosides • Polyphenols • Chromium (in bilberry leaf) • Neomirtilline	*Diabetes:* • α-glucosidase inhibition • May stimulate insulin secretion • Inhibits glucose uptake • Antioxidant activity • Anti-inflammatory effects	• Abdominal upset • Possible hypotension • Possible hypoglycemia • Possible bleeding
Diabetes, Hypertension, Diabetic Retinopathy; Hypertensive Retinopathy; Prediabetes, Metabolic Syndrome:		*Hypertension, Diabetic Retinopathy:* • Vasorelaxation • Antioxidant activity • Anti-inflammatory effects • Improved ocular blood flow	*Drug interactions:*[1] • Possible bleeding with antiplatelets/anti-coagulants • Additive glucose-lowering effects with sulfonylureas and insulin
Insufficient Reliable Evidence to Rate			

Note: Reference numbers correspond to the subject's references in the text

(Continued)

Table 1 *continued*

Product & Natural Medicines Rating	Chemical Constituents	Mechanism of Action	Side Effects & Drug Interactions
Bitter melon *Diabetes, Prediabetes:* Insufficient Reliable Evidence to Rate	Various ingredients[1-4] • Momordin • Charantin • Momordicin • Polypeptide-P • Vicine	Various mechanisms[1-8] *Diabetes:* • Tissue glucose uptake; glycogen synthesis • Enhanced glucose oxidation of Glucose-6-phosphate-dehydrogenase (G6PDH) pathway • AMPK pathway activation • α-glucosidase inhibition • PPARγ receptor activation • GLUT 4 translocation	*Side effects:*[1-3] • Gastrointestinal (GI) discomfort • Hypoglycemic coma • Favism • Hemolytic anemia in persons with G6PDH deficiency • Contains known abortifacients (α and β momorcharin) • Seeds have produced severe hypoglycemia, vomiting, death in children *Drug interactions:*[1,9] • Additive glucose-lowering effects with sulfonylureas and insulin • Increased concentrations of drugs metabolized by p-glycoprotein pathway (linagliptin, diltiazem, verapamil, rivoraxaban, apixaban, vincristine, vinblastine, protease inhibitors) due to inhibition of p-glycoprotein efflux

Chia	Various Ingredients[1,3,5]	Various mechanisms[1,3,5]	Side effects:[1,8-10]

Diabetes, Blood Pressure, Metabolic Syndrome:	• α-linolenic acid
	• Fiber
	• Protein
	• Calcium, Phosphorous, Magnesium, Iron
	• Antioxidants:
	  – Chlorogenic acid
	  – Caffeic acid
	  – Quercetin
	  – Kaempferol
	  – Myricetin
		Diabetes:
		• Fiber decreases postmeal glucose
		
		Hypertension:
		• Angiotensin converting enzyme inhibition by some constituents
			• Gastrointestinal (GI) discomfort
			• Allergic reactions
			• Possible increase in triglycerides
			• Possible increased risk for prostate cancer (α-linolenic acid consumption)

Insufficient Reliable Evidence to Rate			*Drug interactions:*[1] • None reported
Obesity:			
Possibly Ineffective			

Note: Reference numbers correspond to the subject's references in the text

(Continued)

Table 1 *continued*

Product & Natural Medicines Rating	Chemical Constituents	Mechanism of Action	Side Effects & Drug Interactions
Chromium *Diabetes,* *Hyperlipidemia:* Possibly Effective *Obesity, Prediabetes:* Possibly Ineffective	Trivalent chromium[1,2]	Various mechanisms[1-8] *Diabetes:* • May enhance cellular effects of insulin • May increase number of insulin receptors • May increase insulin binding or insulin activation • Increased tyrosine kinase activity at insulin receptor • GLUT 4 translocation • Increased AMPK activity • Inhibits acetyl-Coenzyme A carboxylase, resulting in decreased malonyl Coenzyme A *Hyperlipidemia* • Suppression of sterol regulatory element binding protein • Affects lipid metabolism modulation in peripheral tissues • May inhibit 3-hydroxy-3-methyl-glutaryl-CoA reductase (HMG-Co-A reductase inhibition)	*Side effects:*[1,8,12,15] • Gastrointestinal upset • Excessive intake may lead to renal toxicity, severe systemic illness • Dermatologic reactions *Drug interactions:*[1,8-15] • Additive glucose-lowering effects with sulfonylureas and insulin • Chromium is depleted by steroids • Histamine blockers and proton pump inhibitors may block chromium absorption • Coadministration with zinc depletes absorption of both chromium and zinc • Increased insulin sensitivity, adiponectin if combined with Vit C or Vit E • Vit C, NSAIDs increase absorption • Complexes with ferritin and produces ferritin deficiency • Decreases levothyroxine levels • When combined with biotin, decreased hepatic glucose output and gluconeogenesis

Cinnamon	Various Ingredients[1-5]	Various mechanisms[1-9]	Side effects:[1]
Diabetes: Possibly Effective	• Cinnamaldehyde	*Diabetes:*	• Irritation or dermatitis if used topically
Prediabetes, Obesity: Insufficient Reliable Evidence to Rate	• Eugenol	• Increased insulin receptor phosphorylation and improved insulin signaling	• High coumarin content in certain species or products may result in hepatotoxicity, per animal models
Hyperlipidemia, Hypertension: Not Rated by Natural Medicines	• Coumarins	• Increased insulin sensitivity and action	*Drug interactions:*[1]
		• Increased cell/tissue glucose uptake	• Additive glucose-lowering effects with sulfonylureas and insulin
		• Promotes glycogen synthesis	• Due to a coumarin ingredient, it may theoretically result in bleeding if combined with antiplatelets/anticoagulants
		• α-glucosidase inhibition	• Possible additive hepatotoxicity if combined with hepatotoxins (acetaminophen, methotrexate, comfrey, chaparral)
		• Peroxisome proliferator-activated receptor activation	
		• May help delay gastric emptying and reduce excess postprandial glucose and triglyceride levels	
		• GLUT 4 translocation	
		• AMPK activation	
		• GLP-1 activity	
		Hyperlipidemia:	
		• For lipid lowering: inhibiting hepatic-3-hydroxy-methylglutaryl CoA reductase activity	
		Hypertension:	
		• Peripheral vasodilation	

Note: Reference numbers correspond to the subject's references in the text

(Continued)

Table 1 *continued*

Product & Natural Medicines Rating	Chemical Constituents	Mechanism of Action	Side Effects & Drug Interactions

Fenugreek
 	
Diabetes:
Possibly Effective
Prediabetes,
  Hyperlipidemia,
  Obesity:
Insufficient Reliable Evidence to Rate
	Various ingredients[1-5]
	• Saponins (Diosgenin)
	• Glycosides
	• Seeds contain:
	  – alkaloids (including trigo-nelline)
	  – 4-hydroxyisoleucine
	  – fenugreekine
		Various mechanisms[1-7]
		Diabetes:
		• Delayed gastric emptying
		• Slowed carbohydrate absorption
		• Glucose transport inhibition
		• Increased number of insulin receptors
		• Possible stimulation of glucose-dependent insulin secretion
		• Improved peripheral glucose utilization
		
		Hyperlipidemia:
		• Saponins may increase biliary cholesterol secretion, leading to decreased serum lipids.
			Side effects:[1-3,8]
			• Diarrhea, gas
			• Uterine contractions; possible miscarriage
			• Teratogenicity (cleft palate, spina bifida, hydrocephalus, anencephaly.
			• Allergic reactions
			
			Drug interactions:[1,9]
			• Additive glucose-lowering effects with sulfonylureas and insulin
			• May increase anticoagulant effects of antiplatelets/anticoagulants
			• Decreased effect of theophylline by decreasing its serum concentrations

Flaxseed	Various ingredients[1-3]	Various mechanisms[1-3,5,8]	Side effects:[1]
Diabetes, *Hyperlipidemia, Hypertension, Obesity:* Possibly Effective	• Lignans, including secoisolariciresinol diglucoside, and matairesinol • Linoleic acid • Soluble fiber in seed and oil • α-linolenic acid, a plant omega-3 fatty acid	*Diabetes:* • Soluble fiber slows gastric emptying • Fiber decreases glucose absorption and postprandial glucose *Hyperlipidemia:* • Fiber in flaxseed increases fecal bile acid elimination • Modulation of 7 α–hydroxylase and acyl CoA cholesterol transferase • Decreased production of proinflammatory eicosanoids *Hypertension:* • Alteration of circulating oxylipins	• Gastrointestinal upset • Flax hypersensitivity • Uncooked flaxseed contains cyanogenic glycosides • May exert estrogenic effects in pregnancy • Possible increased risk for prostate cancer (α-linolenic acid consumption)
Prediabetes, Metabolic Syndrome, NAFLD: Insufficient Reliable Evidence to Rate			*Drug interactions:*[1] • Bleeding if combined with antiplatelets/ anticoagulants • Additive glucose-lowering effects with sulfonylureas and insulin • Possible hypotension if combined with antihypertensives. • Possible additive estrogenic or antiestrogenic effect with estrogens. • May decrease absorption of certain medications, such as acetaminophen, furosemide, or other medications. • Antibiotics may affect conversion of Secoisolariciresinol diglucoside (SDG) to certain metabolites that may affect flaxseed activity.

Note: Reference numbers correspond to the subject's references in the text

(Continued)

Table 1 *continued*

Product & Natural Medicines Rating	Chemical Constituents	Mechanism of Action	Side Effects & Drug Interactions
Ginseng	Various ginsenosides[1-9]	Various mechanisms[1-10]	*Side effects:*[1,2]
	• Protopanaxadiol	*Diabetes:*	• Insomnia, headache, restlessness
Panax Ginseng	– Rb1	• Enhance β-cell function	• Increased blood pressure (inconsistent effect) or increased heart rate
Diabetes,	– Rb2	• Modulation of insulin secretion	• Mastalgia
Hypertension,	– Rc	• May decrease carbohydrate absorption in portal circulation	• Mood changes, nervousness
Prediabetes:	– Rd	• May decrease glucose transport and uptake and disposal	• Possible teratogenicity
Insufficient Reliable Evidence to Rate	• Protopanaxatriol	*Hyperlipidemia:*	*Drug interactions:*[1,2]
Hyperlipidemia:	– Rg1	• May increase lipoprotein lipase activity	• Decreased warfarin, diuretic, antihypertensive effectiveness
Not Rated by Natural Medicines	– Re	*Hypertension:*	• Additive estrogenic effects
	– Rf	• *In vitro* may inhibit angiotensin converting enzyme activity	• Possible increased effects of certain analgesics and antidepressants
American Ginseng			• Additive glucose-lowering effects with sulfonylureas and insulin
Diabetes:			
Possibly Effective			
Hypertension:			
Insufficient Reliable Evidence to Rate			
Hyperlipidemia:			
Not Rated by Natural Medicines			

Gymnema sylvestre	Various ingredients[1-10]	Various mechanisms[1,3-10]	Side effects:[1,10]
Diabetes, Metabolic Syndrome, Weight Loss:	• Gymnemic acids (gymnemosides)	Diabetes:	• May cause hypoglycemia
	• Gymnemasaponins	• Impairs ability to discriminate "sweet" taste	• Toxic hepatitis (per case report)
Insufficient Reliable Evidence to Rate	• Gurmarin	• Blocks glucose absorption in small intestine	Drug interactions:[1]
	• Stigmasterol	• Increases number of enzymes promoting glucose uptake	• Additive glucose-lowering effects with sulfonylureas and insulin
	• Betaine	• May increase and stimulate β-cells	• May induce or inhibit CYP450 2C9 (may affect serum concentration of warfarin or ibuprofen)
	• Choline	• May increase insulin release by promoting cell permeability to insulin	• May inhibit CYP 450 1A2 system (may affect serum concentration of some psychiatric medications—some antipsychotics and antidepressants)
			• Conflicting information on CYP 450 3A4 inhibition. Some reports state it may inhibit this enzyme and thus increase serum concentrations of some medications (calcium channel blockers, antibiotics); other reports state there is no impact

(Continued)

Note: Reference numbers correspond to the subject's references in the text

Table 1 continued

Product & Natural Medicines Rating	Chemical Constituents	Mechanism of Action	Side Effects & Drug Interactions
Holy Basil	Various ingredients[1,2,6-8]	Various mechanisms[1,2,6-8]	*Side effects:*[1]
Diabetes, Obesity:	• Eugenol	*Diabetes:*	• May lower thyroxine (worsens hypothyroidism)
Insufficient Reliable Evidence to Rate	• Ursolic acid	• May improve pancreatic β-cell function and thus enhance insulin secretion	• May cause bleeding
	• Apigenin		• Decreased sperm count and fertility
	• Polyphenols	• Enhanced activity of enzymes involved in carbohydrate metabolism	*Drug interactions:*[1]
	• Caffeic acid	– glucokinase	• Additive glucose-lowering effects with sulfonylureas and insulin
	• Chicoric acid	– hexokinase	• Possible bleeding with anticoagulants/antiplatelets
	• P-coumaric acid compound	– phosphofructokinase	• Sedation with phenobarbital sedatives
	• Zinc	• Zinc content may help decrease insulin resistance	

Honey	Various ingredients[1-5]	Various mechanisms[1-7]	Side effects:[1]
Diabetes, Hyperlipidemia, Obesity:	• Fructose	*Diabetes:*	• Allergic reactions
Insufficient Reliable Evidence to Rate	• Glucose	• Fructose:glucose ratio	• Possible botulism
Diabetic Foot Ulcers:	• Oligosaccharides (such as palatinose)	• Fructose may help stimulate insulin release and secretion	• Cardiac toxicity if honey source is rhododendrons (grayanotoxins)
Possibly Effective	• Phenolic acids	• Hepatic glucose uptake by glucokinase and glycogen synthase activation to promote glycogen synthesis and storage	• Infection if topical honey is applied to dialysis tubing exit sites
	• Flavonoids	• Pancreatic antioxidant effects (which may improve pancreatic β-cell function and help decrease lipids)	*Drug interactions:*[1]
	• Proteins	• Prebiotic activity	• Additive effects with anticoagulants/antiplatelets
	• Amino acids	*Obesity:*	• Increased absorption of phenytoin
	• Enzymes	• Modulates ghrelin and peptide YY	
	• Vitamins	*Diabetic Foot Ulcers*	
	• Fatty acids	• Antimicrobial, anti-inflammatory effects	
		• 5,8-kDa stimulates immune cell activity	

Note: Reference numbers correspond to the subject's references in the text

(Continued)

Table 1 continued

Product & Natural Medicines Rating	Chemical Constituents	Mechanism of Action	Side Effects & Drug Interactions
Ivy Gourd *Diabetes:* Possibly Effective *Other Uses:* Insufficient Reliable Evidence to Rate	Various ingredients[1,3-4] • Beta-carotene • Triterpenes (leaves) • Pectin (fruit) • Fiber • Protein • Calcium • Alkaloids	Various mechanisms[1,3-4] *Diabetes:* • Insulin-like activity • Suppresses elevated levels of enzymes involved in glucose production (glucose-6-phosphatase and lactate dehydrogenase) • May restore lipoprotein lipase activity	*Side effects:* [1,5] • GI upset • Drowsiness • Hypoglycemia • Possible allergic reactions *Drug interactions:* [1] • Additive glucose-lowering effects with sulfonylureas and insulin

Magnesium	Various salts[1,2,5,9]	Various mechanisms[1,2,5,9,10]	Side effects:[1]
Diabetes, *Hyperlipidemia,* *Metabolic Syndrome:* Possibly Effective *Hypomagnesemia:* Effective	• Sulfate • Citrate • Hydroxide • Oxide • Chloride	*Diabetes:* • Cofactor for enzymes in glucose metabolic pathways and phosphorylation reactions • Low dietary magnesium may contribute to insulin resistance and type 2 diabetes *Hypomagnesemia:* • Deficiency may be due to diminished insulin action, insulin resistance related to reduced tyrosine kinase at the insulin receptor • impaired insulin action due to impaired insulin signaling.	• GI upset, nausea, vomiting, diarrhea • In diminished renal function, hypermagnesemia may occur *Drug interactions:*[1,2] • Many medications may deplete magnesium levels: diuretics, proton pump inhibitors, digoxin, β-2 agonists, steroids, cyclosporine, tacrolimus, and others • With magnesium supplementation: additive hypotension with calcium channel blockers or hypermagnesemia with potassium sparing diuretics (spironolactone) • Concomitant magnesium administration may impair absorption of certain antibiotics, calcium, bisphosphonates • Additive glucose-lowering effects with sulfonylureas and insulin

Note: Reference numbers correspond to the subject's references in the text

(Continued)

Table 1 *continued*

Product & Natural Medicines Rating	Chemical Constituents	Mechanism of Action	Side Effects & Drug Interactions
Milk thistle	Various ingredients:[1,3,5,8]	Various mechanisms[1-2,5,7-9,17]	*Side effects:*[1]
	• Silymarin, a dry mixture of flavonolignans including:	*Diabetes:*	• Diarrhea, weakness, sweating
Diabetes:	– silybin A & B	• Antioxidant, anti-inflammatory effects (helps with glucose reduction and prevents complications)	• Possible allergic reactions if also allergic to ragweed, marigolds, daisies, chrysanthemums
Possibly Effective	– isosilibin A & B	• Inhibits hepatic glucogenesis	• May have estrogenic effects, so women with breast or uterine cancer should avoid its use

Hyperlipidemia, Diabetic Nephropathy, NAFLD, Nonalcoholic Steatohepatitis (NASH):	– silychristine
	  – isosilychristine
	  – taxifolin
	  – silidianin
		• Decreased insulin resistance, possibly through cytoprotection
		• Decreases malondialdehyde
		• Peroxisome proliferator activated receptor-γ agonist
		• Inhibits aldose reductase
			Drug interactions:[1,11]

			• Phosphatidylcholine enhances bioavailability
		Hyperlipidemia:	• Beneficial interactions with hepatotoxic agents such as acetaminophen, antipsychotics, alcohol
Insufficient Reliable Evidence to Rate		• Decreases cholesterol synthesis • Decreases oxidized LDL • May diminish HMG-Co-A reductase	• Increases concentrations of glucuronidated drugs (acetaminophen, haloperidol, lamotrigine)
		Diabetic Nephropathy	• Increases absorption of chemotherapy drugs, calcium channel blockers, and some antibiotics
		• May decrease interleukins, as well as TNF-α and TNF-β, a marker of fibrosis	• May increase concentrations of raloxifene, tamoxifen
			• May decrease concentration of antiretrovirals
			• Additive glucose lowering effects with sulfonylureas and insulin

	Various ingredients[1,3-4]	Various mechanisms[1,3-5]	Side effects:[1,6-7]
Mulberry *Diabetes:* Possibly Effective *Hyperlipidemia:* Insufficient Reliable Evidence to Rate	• 1-deoxnojirimicin • Fagomine	*Diabetes:* • α-glucosidase inhibition • Increased Insulin secretion • May decrease insulin resistance by activating phosphatidylinositol-3-kinase/protein kinase B, glycogen synthase kinase-3β signaling pathways • Modulate glucose transporter-4 translocation *Hyperlipidemia* • Antioxidant affects may decrease lipid peroxidation (increased LDL resistance to oxidative changes)	• GI upset, including nausea, vomiting, abdominal fullness • Headache • Cough • Increased serum creatinine *Drug interactions:*[1] • Phosphatidylcholine enhances bioavailability • Additive glucose-lowering effects with sulfonylureas and insulin
Nopal *Diabetes:* Possibly Effective *Hyperlipidemia,* *Metabolic Syndrome,* *Weight Loss, BPH,* *Alcohol Hangover:* Insufficient Reliable Evidence to Rate	Various ingredients[1,3-4,6] • Fibrous polysaccharides • Phytochemicals, such as pectin • Phenolic compounds • Flavonoids • Betalains • Chromium	Various mechanisms[1,3-4,6-7] *Diabetes:* • Slows carbohydrate absorption • Possibly increases insulin sensitivity • Chromium content may improve glucose metabolism *Hyperlipidemia:* • Fiber content decreases lipid and fat absorption in the gut	Side effects:[1,5,11] • Diarrhea, nausea, abdominal fullness, increased stool volume • Headache • Hypoglycemia *Drug interactions:*[1,11] • Additive glucose-lowering effects with sulfonylureas and insulin

Note: Reference numbers correspond to the subject's references in the text

(Continued)

Table 1 *continued*

Product & Natural Medicines Rating	Chemical Constituents	Mechanism of Action	Side Effects & Drug Interactions
Probiotics (Lactobacillus species and Others) *Diabetes, Hyperlipidemia:* Possibly Effective *Obesity:* Insufficient Reliable Evidence to Rate	Numerous species, including:[1-5,25] • Lactobacillus species • Bifidobacterium species • Streptococcus thermophilus • Saccharomyces boulardii • Akkermansia muciniphila • Clostridium species • Anaerobutyricum hallii	*Diabetes (theoretical):*[1-5,25] • Possible enhanced incretin action • Release of beneficial organic and free fatty acids that act against pathogenic microbes • Decreased inflammation • Decreased insulin resistance • Antioxidant activity	*Side effects:*[2,9] : • GI upset • Constipation • Possible systemic infections in immuno-compromised or those on chemotherapy or radiation treatment. *Drug interactions:*[2,14] • Antibiotics, antifungals: decreased probiotic effects • Immunosuppressants (cyclosporine, methotrexate, etc): weakened state may lead to infections due to probiotic microbes

Psyllium	Various ingredients[1-3]	Various mechanisms[1-6]	Side effects:[1]
Diabetes,	• Soluble viscous gel-forming fiber	*Diabetes:*	• Allergies
Hypertension:	• Mix of acidic and neutral polysaccharides with galacturonic acid	• Formation of viscous gel that slows intestinal glucose absorption, thus lowering postprandial glucose	• Cough
Possibly Effective	• Polysaccharides: D-xylose, L-arabinose, pentosanes	• Delayed gastric emptying	• Swallowing disorders
Hyperlipidemia:		• Carbohydrate sequestering	• Flatulence
Likely Effective		• "Second meal effect"	• "Sugar-free" products may contain aspartame so persons with phenylketonuria may have issues
Obesity:		*Hyperlipidemia:*	
Insufficient Reliable Evidence to Rate		• Prevents reabsorption of bile salts and enhanced elimination in fecal bile acids	*Drug interactions:*[1]
		• Lowers dietary fat absorption	• Additive glucose-lowering effects with sulfonylureas and insulin
		• Reduced cholesterol synthesis due to reduced insulin stimulation (due to lower glucose)	• Binding reactions: decreased absorption of many other drugs (anticonvulsants, metformin, iron, some psychiatric meds)
		Obesity:	• Additive blood pressure or lipid lowering with antihypertensives and antihyperlipidemics
		• May decrease appetite	

Note: Reference numbers correspond to the subject's references in the text

(Continued)

Table 1 *continued*

Product & Natural Medicines Rating	Chemical Constituents	Mechanism of Action	Side Effects & Drug Interactions
Tea	Various ingredients:[1-3,5,8]	Various mechanisms:[1,4-5,8-11]	*Side effects:*[1,12]
Diabetes,	• Green tea	*Diabetes:*	• Possible hepatoxicity
Metabolic Syndrome,	– Epigallocatechin gallate (EGCG)	• Inhibition of hepatic gluconeogenesis	• GI upset
NAFLD, Obesity:	– Tannins	• Enhanced insulin activity	• Caffeine content may cause insomnia, anxiety, tachycardia
Insufficient Reliable Evidence to Rate	– Epigallocatechin	• Decreased insulin resistance	• Miscarriage if caffeine content is higher than 300 mg/day
	– Epicatechin	• Tyrosine phosphorylation of insulin receptor and receptor substrate	*Drug interactions:*[1,8]
Hyperlipidemia, Hypertension:	– Epicatechin gallate	• Suppresses phosphoenolpyruvate carboxykinase (gluconeogenic enzyme)	• Sympathomimetics or amphetamines may cause toxicity due to caffeine content
Possibly Effective	– Gallocatechin gallate	• Modulates glucose-6-phosphatase	• Increased blood pressure, heart rate with MAO inhibitors
	– has more Catechins (polyphenols) than oolong and black tea	• Improves cytokine-induced β-cell damage	• May antagonize antiplatelet effects of warfarin (Vit K content)
	• Oolong and black tea	• Regulates gene expression involved in insulin signal transduction pathways	• Decreased concentrations of nadolol
	– Theaflavins	• Antioxidant effects	• Negates calming effects of barbiturates
	– Thearubigins	• α-glucosidase and α-amylase inhibition	• Diminished absorption of iron and folic acid (may impact pregnant women)
			• Additive glucose-lowering effects with sulfonylureas and insulin

Tea (continued)

Hyperlipidemia:

- Decreased LDL oxidation
- Enhanced gene expression of enzymes that stimulate bile acid production and decrease hepatic cholesterol concentration
- Upregulation of hepatic LDL receptors

Hypertension:

- NADPH oxidase activity suppression
- Reduces reactive oxygen species

Obesity:

- Thermogenesis
- Decreased carbohydrate absorption
- Stimulate the sympathetic nervous system
- Appetite suppression
- Suppresses ghrelin
- Increases adiponectin

Note: Reference numbers correspond to the subject's references in the text

(Continued)

Table 1 *continued*

Product & Natural Medicines Rating	Chemical Constituents	Mechanism of Action	Side Effects & Drug Interactions
Turmeric	Various ingredients[1-3]	Various mechanisms[1,4-6]	*Side effects:*[1,9]
Diabetes, Metabolic Syndrome, Obesity: Insufficient Reliable Evidence to Rate	• Curcumin • Diferuloylmethane • Demethoxycurcumin • Bisdemethoxycurcumin • Cyclocurcumin	*Diabetes:* • Antioxidant • Anti-inflammatory • Improved β-cell function • α-glucosidase inhibitor activity • Inhibits TNF-α • Inhibits NF-κB activation • Lowers TBARS (thiobarbiturate acid reactive substance) • PPARγ activation • Activates hepatic enzymes involved with gluconeogenesis • GLP-1 effects • Microbiome modulation	• GI upset • Pruritus, allergic dermatitis • Root products have higher lead concentrations than curcuminoid extracts • Antiplatelet properties • May inhibit iron absorption
Hyperlipidemia, NAFLD: Possibly Effective			*Drug interactions:*[1,3,6,10] • Additive effects with antiplatelets/anticoagulants • Inhibits CYP450 1A2, 2B6, 2C9, 2C19, 2D6, 2E1, 3A4, so may increase concentrations of several drugs: secretagogues, some statins, antihypertensives, warfarin, others
Diabetic Nephropathy; Neuropathy; Retinopathy: Not Rated by Natural Medicines		*Hyperlipidemia:* • Increased lipoprotein lipase • Inhibits lipid peroxidation, protein carbonyl and lysosomal enzyme activities • Decreases oxidized LDL levels • Activates hepatic cholesterol α hydroxylase, stimulating conversion of cholesterol to bile acids • Inhibits HMG CoA reductase	• May inhibit OAT-P and decrease clearance of meds that use these transporters (pioglitazone, repaglinide) • Additive glucose-lowering effects with insulin or secretagogues • Complexed with zinc or coadminsitered with piperidine to improve absorption and bioavailability

Turmeric
(continued)

Obesity:

- Down regulates Janus kinase

Diabetic Nephropathy:

- Decreases renal inflammation by suppressing NF-κB and IκBα action
- Decreases TGF beta-1 regulation, monocyte chemoattract protein-1, ICAM-1

Diabetic Neuropathy:

- Decreases neuroinflammatory lipid peroxidation

Diabetic Retinopathy:

- Stops retinal expression of proinflammatory cytokines, TNF-α, VEGF, and ICAM-1

Note: Reference numbers correspond to the subject's references in the text

(Continued)

Table 1 *continued*

Product & Natural Medicines Rating	Chemical Constituents	Mechanism of Action	Side Effects & Drug Interactions
Vinegar	Various ingredients[1,2]	Various mechanisms[1,3-6]	*Side effects:*[1,7-10]

Diabetes, Obesity: Insufficient Reliable Evidence to Rate	• Acetic acid
	• Mineral salts
	• Amino acids
	• Polyphenols
	  – Galic acid
	  – Catechin
	  – Caffeic acid
	  – Ferulic acid
		Diabetes:
		• Delays gastric emptying
		• Suppresses disaccharidases
		• Promotes muscle glucose uptake
		• Suppresses hepatic glucose production
		• Increases peripheral tissue glucose utilization
			• GI upset
			• Hypoglycemia in persons with gastroparesis
			• Oropharyngeal inflammation; caustic esophageal injury
			• Hypokalemia

Hyperlipidemia: Not Rated by Natural Medicines	• Organic acids
	  – Tartaric
	  – Citric
	  – Malic
	  – Lactic
		• Enhances flow-mediated vasodilation
		• Facilitates insulin secretion
		• Binds to free fatty-acid receptors, which may increase GLP-1 secretion
		• Stimulates 5'AMP-activated protein kinase (AMPK) activation
		• GLUT-4 mobilization
			Drug interactions:[1,10]
			• Hypokalemia with potassium depleters (diuretics or certain supplements) or digoxin toxicity (if hypokalemia occurs)
			• Additive glucose-lowering effects with insulin or secretagogues

		Hyperlipidemia: • AMPK activation • Decreased sterol regulatory element binding protein-1	

Vinegar (continued)

Obesity:

- Decrease visceral fat accumulation
- Decreased lipogenesis
- Increased lipolysis
- Increased oxygen consumption via AMPK activation
- Increased energy expenditure via PPAR-α gene
- Satiety due to increases in Peptide Y-Y and oxyntomodulin and decreased ghrelin

Note: Reference numbers correspond to the subject's references in the text

(Continued)

Table 1 *continued*

Product & Natural Medicines Rating	Chemical Constituents	Mechanism of Action	Side Effects & Drug Interactions
Zinc *Diabetes:* Possibly Effective	Various Salts[1] • Sulfate • Gluconate • Chloride • Acetate • Others	Various mechanisms[1-3] *Diabetes:* • Antioxidant (decreases TBARS) • Increases depleted antioxidant enzymes (glutathione peroxidase, super oxide dismutase, catalase) • Increases glycolytic enzyme activity (phosphofructose and pyruvate kinase) • Enhances phosphorylation reactions to activate insulin signaling cascade • Mobilizes GLUT-4 transporters • Protects β-cells by inhibiting activity of destructive amyloid polypeptides, proinflammatory molecules • Zinc transporters have role in pancreatic islet cells and regulate insulin production • α-glucosidase inhibition • Due to antioxidant effects, helps decrease microvascular complications	*Side effects:[1]* • GI upset (nausea, vomiting) • Metallic taste • At higher doses, may cause copper deficiency and affect iron absorption • At > 50 mg/day, may lower HDL • Worsening prostate function *Drug interactions:[1]* • Competes with chromium for absorption • Iron and zinc may interfere with each other's absorption • High magnesium intake may decrease zinc absorption • Taking with black coffee decreases zinc absorption • May interfere with absorption of certain antibiotics: Ciprofloxacin, cephalexin, certain tetracyclines) • Some medications may decrease zinc levels: Lisinopril, cholestyramine, steroids, some estrogens, proton pump inhibitors, some anticonvulsants: Phenytoin, divalproex sodium

Table 2—Botanical and Nonbotanical Products Used for Diabetes Comorbidities

Product & Natural Medicines Rating	Chemical Constituents	Mechanism of Action[1-8]	Side Effects & Drug Interactions
α-Lipoic Acid *Diabetes, Diabetic Neuropathy, Hyperlipidemia, Obesity:* Possibly Effective *Diabetic Retinopathy;* *Diabetic Nephropathy:* Possibly Ineffective	Various ingredients:[1,3-7] • Dihydrolipoic acid (DHLA) • R and S enantiomer	Various mechanisms[1-8] *Diabetes:* • Promotes tyrosine phosphorylation of insulin receptor • Promotes GLUT1 and GLUT4 activity to enhance glucose uptake *Diabetic Complications (Neuropathy, Retinopathy, Nephropathy):* • Antioxidant activity • Catalytic agent associated with pyruvate dehydrogenase and α-ketoglutarate dehydrogenase enzyme complexes • Interacts with pyrophosphatases to convert pyruvic acid to acetyl-coenzyme A (in the Krebs cycle) to produce energy in the form of ATP • Augments/maintains glutathione (GSH) • Increases levels of Nrf2 • Reactive oxygen species and reactive nitrogen species scavenger • Helps regenerate endogenous Vit E and Vit C	*Side effects:*[1] • Nausea, vomiting, vertigo • Possible allergic skin reactions • Malodorous urine • Thyroid dysfunction • IV: headache, pain, injection site reactions *Drug interactions:*[1,2] • May attenuate benefit of chemotherapy • Binds antacids if given at same time • Food decreases bioavailability • May decrease conversion of thyroxine to active T3 form • Additive glucose-lowering effects with insulin and sulfonylureas

(Continued)

Note: Reference numbers correspond to the subject's references in the text

Table 2 continued

Product & Natural Medicines Rating	Chemical Constituents	Mechanism of Action	Side Effects & Drug Interactions
α-Lipoic Acid (continued)		*Diabetic Complications (Neuropathy, Retinopathy, Nephropathy):* • Inhibits NF-κB activation • Anti-inflammatory: decreases TNF-α, interleukin-6, and C-reactive protein *Obesity:* • Increases energy expenditure • Suppresses hypothalamic AMP-activated protein kinase.	

Benfotiamine	Various ingredients[1,2]	Various mechanisms[1-4]	Side effects:[1]

Diabetic Neuropathy:
Possibly Effective
Diabetic Nephropathy:
Possibly Ineffective
Peripheral
Neuropathy:
"Possibly Ineffective"
	• Thiamine prodrug	*Diabetic Complications (Neuropathy, Nephropathy, Retinopathy):*
		• Enhanced transketolase activity
		  – Inhibits diacylglycerol protein kinase C pathway
		  – Inhibits advanced glycation end product formation pathway
		  – Inhibits hexosamine pathway
		• Inhibits activation of NK-κB
		• Modulates Vascular Endothelial Growth Factor Receptor 2
		• Activates Protein Kinase B to prevent hyperglycemia-induced apoptosis
		• Anti-inflammatory: inhibits activation of Mitogen-Activated Protein Kinases (MAPK)
		• Decreases Glycogen Synthase Kinase-3 β (modulates cell survival)
			• Possible skin rashes
			
			Drug interactions:[1,2]
			• Drugs/plants that decrease thiamine activity
			  – Metformin
			  – Betel nut
			• Plants that Cause Thiamine Deficiency
			  – Horsetail
			• Drugs that decrease thiamine levels in body
			  – Antibiotics
			  – Oral contraceptives
			  – Diuretics
			  – Some anticonvulsants
			  – Chemotherapy drugs

Note: Reference numbers correspond to the subject's references in the text

(Continued)

Table 2 *continued*

Product & Natural Medicines Rating	Chemical Constituents	Mechanism of Action	Side Effects & Drug Interactions
Coenzyme Q10	Various ingredients[1,2]	Various mechanisms[1-7]	*Side effects:*[1,8]
Congestive Heart Failure, Diabetic Neuropathy:	• Benzoquinone nucleus • Polyisoprenoid tail (10 Units) • Ubiquinone (fully oxidized) form • Ubiquinol (reduced form)	*Metabolic Functions:* • Co-factor in electron transport chain involved with ATP production • Direct membrane stabilizer • Antioxidant (free radical scavenger)	• Abdominal upset • Anorexia • Dizziness • Headache
Possibly Effective			*Drug interactions:*[1,8-13]
Diabetes:		*Diabetes:*	• Warfarin – may see decreased INR
Possibly Ineffective		• Increases activity of glycerol-3-phosphate dehydrogenase and thus improves glucose-stimulated insulin secretion • Improved endothelial dysfunction	*Drugs that decrease CoQ10:*
Hypertension, Hyperlipidemia, NAFLD,			• Statins • Red yeast rice • Omega-3 Fatty Acids • Amitriptyline • Antihypertensives
Statin-Induced Myalgia,		*Heart failure:* • Helps with myocardial ATP production • Overcoming reactive oxygen species	*Disease states associated with lower CoQ10 levels:*
Statin-Induced Myopathy:		*Hypertension:* • Vasodilation, which decreases peripheral resistance	• Heart failure (due to statin use) • Diabetes
Insufficient Reliable Evidence to Rate		*Statin-Associated Muscle Symptoms:* • May correct mitochondrial dysfunction	*Beneficial CoQ10 Interactions:* • Doxorubicin: CoQ10 diminishes cardiotoxicity (but also may diminish cancer benefits)

Fish Oil	Various ingredients[1,3]	Various mechanisms[1,3,4]	Side effects:[1,3]
High Triglycerides: Effective	• EPA (Eicosapentanoic acid) • DHA (Docosahexanoic acid)	*Hypertriglyceridemia:* • Decreased lipogenesis and intestinal cholesterol absorption. • Inhibits gene transcription for sterol regulatory element binding program • Inhibits hepatic diacyl-glycerol acyl transferase • PPAR-α modulation • Increased triglyceride clearance by upregulating lipoprotein lipase • Intracellular degradation of apolipoprotein B, thus interfering with VLDL secretion	• Gastrointestinal upset (loose stools, nausea, heartburn) • Halitois • Allergies • Fishy taste • Bleeding at doses > 3 g/day
Heart Failure, Hypertension: Possibly Effective			*Drug interactions:*[1]
Diabetes, Prediabetes, NAFLD, Obesity; Diabetic Nephropathy:			• Warfarin; may see increased INR • Additive effects with antihypertensives, hypoglycemics, anticoagulants, statins • Decreases hypertensive effect of cyclosporine
Diabetic Retinopathy: Likely Ineffective		*Anti-inflammatory Effects:* • Decreases TNF-α • Inhibits activation of NF-κB • Inhibits different interleukins (IL-6 and IL-1β) • Downregulates mitogen-activated protein kinases • Decreases adhesion molecules (VCAM-1), E-selectin, others • Modulate PPAR-α	**Drugs that increase triglycerides: estrogens** *Disease State Interactions (due to increased triglycerides:* • Pancreatitis • Diabetes

Note: Reference numbers correspond to the subject's references in the text

(Continued)

Table 2 continued

Product & Natural Medicines Rating	Chemical Constituents	Mechanism of Action	Side Effects & Drug Interactions
Fish Oil (continued)		*Anti-thrombotic effects:* • Inhibits prothrombotic and vasoconstrictive mediator production (thromboxane A2 and thromboxane B2) • Promotes thromboxane A3 production *Vasodilation:* • Promotes prostacyclin synthesis *Anti-arrhythmic Effects:* • Cardiac membrane stabilization by regulating calcium channels and intracellular calcium activity	
Garcinia cambogia *Obesity:* Insufficient Reliable Evidence to Rate	Various ingredients[1,2] • Hydroxycitric acid	Various mechanisms[1,2] *Obesity:* • Inhibition of adenosine triphosphate citrate lyase, decreasing acetyl-CoA levels; leads to decreased fatty acid synthesis • Decreased lipogenesis, which may decrease food intake • Decreased conversion of Acetyl-CoA to malonyl-CoA • Decreased hepatic glycogen synthesis and glucoreceptors (may help increase satiety) • Increased brain serotonin reuptake activity	*Side effects:*[1-3] • GI upset • Headache • Pancreatitis • Increased blood pressure • Acute necrotizing eosinophilic myocarditis • Affects platelet aggregation • Hepatotoxicity (liver transplantation) *Drug interactions:*[1] • Additive glucose-lowering effects with sulfonylureas and insulin • Additive hepatotoxicity with hepatotoxins • Serotonin syndrome in combination with SSRIs or other serotonergic drugs

Garlic	Various ingredients[1,2]	Various mechanisms[1-7]	Side effects:[1]
Hypertension, Hyperlipidemia, Diabetes: Possibly Effective	• Alliin • Allicin • Ajoene • S-allyl-L-cysteine • S-allylmercapto-cysteine • Diallyldisulfide • Dimethyltrisulfide	*Hypertension:* • Nitric oxide, hydrogen sulfide production • Decreased production of endothelin 1 and angiotensin II *Hyperlipidemia:* • Decreased activity of enzymes involved in cholesterol synthesis (glucose-6-phosphate-dehydrogenase) • Decreased fatty acid synthetase (catalyzes fatty acid synthesis) • HMG-Co-A reductase inhibition • Suppressed LDL oxidation *Diabetes:* • Increased endogenous insulin production • Increased insulin sensitivity • Enhanced β-cell regeneration • Inhibition of carbohydrate absorption • Decreased oxidative stress	• Gastrointestinal (GI) discomfort • Allergic reactions • Burns (topical use) • Bleeding *Drug interactions:*[1] • Additive effects with antiplatelets/anticoagulants • CYP3A4 inducer, thus lowering efficacy of protease inhibitors, some statins, certain anticonvulsants • Decreases isoniazid levels 65% • Increased ethanol, acetaminophen concentrations • Additive hypotension with antihypertensives • Additive glucose-lowering effects with sulfonylureas and insulin

Note: Reference numbers correspond to the subject's references in the text

Table 2 *continued*

Product & Natural Medicines Rating	Chemical Constituents	Mechanism of Action	Side Effects & Drug Interactions
Ginkgo biloba	Various Ingredients[1,2]	Various mechanisms[1-3]	*Side effects:*[1,4]
Diabetic Retinopathy, Glaucoma, Peripheral Arterial Disease:	• Flavone glycosides	*Diabetic Complications (Diabetic Retinopathy, Glaucoma, Peripheral Arterial Disease):*	• Gastrointestinal upset
Likely Ineffective	– Quercetin	• Antioxidant activity	• Headache
Diabetes:	– Kaempferol	• Inhibits platelet aggregation	• Allergic reactions
Not Rated by Natural Medicines	– Isorhamnetin	• Improves circulation	• Seizures
	• Terpenoids	• Inhibits platelet-activating factor	• Bleeding
	– Ginkgolides	• Increases ocular blood flow	*Drug interactions:*[1,5]
	– Bilobalides		• Additive effects with antiplatelets/anticoagulants
		Diabetes:	• Hypomania (with melatonin, St John's wort, some antidepressants)
		• May increase insulin secretion	• Increased serum drug concentrations
			– Antipsychotics
			– Antidepressants
			– Cardiac medications
			– Sulfonylureas
			• Decreased serum drug concentrations
			– Anticonvulsants (phenytoin)
			– Some statins
			– Cyclosporine
			– Diltiazem

Glucomannan	Various Ingredients[1,2]	Various mechanisms[1-5]	Side effects:[1,2]
Hyperlipidemia, Diabetes: Possibly Effective *Hypertension, Obesity:* Insufficient Reliable Evidence to Rate	• Fiber • Polysaccharide: – D-glucose – D-mannose (these are linked by β-1,4 glycosidic bonds)	*Hyperlipidemia:* • Inhibits cholesterol absorption in jejunum • Inhibits bile acid absorption in ileum • Inhibits HMG-CoA-reductase *Diabetes:* • Increased viscosity and slowed food absorption in small intestine • Decreased postprandial glucose: Blocks carbohydrate hydrolyzing enzymes • Prebiotic effects *Obesity:* • Fecal energy loss • Prolonged gastric emptying • Satiety • Increased chewing time	• Gastrointestinal upset • Esophageal/intestinal obstruction • Choking *Drug interactions:*[1] • May bind other medications; do not administer at same time • Binds vitamins A, D, E, K • Additive glucose-lowering effects with sulfonylureas and insulin • Additive lipid-lowering effects with anti-hyperlipidemics

Note: Reference numbers correspond to the subject's references in the text

(Continued)

Table 2 *continued*

Product & Natural Medicines Rating	Chemical Constituents[1-4]	Mechanism of Action	Side Effects & Drug Interactions
Hibiscus	Various Ingredients[1-4]	Various mechanisms[1-7]	*Side effects:*[1,8]

Hypertension: Possibly Effective	• Organic acids
	  – Malic
	  – Hibiscus
	  – Citrus
		Hypertension:
		• Angiotensin converting enzyme inhibition
		• Diuresis
		• Vasorelaxation
			• Gastrointestinal upset (abdominal distention, constipation)
			• Dysuria
			• Headache
			• Tinnitus

Hyperlipidemia, Obesity: Insufficient Reliable Evidence to Rate	• Anthocyanins
	  – Delphinidin-3-sambubioside
	  – Cyanidin-3-sambubioside
	• Polyphenols
		Hyperlipidemia:
		• Inhibition of LDL-C oxidation
		
		Obesity:
		• Inhibits fat accumulation
			• Hepatotoxicity
			• Abortifacient properties
			• May adversely affect fluid intake during lactation

Diabetes: Not Rated by Natural Medicines	• Flavonoids
	  – Gossypetine
	  – Hibiscetin
	  – Various glycosides
		• Decreases adipogenesis
		
		Diabetes:
		• α-glucosidase inhibition
			Drug interactions:[1,10]
			• Decreased chloroquine efficacy
			• Decreased simvastatin efficacy
			• Additive glucose lowering effects with sulfonylureas and insulin
			• Hypotension with antihypertensives

Pine Bark Extract	Various ingredients[1-3]	Various mechanisms[1-3]	Side effects:[1,3]
Chronic Venous Insufficiency: Possibly Effective	• Procyanidins (70±5%)	*Chronic Venous Insufficiency; Diabetic Retinopathy, Diabetic Foot Ulcers:*	• Gastrointestinal upset
	• Catechin	• Antioxidant	• Diarrhea
Diabetic Retinopathy, Diabetes, Diabetic Foot Ulcers:	• Taxifolin	• Anti-inflammatory	• Headache
	• Phenolic acids:	• Enhances endothelial production of nitric oxide from L-arginine via nitric oxide synthase (enhances blood flow to retina, kidneys, peripheral circulation)	• Rash
Insufficient Reliable Evidence to Rate	– Benzoic		*Drug interactions:*[1]
	– Cinnamic (includes gallic, caffeic, ferulic)	*Hypertension:*	• Additive glucose-lowering effects with sulfonylureas and insulin
Hyperlipidemia: Possibly Ineffective		• Enhanced endothelial function, vasodilation	• Bleeding with antiplatelets or blood thinner
		• ACE inhibition	• Antagonizes immunosuppressants (steroids, cyclosporine)
		• Anti-thrombotic effect	
		Diabetes:	
		• α-glucosidase inhibition	
		Hyperlipidemia:	
		• Mitigates LDL oxidation	

Note: Reference numbers correspond to the subject's references in the text

(Continued)

Table 2 continued

Product & Natural Medicines Rating	Chemical Constituents	Mechanism of Action	Side Effects & Drug Interactions
Red Yeast Rice (RYR) *Hyperlipidemia:* Likely Effective	Various ingredients:[1,3-4] • Unsaturated fatty acids • Polyketides • Phytosterols • Pigments (rubropunctamine, monascorubramine) • Monacolin M, L, J, X, K, others	Various mechanisms:[1,3,5] *Hyperlipidemia:* • HMG-CoA reductase inhibition	*Side effects:*[1,3,5] • Gastrointestinal upset • Allergic reactions • Myalgias • Renal toxicity if citrinin inadvertently produced • Teratogenicity • Increased liver function tests *Drug interactions:*[1,3] • Increased serum drug concentrations and possible toxicity of RYR: grapefruit, macrolides, azole antifungals, protease inhibitors, nefazodone • Decreased serum drug concentrations and possible sub-therapeutic effect of RYR: St. John's wort, some anticonvulsants • Gemfibrozil: rhabdomyolysis • Niacin: myopathy, liver toxicity • Thyroid supplements: possible thyroid function abnormalities

St. John's wort	Various ingredients[1]	Various mechanisms[1,2]	Side effects:[1,3]
Depression: Likely Effective	• Hyperforin • Adhyperforin • Hypericin • Naphthodianthrones • Flavonoids	*Depression:* • Selective serotonin reuptake inhibition • Prevents reuptake of norepinephrine and dopamine • May affect GABA and glutamate	• Phototoxicity, photosensitivity • Gastrointestinal upset • Sleep difficulties • Withdrawal symptoms if stopped abruptly *Drug interactions:*[1,2] • Potent CYP 450 inducer of 3A4: Decreased cyclosporine, protease inhibitor, oral contraceptive, antihypertensive, statin, digoxin effectiveness • Potent CYP 450 inducer of 2C9: Decreased warfarin effectiveness • Additive serotonergic effects with other serotonergic drugs (serotonin syndrome possible) • Possible increased sedation with narcotics and certain analgesics

Note: Reference numbers correspond to the subject's references in the text

(Continued)

Table 2 *continued*

Product & Natural Medicines Rating	Chemical Constituents[1,4]	Mechanism of Action	Side Effects & Drug Interactions
Vitamin D *Osteoporosis:* Likely Effective *Diabetes:* Insufficient Reliable Evidence to Rate	Various ingredients[1,4] • Ergocalciferol (vitamin D2) • Cholecalciferol (vitamin D3)	Various mechanisms[1-7] *Osteoporosis:* • Regulates serum calcium and phosphorous concentrations • Regulates bone health, muscle strength • Anti-inflammatory: interferes with cytokine generation, action Downregulates NF-κB *Diabetes:* • Low Vit D levels (once thought to be associated with impaired pancreatic β-cell function) and insulin resistance	*Side effects:*[1,8] • Toxicity when 25-OH(D) exceeds 150 ng/mL (374.4 nmol/L): Nausea, vomiting, poor appetite, weakness, weight loss, constipation • Possible hypercalcemia with high doses • Bone loss at high doses (4,000 to 10,000 IU/day of Vit D3) *Drug interactions:*[1] • Decreased serum concentrations of vitamin D: Some anticonvulsants (phenobarbital, phenytoin), rifampin, some HIV medications • Steroids: impair Vit D metabolism • Impaired absorption of vitamin D: orlistat, cholestyramine • Arrhythmias: with digoxin, if hypercalcemia • Hypermagnesemia: with magnesium-containing antacids

Index

Note: Page numbers followed by *t* refer to tables.

A

A1C
  aloe, 21–22
  α-lipoic acid, 163
  banaba, 25
  berberine, 29–32
  bitter melon, 40–42
  chia, 46
  chromium, 49–53
  cinnamon, 57–58
  coenzyme Q10 (CoQ10), 174–175
  fenugreek, 63–64
  flaxseed, 69–70
  garlic, 195–196
  ginkgo, 200
  ginseng, 76–78
  gymnema, 83
  holy basil, 88–89
  honey, 92–93
  ivy gourd, 97
  magnesium, 101–103
  milk thistle, 107–108
  mulberry, 113–114
  pine bark extract, 216
  probiotics, 124
  psyllium, 131
  supplement use, 240
  tea, 136–137
  turmeric, 142–143
  vinegar, 149
  vitamin D, 231
  zinc, 155–156
abdominal fullness, 263*t*
abdominal pain, 246*t*
abdominal upset, 248*t*–249*t*, 276*t*
abortifacient, 39, 208, 250*t*
acarbose, 113
acemannan, 20, 246*t*
acetaminophen (Tylenol®), 56, 68, 107, 194, 242, 255*t*, 262*t*, 279*t*
acetate, 272*t*
Acetic acid (vinegar), 147–151, 270*t*–271*t*
acetyl-Coenzyme A (acetyl-CoA), 160, 189, 252*t*, 273*t*, 278*t*
acne, 152, 204
acupuncture, 1
acute hepatitis, 20, 246*t*
acute necrotizing eosinophilic myocarditis (ANEM), 189, 278*t*
acyl CoA cholesterol transferase, 68, 255*t*
adaptogen, 75
addiction, 6, 68
adenosine monophosphate (AMP), 20
adenosine monophosphate activated protein kinase (AMPK), 28, 39, 49, 56
adenosine monophosphate activated protein kinase (AMPK) activation, 147, 246*t*, 248*t*, 250*t*, 252*t*–253*t*, 270*t*–271*t*
adenosine triphosphate (ATP), 160, 170, 273*t*, 276*t*
adenosine triphosphate citrate lyase, 189, 278*t*
adhyperforin, 225, 285*t*

adipogenesis, 282*t*

adiponectin, 46, 50, 135–136, 142, 252*t*, 267*t*

adipose tissue, 152, 208

advanced glycation end product formation pathway, 166, 275*t*

Aegele marmelos (bael tree), 4

aegeline, 4

African American population, 2

aging, 214

Agriculture Improvement Act of 2018, 237

"agua de Jamaica", 211

ajoene, 193, 279*t*

Akkermansia muciniphila, 122, 264*t*

alcohol, 238, 262*t*–263*t*

alcohol hangover, 117, 120, 263*t*

alcoholic cirrhosis, 106

alcohol-related neuropathy, 166

aldose reductase inhibition, 28, 106, 248*t*, 262*t*

algal-derived eicosapentanoic acid (EPA), 180

Aljawad, FH, 174

alkaloid, 62, 96, 254*t*, 260*t*

all-cause mortality, 182, 232

allergic hypersensitivity, 62

allergic reaction
    α-lipoic acid, 161, 273*t*
    benfotiamine, 166
    chia, 45, 251*t*
    cinnamon, 56
    fenugreek, 254*t*
    flaxseed, 68
    garlic, 279*t*
    ginkgo, 198, 280*t*
    honey, 91, 259*t*
    ivy gourd, 260*t*
    milk thistle, 107, 262*t*
    psyllium, 129
    red yeast rice, 219, 284*t*

allergy, 240, 265*t*, 277*t*

allicin, 193, 279*t*

alliin, 193, 279*t*

alliinase, 193

allithiamine. *See* benfotiamine

Allium sativum (garlic). *See* garlic

allopathic medication, 3

aloe (*Aloe vera L.*), 2, 7, 20–23, 246*t*

aloeresin A, 20, 246*t*

Aloe vera L. (aloe). *See* aloe

aloin, 7

α-2 agonist activity, 28, 248*t*

α-adrenergic activity, 28, 248*t*

α-amylase inhibition, 134, 266*t*

α-glucosidase inhibition
    aloe, 20, 246*t*
    berberine, 28, 248*t*
    bilberry, 34, 249*t*
    bitter melon, 39, 250*t*
    cinnamon, 56, 253*t*
    hibiscus, 208, 282*t*
    mulberry, 112–113, 263*t*
    nopal, 117
    pine bark extract, 214, 283*t*
    tea, 134, 266*t*
    turmeric, 141, 268*t*
    zinc, 152, 272*t*

α-ketoglutarate dehydrogenase enzyme complex, 160

α-linolenic acid, 45, 68, 180, 251*t*

α-lipoic acid (ALA), 26, 160–165, 168, 243, 255*t*, 273*t*–274*t*

Alpha Lipoic Acid in Diabetic Neuropathy (ALADIN I and III) trials, 161

α-momorcharin, 39

altitude sickness, 198

Alzheimer's disease, 11, 152, 160, 198

Amanita phalloides poisoning, 106, 160

American blueberry (*Vaccinium corymbosum*), 34

American Botanical Council (ABC), 2

American Diabetes Association (ADA), 25, 100, 186, 238, 240

American ginseng, 2. *See also* ginseng

American Heart Association (AHA) Scientific Advisory, 185

amino acid, 62, 91, 147, 259*t*, 270*t*

amitriptyline, 171, 276*t*

Amorphophallus konjac K. Koch (glucomannan). *See* glucomannan

amphetamine, 135, 266*t*

amyloid polypeptide, 152, 272*t*

anabolic steroid, 4, 7

Anaerobutyricum hallii, 264*t*

analgesic effect, 75, 285*t*

analgesic medication, 76

analgesic properties, 87, 256*t*

anaphylactic reaction, 68

andanamide, 238
Anderson, R, 50
anemia, 138, 153
anencephaly, 62
angina, 136, 183
angiotensin converting enzyme (ACE)
    activity, 75, 208–209, 214, 256*t*
angiotensin converting enzyme (ACE)
    inhibition, 45, 251*t*, 282*t*
angiotensin-converting enzyme (ACE)
    inhibitor, 109, 162, 172, 216, 283*t*
angiotensin II, 193, 279*t*
angiotensin receptor blockers ARBs, 5, 24,
    225
animal data, 87
anorexia, 222, 276*t*
antacid, 100, 161, 230, 273*t*, 286*t*
anthocyanin, 34, 208, 282*t*
anthocyanoside, 35, 249*t*
anthraquinone, 7, 20
anti-aging effect, 134
anti-androgenic properties, 87
anti-arrhythmic properties, 180
antibacterial activity, 193, 225
antibiotic
    benfotiamine, 166, 275*t*
    flaxseed, 69, 255*t*
    garlic, 194
    gymnema, 82
    magnesium, 261*t*
    milk thistle, 107, 262*t*
    probiotics, 264*t*
    vitamin D, 230
    zinc, 153, 272*t*
anticancer treatment, 62
anticoagulant drug
    bilberry, 249*t*
    cannabidiol (CBD) supplement, 238
    cinnamon, 253*t*
    fenugreek, 63, 254*t*
    fish oil (ω-3 fatty acid), 181, 277*t*
    flaxseed, 255*t*
    garlic, 279*t*
    ginkgo, 280*t*
    holy basil, 88, 258*t*
    honey, 92, 259*t*
    supplement use, 240
    turmeric, 142, 268*t*
anticoagulant effect, 171

anticonvulsant agent
    benfotiamine, 275*t*
    cannabidiol (CBD) supplement, 238
    garlic, 194, 279*t*
    ginkgo, 199, 280*t*
    psyllium, 265*t*
    red yeast rice, 221, 284*t*
    vitamin D, 230, 286*t*
    zinc, 153, 272*t*
antidepressant, 8, 76, 221, 226, 243,
    256*t*–257*t*, 280*t*
antidepressant-induced sexual dysfunction,
    198
antifungal, 264*t*
anti-glaucoma product, 36
antihyperlipidemic agent, 129, 204, 221,
    265*t*, 281*t*
antihypertensive action, 68
antihypertensive effect, 208
antihypertensive medication
    banaba, 24, 247*t*
    berberine, 28, 31, 248*t*
    coenzyme Q10 (CoQ10), 171, 276*t*
    fish oil (ω-3 fatty acid), 181, 277*t*
    flaxseed, 69, 255*t*
    garlic, 194, 279*t*
    ginseng, 76, 256*t*
    psyllium, 129, 265*t*
    St. John's wort, 243, 285*t*
    turmeric, 268*t*
antihypertensive properties, 193
anti-inflammatory activity, 106, 238, 242
anti-inflammatory drug, 50, 87, 286*t*
anti-inflammatory effect, 75, 141, 166, 180,
    249*t*, 259*t*, 262*t*, 275*t*, 277*t*
anti-inflammatory properties, 34, 214,
    268*t*, 274*t*, 283*t*
antimicrobial drug, 123, 259*t*
antimicrobial effect, 91
antiobesity treatment, 62
antioxidant
    α-lipoic acid, 160–161, 273*t*
    bilberry, 36, 249*t*
    case study, 242
    chia, 45, 251*t*
    coenzyme Q10 (CoQ10), 170, 276*t*
    fenugreek, 62
    flaxseed, 68
    ginkgo, 198, 201, 280*t*

honey, 91
milk thistle, 106, 262*t*
mulberry, 112, 263*t*
pine bark extract, 214, 283*t*
probiotics, 122, 264*t*
tea, 134, 266*t*
turmeric, 141, 268*t*
zinc, 152, 272*t*
antioxidant response element (ARE), 160
antiplatelet activity, 34, 199
antiplatelet agent
bilberry, 249*t*
cinnamon, 253*t*
fenugreek, 254*t*
flaxseed, 255*t*
garlic, 194, 279*t*
ginkgo, 280*t*
holy basil, 88, 258*t*
honey, 92, 259*t*
pine bark extract, 283*t*
turmeric, 142, 268*t*
antiplatelet effect, 266*t*
antiplatelet properties, 34, 69, 87, 135, 142, 193, 268*t*
antipsychotic medication, 199, 257*t*, 262*t*, 280*t*
antiretroviral drug, 107, 194, 262*t*
antiseptic, 147
antithrombotic effect, 180, 214, 278*t*, 283*t*
antiviral effect, 225
anxiety, 135, 225, 266*t*
anxiolytic, 237
apigenin, 87, 258*t*
apixiban, 40
apolipoprotein B, 181, 205, 277*t*
appetite, 286*t*
appetite suppression, 135, 150, 265*t*, 267*t*
arachidonic acid pathway, 180
Aristolochia serpentaria, 7
arrhythmia, 230, 286*t*
arsenic, 7
Artemisia absinthium, 84
arthritis, 34, 56, 89, 180, 214
artichoke, 26
ASCEND (A Study of Cardiovascular Events in Diabetes) study, 182–183
Asian population, 2
aspartame, 129, 265*t*
aspirin, 34, 87–88, 142, 194, 199

asthma, 62, 82, 91, 198, 214
Astra Zeneca, 184
Atherosclerosis Risk in Communities Study (ARIC), 101
atherosclerotic cardiovascular disease, 186
atherosclerotic lesion, 112
athletic supplementation, 6
atorvastatin, 171, 174, 242
atrial fibrillation, 183
attention deficit hyperactivity disorder (ADHD), 152
Aung, T, 183
autoimmune disease, 230
Ayurvedic medicine, 82, 87
azole antifungal, 221, 284*t*

B

bael tree, 4
banaba (*Lagerstroemia speciosa L*), 24–27, 247*t*
barbituate, 266*t*
benfotiamine (also known as Vitamin Bl, Allithiamines), 166–169, 243, 275*t*
benign prostatic hyperplasia (BPH), 117, 263*t*
benzodiazepine, 238
benzoic acid, 214, 283*t*
benzoquinone nucleus, 170, 276*t*
berberine (*Coptis chinensis [Huanglian or French]*), 6, 26, 28–34, 39, 109, 222, 242, 248*t*
β-1,4 glycosidic bond, 204
β-2 agonist, 100, 261*t*
β agonist, 6
β blocker, 24, 50, 135, 172
beta-carotene, 96, 260*t*
β-cell, 134, 170, 180, 257*t*, 272*t*
β-cell function, 75, 77, 141–142, 152–153, 256*t*, 268*t*
β-cell regeneration, 279*t*
β-cell sensitivity, 49
β-glucan, 131
betaine, 82, 257*t*
betalain, 117, 263*t*
β-momorcharin, 39
betel nut, 166, 275*t*
Bifidobacterium, 91, 122, 264*t*
biguanide, 11

bilberry (*Vaccinium myrtillus L.*), 34–38, 243, 249*t*
bile acid, 28, 135, 204, 267*t*–268*t*, 281*t*
bile salt, 129, 265*t*
biliary cholesterol, 254*t*
bilobalide, 280*t*
bioavailability, 273*t*
biologic agent, 123
biotin, 50, 252*t*
bisdemethoxycurcumin, 141, 268*t*
bisphosphonate, 101, 261*t*
bitter melon (*Momordica charantia*), 39–44, 250*t*
bitter orange, 135
black tea, 134, 137–138, 266*t*
bleeding
  aloe, 20
  bilberry, 34, 249*t*
  case study, 242
  cinnamon, 253*t*
  fish oil (ω-3 fatty acid), 181, 183, 277*t*
  flaxseed, 69, 255*t*
  garlic, 194, 279*t*
  ginkgo, 199, 280*t*
  holy basil, 87–88, 258*t*
  honey, 92
  pine bark extract, 215, 283*t*
  turmeric, 142
blood glucose, 56, 204, 214, 240. *See also* fasting glucose; glucose; postprandial glucose; *under specific supplement*
blood loss, 246*t*
blood pressure. *See also* hypertension; hypotension
  banaba, 24–25
  berberine, 28–31
  case study, 242–243
  chia, 45–47, 251*t*
  chromium, 52
  cinnamon, 56–57
  coenzyme Q10 (CoQ10), 173
  flaxseed, 68–71
  garcinia, 189, 278*t*
  garlic, 194
  ginseng, 75–76, 256*t*
  gymnema, 83
  hibiscus, 209
  pine bark extract, 214, 216
  psyllium, 265*t*

tea, 135, 138, 266*t*
blood thinner, 240, 283*t*
blood-thinning, 63
blood viscosity, 200
bodybuilding supplement, 4, 7
body mass index (BMI), 84, 101, 119, 131, 138, 164, 190, 200, 242
body weight, 119, 150
boldo, 63
bone, 229–230, 286*t*
bone mineral density, 230
botanical product, 1, 12. *See also under specific supplement*
botulism, 92, 259*t*
bread, 46
breast cancer, 107, 230, 262*t*
breastfeeding. *See* lactation
Brewer's yeast, 49, 52
burn, 96, 279*t*
butyrate, 122

C

caffeic acid, 45, 87, 147, 251*t*, 258*t*, 270*t*
caffeine, 134–135, 137, 199, 266*t*
calcidiol, 229
calcitriol, 229
calcium, 45, 96, 101, 229–230, 251*t*, 260*t*–261*t*, 286*t*
calcium channel, 180
calcium channel blocker (CCB), 40, 82, 100, 107, 194, 199, 261*t*–262*t*, 278*t*
calf pain, 200
Camellia sinensis (tea). *See* tea
cancer, 39, 62, 134, 141, 171, 230, 232–233, 240
cancer prevention, 193
Cannabis sativa, 237
captopril, 209
carbamazepine, 129
carbohydrate
  absorption, 75, 117, 135, 193, 254*t*, 256*t*, 263*t*, 267*t*, 279*t*
  honey, 91
  hydrolyzing enzyme, 204, 281*t*
  malabsorption, 113
  metabolism, 77, 87, 160, 258*t*
  sequestering, 129, 265*t*
carbon atom, 180

carcinogen, 7, 20, 49
carcinogenicity, 246t
cardiac
    autonomic function, 162
    cell membrane stabilization, 180
    death, 182
    disease, 170
    drug, 107
    effect, 92
    ion channel, 180
    medication, 199, 280t
    reaction, 4, 28
    toxicity, 259t
    transplantation, 172
cardiovascular death, 172, 183
cardiovascular disease (CVD), 41, 45–46,
    68, 100, 134, 137–138, 170–172, 180–184,
    232–233
cardiovascular event, 194, 232, 243
cardiovascular mortality, 175, 232
cardiovascular risk factor, 103, 119, 220
caryophyllene, 87
case study, 242–243
catalase, 152, 272t
cataract, 36, 160
catechin, 134–135, 147, 214, 266t, 270t,
    283t
catechol-o-methyltransferase enzyme, 135
caustic esophageal injury, 148, 270t
celecoxib, 199
cellular thermogenesis, 135
Center for Drug Evaluation and Research,
    7
central nervous system (CNS) depressant,
    28, 75, 248t
central-nervous-system-stimulant effect, 75
central retinal arteries, 201
cephalexin, 153, 272t
cerebral insufficiency, 198
charantin, 39, 250t
chemotherapy, 91, 122, 264t
chemotherapy drug, 40, 107, 161, 166,
    262t, 273t, 275t
chia (Salvia Hispanica L.), 45–48, 251t
chicoric acid, 87, 258t
chilblain, 198
children, 2, 39, 42, 76, 92, 102–103, 240,
    250t
China, 50–51

China Coronary Secondary Prevention
    Study, 221
Chinese product, 5–6
Chinese subject, 58
chiropractic manipulation, 1
chloride, 261t, 272t
chlorogenic acid, 45, 251t
chloroquine, 208
chlorpropamide, 39, 117
choking, 281t
cholecalciferol (Vitamin D3), 229, 286t
cholesterol
    absorption, 28, 181, 281t
    aloe, 21–22
    α-lipoic acid, 163
    berberine, 31, 248t
    bitter melon, 40
    case study, 243
    chromium, 49–50
    coenzyme Q10 (CoQ10), 174
    fenugreek, 62–63
    flaxseed, 68, 71–72, 255t
    garcinia, 190
    garlic, 195
    glucomannan, 204–205
    holy basil, 88
    ivy gourd, 98
    milk thistle, 106, 262t
    nopal, 119
    pine bark extract, 217
    psyllium, 130
    red yeast rice, 219, 221–222
    synthesis, 193, 265t, 279t
    tea, 136–138
    turmeric, 143–144
    vinegar, 150
    zinc, 154–155
cholestyramine, 153, 230, 272t, 286t
choline, 82, 257t
chromium, 26, 34, 49–55, 153, 249t, 252t,
    263t
cinnamaldehyde, 56, 253t
cinnamic acid, 214, 283t
Cinnamomum burmanii, 25
cinnamon (Cinnamomum cassia) or
    (Cinnamomum zeylanicam), 2, 6–7, 25,
    56–61, 243, 253t
ciprofloxacin, 153, 272t
circulation, 280t

circulatory disorder, 34
cirrhosis, 107
citrate, 261t
citric acid, 270t
citrinin, 219
Citrullus colocynthis, 84
citrus acid, 282t
claudication, 5, 200, 242–243
cleft palate, 62
clenbuterol, 6
clopidogrel, 63, 88, 92, 142
Clostridium species, 264t
clozapine (Clozaril®), 82
coagulation factor, 45
Coccinia indica, Also Known as *Coccinia cordifolia and Coccinia grandis* (ivy gourd). *See* ivy gourd
Cochrane Database, 58
Cochrane Evaluation, 173
Cochrane Review, 41, 163, 171, 196, 200–201, 209, 226
Cochrane Systematic Review, 138
Code of Federal Regulations, 223
coenzyme Q10 (CoQ10), 25, 170–179, 221, 276t
coffee, 272t
cognitive function, 75
cold, 112, 152
colon cancer, 230
coma, 199
compactin, 219
complementary and alternative medicine (CAM), 1–4, 88, 135, 194
complementary health approaches (CHA), 1
congestive heart failure, 276t
constipation, 62, 68, 82, 100, 112, 189, 204, 264t, 286t
consumer information, 10–11
Consumer Lab, 10, 239
Consumer Protection Act, 9
Consumer Reports, 10
consumer safety, 11
Consumers Union, 10
contaminant, 6
cooking spice, 62
copper deficiency, 153, 272t
Coptis chinensis [Huanglian or French] (berberine). *See* berberine

coronary artery disease, 104
coronary heart disease (CHD), 100, 132, 182, 184, 194, 221
coronary revascularization, 183–184, 221
corsolic acid, 24–25, 247t
corticosteroid, 215
cosmetic, 45
cost, 3, 8
Costello, RB, 52–53
cough, 91, 147, 263t, 265t
coumarin, 56, 62–63, 253t
Council for Responsible Nutrition, 126
Cox-2 inhibitor, 199
C-peptide, 84, 142, 199–200
cranberry (*Vaccinium macrocarpum*), 34
C-reactive protein, 46, 160, 274t
creatine kinase, 220
creatine phosphokinase, 219, 222
crepe myrtle, 24
croup, 147
Curcuma longa Linn (turmeric). *See* turmeric
curcumin (diferuloylmethane), 141, 268t
curry powder, 141
cutaneous reaction, 219
cyanide glycoside, 68, 255t
cyanidin-3-sambubioside, 208, 282t
cyclocurcumin, 141, 268t
cyclosporine
    fish oil (ω-3 fatty acid), 181, 277t
    garlic, 194
    ginkgo, 199, 280t
    magnesium, 100, 261t
    pine bark extract, 215, 283t
    probiotics, 123, 264t
    St. John's wort, 225, 285t
CYP 450 1A2, 82, 142, 199, 257t, 268t
CYP 450 2B6, 142, 268t
CYP 450 2C9, 82, 107, 199, 225, 248t, 257t, 268t, 285t
CYP 450 2C19, 142, 199, 268t
CYP 450 2D6, 76, 107, 142, 199, 248t, 268t
CYP 450 2E1, 142, 194, 268t
CYP 450 3A4
    berberine, 248t
    garlic, 194, 279t
    ginkgo, 199
    gymnema, 82, 257t
    milk thistle, 107

red yeast rice, 221
St. John's wort, 225, 285*t*
turmeric, 142, 268*t*
CYP 450 enzyme, 28, 142, 238
CYP 450 isoenzyme, 199
CYP 450 system, 82
cystatin C, 232
cytochrome P450 (CYP450). *See under* CYP450
cytokine, 134, 229, 286*t*
cytokine-induced β-cell damage, 266*t*
cytokine-induced inflammation, 160
cytoprotectant, 106

D

dammarane saponin, 82
dammarane-type triterpene glycoside, 75
"dawn phenomenon", 147
death, 181–184, 250*t. See also* mortality
deep-vein thrombosis (DVT), 242
degludec, 242
delphinidin-3-sambubioside, 208, 282*t*
delta-9-tetrahydrocannabinol (THC), 237
delta-9-tetrahydrocannabivarin (THVC), 238
dementia, 198–199
demethoxycurcumin, 141, 268*t*
depression, 4–5, 141, 225–226, 242
dermatitis, 56, 253*t*, 268*t*
dermatological condition, 50, 152
dermatological reaction, 252*t*
detoxification, 147
dextromethorphan, 191
D glucose, 204
diabetes. *See also under specific type; under specific supplement*
    agent, oral, 30, 42, 57, 63, 88, 112
    comorbidities. *see under specific supplement*
    corticosteroid-induced, 49
    fraud, 11
    management, 6, 75
    medication, 171, 194, 215. *see also* insulin
    persons with diabetes (PWD), 1–5, 9, 11
    statistics, 1
Diabetes Care and Education Specialist, 94
diabetes-induced liver damage, 208

diabetes-related neuropathy, 170
diabetic microangiopathy, 144
diacylglycerol-protein kinase C pathway, 166, 275*t*
diallyldisulfide, 193, 279*t*
dialysis tubing, 259*t*
diaphoresis, 247*t*
diarrhea, 20, 28, 69, 129, 219, 246*t*, 254*t*, 261*t*–263*t*, 283*t*
diastolic blood pressure (DBP)
    chia, 46–47
    cinnamon, 57
    coenzyme Q10 (CoQ10), 173, 175
    flaxseed, 70–71
    garlic, 194
    glucomannan, 205
    gymnema, 83
    hibiscus, 209–210
    nopal, 119
    pine bark extract, 216–217
    tea, 137–138
    zinc, 154, 156
diet, 2
dietary fat, 117, 265*t*
dietary supplement, 1–2, 4, 7–10
Dietary Supplement Health and Education Act (DSHEA) of 1994, 1–2, 8–10
Dietary Supplement Ingredient Advisory List, 11
Dietary Supplement Verification Program, 10
diet therapy, 57
diferuloylmethane, 268*t*
digoxin, 100, 148, 225, 230, 246*t*, 261*t*, 285*t*–286*t*
digoxin toxicity, 20, 270*t*
dihydrolipoic acid (DHLA), 160, 273*t*
diltiazem, 40, 280*t*
dimethyltrisulfide, 193, 279*t*
dipeptidyl peptidase 4 (DPP4) inhibitor, 40
direct oral anticoagulants (DOACs), 40
disaccharidase, 147, 270*t*
distal polyneuropathy, 167
distal symmetric sensorimotor polyneuropathy (DSPN), 161
diuresis, 282*t*
diuretic, 76, 100, 148, 166, 208, 256*t*, 261*t*, 270*t*, 275*t*
divalproex sodium, 153, 272*t*

dizziness, 247t, 276t

D mannose, 204

DNA (deoxyribonucleic acid), 152

docosahexanoic acid (DHA), 6, 47, 180, 182, 277t

Dong, H., 30–31

dopamine, 227, 285t

Doppler flow velocity measurement, 215

dosage, 239

double bond, 180

doxorubicin, 171

doxorubicin-mediated cardiotoxicity, 171, 276t

dropsy, 147

drowsiness, 260t

drug metabolism, 225

dry eye syndrome, 180

dulaglutide, 242

D-xylose, 129, 265t

dyslipidemia, 31, 194

E

economic adulteration, 8

edema, 189

"Effective" rating, 245

eicosanoid, 255t

eicosapentanoic acid (EPA), 6, 47, 180, 182–183, 277t

elderly population, 10, 240

electron transport chain, 276t

ellagitannins, 24, 247t

emmenagogue, 39

endocannabinoid system, 122

endothelial dysfunction, 134, 167, 170, 276t

endothelial function, 283t

endothelial growth factor receptor 2, 275t

endothelial production, 214, 283t

endothelin 1, 193, 279t

endothelium-derived relaxing factor, 170

energy expenditure, 135, 274t

energy harvesting, 122

energy supplement, 4

enzyme, 91, 259t–260t, 267t

EPA ethyl ester, 183

Epanova® (Astra-Zeneca), 185

ephedra, 135

epicatechin, 134, 266t

epicatechin gallate, 134, 266t

Epidiolex®, 237

epigallocatechin gallate (EGCG), 134–135, 266t

epithelialization, 91

ergocalciferol (Vitamin D2), 229, 286t

"ergogenic aids", 75

ergogenic properties, 49, 214

erythrocyte malondialdehyde, 201

erythrocyte rigidity, 200

escitalopram (Lexapro®), 4–5, 242

E-selectin, 180, 277t

esophageal injury, 148

esophageal obstruction, 204, 281t

estimated glomerular filtration rate (eGFR), 231–232

estrogen, 153, 272t, 277t

estrogenic effect, 68–69, 76, 107, 255t–256t, 262t

ethanol, 104, 194, 279t

etoposide, 40

eugenol, 56, 87, 253t, 258t

euglycemic, 131

eye infection, 96, 112

ezetimibe, 222

F

fagomine, 112, 263t

fasting glucose. *See also* glucose

aloe, 21–22

α-lipoic acid, 162–163

banaba, 25

berberine, 29–31

bitter melon, 40–42

chia, 46

chromium, 49–53

cinnamon, 57–58

coenzyme Q10 (CoQ10), 174–175

delta-9-tetrahydrocannabivarin (THVC), 238

fenugreek, 63–64

flaxseed, 69

garlic, 195

ginkgo, 200

ginseng, 77–78

glucomannan, 205

gymnema, 83–84

holy basil, 88

honey, 92–93
ivy gourd, 97
magnesium, 102–103
milk thistle, 107–108
mulberry, 113–114
probiotic, 123–124
psyllium, 131
tea, 136–137
turmeric, 142–143
vinegar, 148–149
vitamin D, 231
zinc, 153–156
fat, 117, 263*t*, 282*t*
fatal kernicterus, 28
fatty acid, 49–50, 91, 189, 193, 259*t*,
  278*t*–279*t*
favism, 39, 250*t*
FDA (Food & Drug Administration), 7–10,
  91, 132, 186, 220, 237, 239, 245
"FDA 101: Health Fraud Awareness", 11
fecal bile acid, 129, 255*t*, 265*t*
fecal energy loss, 204, 281*t*
fecal sterol excretion, 204
fenugreek (*Trigonella foenum-graecum
  Linn.*), 34, 62–67, 254*t*
fenugreekine, 62, 254*t*
ferritin, 50, 252*t*
fertility, 87, 258*t*
ferulic acid, 147, 270*t*
fetal malformation, 65
fetal neurodevelopment, 65
fever, 96
feverfew, 194, 199
fever-reducing properties, 87
fiber
  aloe, 20, 246*t*
  chia, 45, 251*t*
  fenugreek, 62
  flaxseed, 68, 255*t*
  glucomannan, 204, 281*t*
  ivy gourd, 96, 260*t*
  nopal, 117, 263*t*
  psyllium, 265*t*
fibrosis, 106, 109, 262*t*
fibrous polysaccharides, 263*t*
fish, 36
fish oil (ω-3 fatty acid), 45, 68, 171, 180–
  188, 242, 277*t*–278*t*. *See also* omega-3
  fatty acid

fishy taste, 277*t*
5,8-kDa component, 91, 259*t*
5-HT1A serotonin receptor, 238
flatulence, 56, 62, 129, 193, 204, 265*t*
flavone glycoside, 198, 280*t*
flavonoid
  bilberry, 34
  fenugreek, 62
  ginkgo, 198
  hibiscus, 208, 282*t*
  honey, 91, 259*t*
  nopal, 117, 263*t*
  St. John's wort, 225, 285*t*
  supplement use, 6
flavonolignans, 106
flavoring agent, 62
FLAX-PAD study, 70
flaxseed (*Linum usitassimum L.*), 47, 68–
  74, 180, 242, 255*t*
flosin B, 24, 247*t*
flow-mediated vasodilation, 147, 270*t*
flu, 5
fluoroquinolone, 24, 101, 247*t*
fluoxetine (Prozac®), 4, 191, 199, 226
fluvoxamine (Luvox®), 82
folate absorption, 138
folic acid, 26, 135, 266*t*
folk medicine, 45
food absorption, 281*t*
Food and Nutrition Board, 49
foot ulcer, 92–93, 100, 259*t*, 283*t*
4-hydroxyisoleucine, 62, 254*t*
free fatty acid, 122, 141, 147, 264*t*
free fatty acid receptor, 270*t*
free-radical scavenger, 170
fructosamine, 40, 70, 136
fructose, 91, 259*t*
furosemide, 255*t*

G

galacturonic acid, 129, 265*t*
Galega officinalis L. (goat's rue), 11
galic acid, 147, 270*t*
gallocatechin gallate, 134, 266*t*
gamma aminobutyric acid (GABA), 227,
  285*t*
garcinia (*Garcinia cambogia*), 4–5, 189–
  192, 242, 278*t*

Garcinia cambogia (garcinia). *See* garcinia
garlic (*Allium sativum*), 193–197, 199, 243, 279*t*
gas, 254*t*
gastric emptying, 129, 147, 204, 253*t*–255*t*, 265*t*, 270*t*, 281*t*
gastrointestinal (GI) discomfort, 250*t*–251*t*, 279*t*
gastrointestinal (GI) disorder, 39
gastrointestinal (GI) side effect, 161
gastrointestinal (GI) upset
  cannabidiol (CBD) supplement, 238
  chia, 45
  chromium, 252*t*
  cinnamon, 56
  fish oil (ω-3 fatty acid), 277*t*
  flaxseed, 68, 255*t*
  garcinia, 189, 278*t*
  ginkgo, 280*t*
  hibiscus, 281*t*
  honey, 92
  ivy gourd, 96, 260*t*
  magnesium, 261*t*
  mulberry, 263*t*
  pine bark extract, 214, 283*t*
  probiotics, 264*t*
  red yeast rice, 219–220, 222, 284*t*
  St. John's wort, 225, 285*t*
  tea, 135, 266*t*
  turmeric, 268*t*
  vinegar, 148, 270*t*
  zinc, 272*t*
gastrointestinal bleeding, 232
gastrointestinal inflammatory disorder, 141
gastroparesis, 148, 270*t*
gemfibrozil, 221, 284*t*
genital wart, 134
gestational diabetes mellitus (GDM), 53, 122–124, 152–153
ghrelin, 135, 147, 259*t*, 267*t*, 271*t*
ginger, 194, 199
Gingko biloba L. (ginkgo). *See* ginkgo
ginkgo (*Gingko biloba L.*), 2, 5–6, 34, 194, 198–203, 243, 280*t*
ginkgolide, 280*t*
ginseng (*Asian or Korean [Panax ginseng C.A. Meyer] and American [Panax quinquefolius L.]*), 75–81, 256*t*
ginsenoside, 75

Gissi (Gruppo Italiano per lo Studio della Sopravvivenza nell'Infarto miocardico) study, 181
glaucoma, 160, 198, 201, 280*t*
glibenclamide (glyburide), 41, 88–89, 108, 113
gliclazide, 58, 123
glipizide, 117, 199
glucagon-like peptide-1 (GLP-1)
  berberine, 28, 248*t*
  case study, 242
  cinnamon, 56, 253*t*
  hibiscus, 210
  probiotics, 122
  turmeric, 141, 268*t*
  vinegar, 147, 270*t*
glucokinase activation, 87, 91, 258*t*–259*t*
glucomannan (*Amorphophallus konjac K. Koch*), 191, 204–207, 281*t*
gluconate, 272*t*
gluconeogenesis, 141, 152, 252*t*, 268*t*
glucoreceptor, 189, 278*t*
glucose. *See also* blood glucose; fasting glucose; postprandial glucose
  absorption, 68, 82, 117, 134, 204, 246*t*, 255*t*, 257*t*, 265*t*
  aloe, 246*t*
  α-lipoic acid, 162–163
  area under curve (AUC), 36
  banaba, 247*t*
  bilberry, 36
  case study, 242
  chromium, 49
  control, 49
  disposal, 256*t*
  fenugreek, 254*t*
  fish oil (ω-3 fatty acid), 181
  flaxseed, 68–70, 255*t*
  garcinia, 189
  ginkgo, 200
  ginseng, 75–76, 256*t*
  glucomannan, 204
  gymnema, 82, 84, 257*t*
  hibiscus, 208
  homeostasis, 256*t*
  honey, 91, 259*t*
  ivy gourd, 260*t*
  loading, 200
  lowering, botanical and nonbotanical

products, 12. *see also under specific supplement*
lowering agent, 204, 215
lowering effect, 91, 247t
magnesium, 261t
metabolic pathway, 261t
metabolism, 263t
mulberry, 263t
nopal, 117, 119
pine bark extract, 215
probiotics, 124
production, 260t
psyllium, 265t
regulation, 152
tea, 134, 136
transport, 247t, 254t, 256t
uptake, 39, 56, 134, 160, 250t, 253t, 256t–257t, 273t
uptake inhibition, 34, 249t
uptake stimulation, 91, 152, 247t
utilization, 62
zinc, 152
glucose-6-phosphatase, 96, 134, 260t, 266t
glucose-6-phosphate-dehydrogenase (G6PDH), 39, 250t, 279t
glucose dependent insulinotropic peptide (GIP), 119
glucose-stimulated insulin secretion, 248t, 276t
glucose tolerance factor (GTF), 49
glucose transporter GLUT1 activity, 273t
glucose transporter GLUT1 transport, 160
glucose transporter GLUT4 activity, 273t
glucose transporter GLUT4 mobilization, 147, 270t
glucose transporter GLUT4 translocation, 28, 39, 56, 112, 248t, 250t, 252t–253t, 263t
glucose transporter GLUT4 transport, 49, 152, 160, 272t
Glucosol™, 25
glucuronidated drug, 262t
glucuronidation, 107
glutamate, 227, 285t
glutathione (GSH) level, 160, 273t
glutathione peroxidase (GPx), 152, 272t
glyburide, 41, 88, 199
glycemic index, 148
glycemic management, 114

glycemic value, 154–155, 164
glycerol-3-phosphate dehydrogenase, 170, 276t
glycogen synthase activation, 91, 259t
glycogen synthase kinase-3β (GSK-3β), 166
glycogen synthase kinase-3 b signaling pathway, 112, 275t
glycogen synthesis, 39, 56, 250t, 253t, 259t
glycolysis, 141, 147, 152
glycolytic enzyme activity, 152, 272t
glycoside, 282t
glycosides momordin, 39, 254t
goat's rue, 11
goldenseal, 28
Good Manufacturing Practices, 9
gossypetine, 282t
Grading of Recommendations Assessment, Development, and Evaluation (GRADE), 175
grapefruit, 221, 284t
GRAS (generally recognized as safe), 65
grayanotoxins, 92
green tea, 4, 134–135, 137–138, 266t
guar gum, 131
gurmarin, 82, 257t
gut microbiota, 28, 122–123, 246t, 248t
gymnema (*Gymnema sylvestre R. Br.*), 34, 39, 82–86, 257t
gymnemasaponin, 82, 257t
gymnemaside saponin, 82
Gymnema sylvestre R. Br. (gymnema). *See* gymnema
gymnemic acid, 82, 257t

H

halitosis, 277t
haloperidol (Haldol®), 107
Hamilton Depression Scale score, 226
Harris Poll, 9
hazard ratio (HR), 172
HDL cholesterol
  aloe, 22
  α-lipoic acid, 163
  berberine, 31
  bilberry, 36
  chromium, 50, 52
  cinnamon, 59
  coenzyme Q10 (CoQ10), 174

fenugreek, 64–65
flaxseed, 69, 71–72
garcinia, 190
garlic, 195
glucomannan, 205
hibiscus, 210
honey, 91
magnesium, 103
milk thistle, 108
mulberry, 113
nopal, 119
pine bark extract, 217
red yeast rice, 221–222
tea, 137–138
turmeric, 143
vinegar, 150
zinc, 153–156, 272*t*
headache
    α-lipoic acid, 273*t*
    berberine, 248*t*
    coenzyme Q10 (CoQ10), 276*t*
    garcinia, 189, 278*t*
    ginkgo, 280*t*
    ginseng, 76, 256*t*
    mulberry, 263*t*
    pine bark extract, 283*t*
Health Canada, 245
health care provider, 5, 11–12, 239–240
heartburn, 277*t*
heart disease, 163
heart failure (HF), 104, 170–172, 194, 233,
    276*t*–277*t*
heart rate, 76, 135, 173, 210, 256*t*, 266*t*
hemolysis, 50
hemolytic anemia, 39, 250*t*
hemorrhoid, 189
hempbased cannabidiol (CBD)
    supplement, 237
hepatic
    cholesterol, 135, 267*t*
    cholesterol α hydroxylase, 268*t*
    cholesterol production, 147
    cholesterol synthesis, 129
    disorder, 106
    dysfunction, 50
    enzyme, 141, 268*t*
    function, 97
    glucogenesis, 262*t*
    gluconeogenesis, 20, 106, 134, 147, 266*t*

glucose output, 252*t*
glucose production, 147, 270*t*
glucose uptake, 91, 259*t*
glycogen synthesis, 189, 278*t*
LDL receptor, 135, 267*t*
hepatic-3-hydroxy-methylglutaryl CoA
    reductase activity, 56, 253*t*
hepatic diacyl-glycerol acyl transferase,
    181, 277*t*
hepatic glucose-6-phosphate
    dehydrogenase, 193
hepatitis, 20, 246*t*
hepatotoxic agent, 262*t*
hepatotoxic effect, 106
hepatotoxicity, 4, 7, 56, 135, 189, 208, 253*t*,
    266*t*, 278*t*
hepatotoxic supplement, 56
herb, 1–4, 63. *See also under specific type*
hexokinase, 87, 258*t*
hexosamine pathway, 166, 275*t*
hibiscetin, 282*t*
hibiscus (*Hibiscus sabdariffa L.*), 208–213,
    282*t*
Hibiscus sabdariffa L. (hibiscus). *See*
    hibiscus
high carbohydrate breakfast (HCB),
    118–119
high soy protein breakfast (HSPB), 118–
    119
Hippocrates, 147
Hispanic population, 2, 22, 211
histamine blockers (famotidine), 50, 252*t*
HIV (human immunodeficiency virus), 39,
    230, 240, 286*t*
HMG-CoA reductase, 106, 193, 262*t*, 268*t*,
    279*t*, 281*t*, 284*t*
Hodgkin's lymphoma, 230
holy basil (*O tenuiflorum L.; Formerly
    known as Ocimum sanctum L.*), 87–90,
    258*t*
homeopathy, 2
homeostatic model assessment (HOMA),
    153
homeostatic model assessment of insulin
    resistance (HOMA-IR)
    coenzyme Q10 (CoQ10), 175
    flaxseed, 69–70
    ginseng, 77
    magnesium, 102–103

milk thistle, 108
probiotics, 123–124
psyllium, 131
tea, 137
turmeric, 142–143
zinc, 154
honey (sometimes known as manuka
  honey), 91–95, 147, 259*t*
hormone, 62, 229
horsetail plant, 166, 275*t*
Huang, H, 52–53
huckleberry (*Vaccinium ovatum*), 34
human microbiome, 122
hydrocephalus, 62
hydrochlorothiazide, 209
hydrocolloidal dietary fiber polysaccharide,
  204
hydrogen, 113
hydrogen sulfide, 193, 279*t*
hydroxide, 261*t*
hydroxy- 3-methyl-glutaryl CoA reductase
  (HMG-CoA-reductase), 204
hydroxycitric acid (HCA), 189, 278*t*
hypercalcemia, 230–231, 286*t*
hyperforin, 8, 225, 285*t*
hyperglycemia, 35, 58, 129
hyperglycemia-induced apoptosis, 166,
  275*t*
hypericin, 8, 225
Hypericum perforatum L. (St. John's wort).
  See St. John's wort
hyperlipidemia
  aloe, 20, 246*t*
  α-lipoic acid, 273*t*
  banaba, 24
  berberine, 29–30, 32, 248*t*
  case study, 242
  chromium, 53, 252*t*
  cinnamon, 253*t*
  coenzyme Q10 (CoQ10), 170–171, 173,
    276*t*
  fenugreek, 62, 254*t*
  flaxseed, 68, 255*t*
  garlic, 193, 279*t*
  ginseng, 256*t*
  glucomannan, 204, 281*t*
  gymnema, 82
  hibiscus, 208, 282*t*
  honey, 91, 259*t*

Lactobacillus, 122
magnesium, 261*t*
milk thistle, 106, 262*t*
mulberry, 112, 263*t*
nopal, 117, 263*t*
pine bark extract, 217, 283*t*
probiotics, 264*t*
psyllium, 129, 265*t*
red yeast rice, 219–220, 222, 284*t*
tea, 136–137, 266*t*–267*t*
turmeric, 141–142, 268*t*
vinegar, 147, 270*t*
zinc, 152
hypermagnesemia, 100, 230, 261*t*, 286*t*
hypersensitivity, 62, 255*t*
hypertension. *See also* antihypertensive
  medication; blood pressure
  berberine, 29–30, 248*t*
  bilberry, 34, 249*t*
  case study, 242
  chia, 45–46, 251*t*
  cinnamon, 253*t*
  coenzyme Q10 (CoQ10), 170–171, 173,
    276*t*
  fish oil (ω-3 fatty acid), 277*t*
  flaxseed, 68, 255*t*
  garlic, 193–195, 279*t*
  ginseng, 256*t*
  glucomannan, 281*t*
  hibiscus, 208–210, 282*t*
  magnesium, 103
  pine bark extract, 216, 283*t*
  psyllium, 129, 265*t*
  tea, 137, 266*t*–267*t*
hypertensive effect, 75, 277*t*
hypertensive retinopathy, 249*t*
hypertriglyceridemia, 180, 277*t*
hyperzincuria, 152
hyphema, 199
hypoglycemia
  aloe, 20
  α-lipoic acid, 161
  banaba, 24
  berberine, 28
  bilberry, 34, 249*t*
  bitter melon, 39, 250*t*
  case study, 242
  chromium, 50
  coma, 250*t*

fenugreek, 62–63
flaxseed, 69
garcinia, 189
garlic, 194
ginseng, 76
gymnema, 82
gymnema sylvestre, 257*t*
hibiscus, 208
holy basil, 87–88
honey, 91
ivy gourd, 96, 260*t*
magnesium, 101
milk thistle, 107
mulberry, 112
nopal, 117, 263*t*
tea, 135
turmeric, 142
vinegar, 148, 270*t*
hypoglycemic agent, 129, 181, 277*t*
hypoglycemic agent, oral, 3, 30–31, 84
hypokalemia, 20, 148, 246*t*, 270*t*
hypomagnesemia, 100, 102–103, 261*t*
hypomania, 199, 280*t*
hypotension
  banaba, 24, 247*t*
  berberine, 28, 248*t*
  bilberry, 34, 249*t*
  case study, 242
  flaxseed, 69, 255*t*
  garlic, 194, 279*t*
  hibiscus, 208
  magnesium, 100, 261*t*
hypotensive effect, 75
hypothalamic AMP-activated protein
  kinase, 160, 274*t*
hypothyroidism, 87, 258*t*
hypozincemia, 152

I

ibuprofen, 50, 82
icosapent ethyl (Vascepa®), 183, 243
immune cell activity, 91, 259*t*
immune response, 76
immune system, 75, 153, 214
immunocompromised state, 122, 264*t*
immunomodulation, 75, 230
immunosuppressive medication, 123, 215,
  264*t*, 283*t*

impaired fasting glucose (IFG), 77
impaired glucose tolerance (IGT), 25,
  35–36, 49, 51, 77–78, 114, 123, 200
impaired renal function, 24
incremental area under the curve (IAUC),
  118–119
incretin action, 264*t*
incretin activity, 122
incretin effect, 242
Indian cuisine, 87
indigestion, 219
"Ineffective" rating, 245
infant, 28, 63, 76, 230
infection, 75, 82, 87, 259*t*, 264*t*
inflammation, 122, 229, 264*t*
inflammatory cell propagation, 91
inflammatory cytokine, 122
inflammatory disorder, 34, 68, 89, 180, 214
inflammatory eye disorder, 141
inflammatory lipopolysaccharide, 122
inflammatory marker, 70
ingredient, 239–240
injection site reaction, 273*t*
insect bite, 96
insomnia, 76, 135, 256*t*, 266*t*
Institute of Medicine, 49
"Insufficient Reliable Evidence to Rate"
  rating, 245
insulin
  action, 49, 100, 253*t*, 261*t*
  activation, 252*t*
  activity, 134, 152, 266*t*
  aloe, 246*t*
  α-lipoic acid, 161, 273*t*
  area under curve (AUC), 149, 200
  banaba, 247*t*
  berberine, 248*t*
  bilberry, 249*t*
  binding, 252*t*
  bitter melon, 250*t*
  chromium, 50, 252*t*
  cinnamon, 56, 253*t*
  complementary and alternative
    medicine (CAM), 3
  fasting, 78
  fenugreek, 63–64, 254*t*
  flaxseed, 69, 255*t*
  garcinia, 278*t*
  garlic, 193, 279*t*

ginseng, 76–78, 256*t*
glucomannan, 281*t*
gymnema, 82–84, 257*t*
holy basil, 88, 258*t*
honey, 91
ivy gourd, 260*t*
L-aspartate, 107
L-ornithine, 107
magnesium, 101, 261*t*
milk thistle, 107–108, 262*t*
mulberry, 263*t*
nopal, 118–119, 263*t*
pine bark extract, 283*t*
postprandial response grain product, 36
probiotics, 124
production, 272*t*, 279*t*
psyllium, 265*t*
receptor, 49, 56, 62, 100, 134, 252*t*, 254*t*,
    261*t*, 266*t*, 273*t*
receptor β-subunit, 247*t*
receptor expression, 28, 248*t*
receptor phosphorylation, 24, 253*t*
receptor substrate, 134, 160, 266*t*
release, 257*t*, 259*t*
secretagogue, 101, 135, 142
signaling, 122, 253*t*, 261*t*
signaling cascade, 152, 272*t*
signal transduction pathway, 134, 266*t*
stimulation, 265*t*
tea, 135, 137, 266*t*
turmeric, 142, 268*t*
vinegar, 148–149, 270*t*
insulin-like activity, 96, 247*t*, 260*t*
insulin resistance
    aloe, 20, 246*t*
    cannabidiol (CBD) supplement, 238
    chromium, 49
    ginkgo, 200
    ginseng, 77
    holy basil, 87, 258*t*
    human microbiome, 122
    magnesium, 100, 103, 261*t*
    milk thistle, 106, 262*t*
    mulberry, 112, 263*t*
    probiotics, 123, 264*t*
    tea, 134, 266*t*
    turmeric, 141
    vitamin D, 229, 286*t*
    zinc, 153

insulin secretion
    berberine, 28, 31
    bilberry, 34, 249*t*
    fenugreek, 62, 254*t*
    ginkgo, 198, 280*t*
    ginseng, 75, 256*t*
    gymnema, 82
    holy basil, 87, 258*t*
    honey, 259*t*
    mulberry, 112, 263*t*
    tea, 134
    vinegar, 147, 270*t*
    vitamin D, 231
insulin sensitivity
    banaba, 25
    chromium, 50, 252*t*
    cinnamon, 253*t*
    flaxseed, 70
    garlic, 193, 279*t*
    ginseng, 77
    gymnema, 84
    magnesium, 102
    nopal, 117, 263*t*
    probiotics, 123
    tea, 134
    vitamin D, 231
    zinc, 153
integrative health, 1
intent to treat (ITT), 52
intercellular adhesion molecule (ICAM-1),
    141, 269*t*
interleukin, 106, 262*t*
interleukin-1β, 180, 277*t*
interleukin-6, 160, 274*t*, 277*t*
interleukin IL-6, 180
International Lipid Expert Panel (ILEP),
    220
international normalized ratio (INR), 63,
    171, 277*t*
International Probiotics Association, 126
intestinal cholesterol absorption, 181, 277*t*
intestinal lumen L-cell, 147
intestinal obstruction, 204, 281*t*
intestinal parasite, 189
intracellular calcium activity, 180, 278*t*
intracellular lipid accumulation, 208
intraocular pressure, 36
iron
    chia, 45, 251*t*

chromium, 50
psyllium, 129, 265*t*
tea, 135, 266*t*
turmeric, 142, 268*t*
zinc, 153, 272*t*
iron deficiency anemia, 138
irradiation, 91
irritable bowel syndrome, 129
ischemic reperfusion injury, 160
isoniazid, 194, 279*t*
isoprenoid tail, 170
isoquinoline alkaloid, 28, 248*t*
isorhamnetin, 198, 280*t*
isosilibin, 262*t*
isosilychristine, 262*t*
Italian Surveillance System of Natural
Health Products, 219
ivy gourd (*Coccinia indica, also known as Coccinia cordifolia and Coccinia grandis*), 96–99, 260*t*
Ixba action, 141, 269*t*

J

Janus kinase, 141, 269*t*
Japanese product, 5–6

K

kaempferol, 45, 198, 251*t*, 280*t*
"karkade", 208
kernicterus, 248*t*
Khalesi, S, 71
kidney, 214, 229
kidney disease, 232
kidney function, 97
kidney injury molecule (KIM-1), 168
kidney stone, 232
killer cell activity, 214
kinase, 20, 24
konjac (glucomannan), 131
kratom, 6

L

label, 5–6, 10
lactate dehydrogenase, 96, 260*t*
lactation
aloe, 20
berberine, 28

bitter melon, 42
coenzyme Q10 (CoQ10), 176
fenugreek, 62–63
garlic, 194
ginseng, 76
hibiscus, 208
honey, 92
red yeast rice, 219
supplement use, 240
lactic acid, 270*t*
lactic acidosis, 24, 247*t*
Lactobacillus, 122, 264*t*
Lagerstroemia speciosa L (banaba), 25. *See* banaba
lagerstroemin, 24, 247*t*
lamotrigine (Lamictal®), 107
Langerhans cell, 84
L-arabinose, 129, 265*t*
L-arginine, 283*t*
laxative, 20
LDL cholesterol
aloe, 21–22
α-lipoic acid, 163
berberine, 28–29, 31, 248*t*
chromium, 52
cinnamon, 57, 59
coenzyme Q10 (CoQ10), 173–174
fenugreek, 63–64
fish oil (ω-3 fatty acid), 181, 183
flaxseed, 68–69, 71–72
garlic, 195
glucomannan, 205
hibiscus, 210
magnesium, 103
milk thistle, 106, 108, 262*t*
mulberry, 112–113
nopal, 119
pine bark extract, 216–217
psyllium, 130
red yeast rice, 220–222
tea, 136–138
turmeric, 143–144
vinegar, 150
zinc, 154–156
LDL-C oxidation, 208, 282*t*
LDL oxidation, 135, 193, 214, 267*t*–268*t*, 279*t*, 283*t*
lead, 7, 268*t*
left ventricular ejection fraction (LVEF),

levothyroxine, 50, 252t
Liang, Y., 30
lifestyle modification, 30, 35
lignan, 68–69, 255t
"Likely Effective" rating, 245
"Likely Ineffective" rating, 245
linagliptin, 40
linamarin, 68
linoleic acid, 68, 255t
Linum Usitassimum L. (flaxseed). *See*
  flaxseed
linustatin, 68
lipid
    absorption, 117, 135
    aloe, 246t
    α-lipoic acid, 162–164
    banaba, 25
    berberine, 28, 30
    bilberry, 36
    case study, 242
    chia, 45–46
    chromium, 49–50, 252t
    cinnamon, 56–58, 253t
    coenzyme Q10 (CoQ10), 173, 175
    delta-9-tetrahydrocannabivarin
      (THVC), 238
    fenugreek, 62, 64, 254t
    fish oil (ω-3 fatty acid), 180–181
    flaxseed, 68–69, 71–72
    garcinia, 190
    garlic, 195
    ginseng, 75
    glucomannan, 204, 281t
    gymnema, 83–84
    hibiscus, 208, 210
    honey, 92
    magnesium, 103
    management, 114
    milk thistle, 108
    mulberry, 113
    nopal, 263t
    oxidation, 189
    peroxidation, 112, 141, 263t, 268t
    pine bark extract, 214, 217
    psyllium, 129–130, 265t
    red yeast rice, 219–220
    tea, 138
    turmeric, 143
    zinc, 153–155
lipid-lowering activity, 193
lipid-lowering agent, 129, 183
lipogenesis, 147, 181, 189, 271t, 277t–278t
lipolysis, 147, 271t
lipoprotein lipase activity, 75, 96, 141, 181,
  256t, 260t, 268t, 277t
lisinopril, 153, 209, 272t
lithium, 129
liver
    α-lipoic acid, 160
    enzyme, 238
    function enzyme, 41
    function test, 107, 219, 284t
    injury, 4
    toxicity, 221, 284t
    transaminase, 222
    transplantation, 4, 189, 278t
Liver Disease Research Branch of the
  National Institute of Diabetes and
  Digestive and Kidney Diseases (NIDDK),
  4
LiverTox website, 4
lorcaserin (Belviq®), 7
losartan, 242
lovastatin, 219–221
Lovaza® (GlaxoSmithKline), 185
lupus, 215
lysine, 156
lysosomal enzyme activity, 141, 268t

M

macrolide, 194, 221, 284t
macrolide antibiotic, 238
macrophage infiltration, 141
macular degeneration, 152, 198, 201
macular edema, 163, 215
magnesium, 45, 100–105, 153, 155, 251t,
  261t, 272t, 286t
major adverse cardiovascular events
  (MACE), 172
malic acid, 270t, 282t
malondialdehyde (MDA) concentration,
  106–107, 109, 262t
malonyl-CoA, 50, 189, 278t
mania, 76, 189
Manuka honey, 91, 93. *See also* honey
maple syrup, 62

marijuana, 237
massage therapy, 1
mastalgia, 76, 256*t*
matairesinol, 68, 255*t*
mechanical assist implantation, 172
medication. *See also under specific name;
    specific type*
    drug interaction, 4–5, 21, 28
    oral, 21, 118
    oral diabetes agent, 24, 30, 42, 57, 63,
        88, 112
    prescription, 4–5, 7–8, 65, 166, 183,
        185–186, 209, 237–239
medicinal herb, 96
Mediterranean ancestry, 39
melatonin, 199
melon, 39
membrane stabilization, 170, 180, 276*t*
men's health supplement, 4
menstrual disorder, 106, 189
menstruation, 39
mental alertness, 134
mercury, 181
metabolic syndrome
    α-lipoic acid, 163
    berberine, 28, 248*t*
    bilberry, 34, 249*t*
    chia, 45, 251*t*
    cinnamon, 58
    coenzyme Q10 (CoQ10), 173
    flaxseed, 68, 255*t*
    gymnema, 82, 84
    gymnema sylvestre, 257*t*
    hibiscus, 209
    magnesium, 103, 261*t*
    nopal, 117, 263*t*
    pine bark extract, 214
    tea, 137, 266*t*
    turmeric, 143, 268*t*
    zinc, 155
metacarpal nerve, 167
metallic taste, 272*t*
Metamucil®, 132
metatarsal nerve, 167
metformin
    aloe, 21
    banaba, 25
    benfotiamine, 166, 275*t*
    berberine, 29

bitter melon, 40–41
    case study, 242
    fenugreek, 65
    Galega officinalis L., 11
    garlic, 195
    ginkgo, 200
    milk thistle, 108
    nopal, 117
    probiotics, 122
    psyllium, 129, 265*t*
methotrexate, 56, 123, 264*t*
methyl eugenol, 87
mevalonate pathway, 170
mevinolin, 219
microbial infection, 123
microbiome dysfunction, 122
microbiome modulation, 268*t*
microcirculation, 36
microvascular complication, 28, 152, 166,
    196, 200, 214, 272*t*
Middle-Eastern ancestry, 39
migraine headache, 100
milk thistle (*Silybum marianum*), 32,
    106–111, 243, 262*t*
mind and body practice, 1
mineral, 1
mineral salt, 147, 270*t*
"miracle cure", 240
Mirtogenol®, 36
miscarriage, 135, 254*t*, 266*t*
mitochondrial ATP production, 170
mitochondrial dysfunction, 171, 276*t*
mitogen-activated protein kinase (MAPK),
    166, 180, 275*t*, 277*t*
Momordica charantia (bitter melon). *See*
    bitter melon
momordicin, 39, 250*t*
momordin, 250*t*
monacolin, 219–221, 284*t*
monascorubramine, 284*t*
Monascus purpureus went (red yeast rice).
    See red yeast rice
monoamine oxidase (MAO) inhibitor, 135,
    266*t*
monocyte chemoattractant protein-1, 141,
    269*t*
monocyte infiltration, 180
monofloral, 91
monosaccharide, 148

mood change, 76, 256*t*
mood disturbance, 50
mortality, 182, 194, 221, 232
Morus alba Linn. (mulberry). *See* mulberry
Mosheni, M, 173
mosquito repellant, 87
motor nerve conduction velocity (MNCV), 162
mucilage, 204
mucin production, 122
mucopolysaccharide soluble fiber, 117
mucositis, 91
mulberry (*Morus alba Linn.*), 112–116, 263*t*
multifloral, 91
multi-infarct dementia, 198
multiple sclerosis, 215, 230
muscle, 152, 176, 222, 229–230, 286*t*
muscle building supplement, 7
muscle glucose uptake, 147, 270*t*
muscle pain, 248*t*
muscle protein kinase, 20
musculoskeletal disorder, 220
myalgia, 219–220, 242, 284*t*
myocardial ATP production, 170, 276*t*
myocardial infarction (MI), 136, 172–173, 181–184, 194, 221, 232
myopathy, 170, 221, 284*t*
myricetin, 45, 251*t*

N

nadolol, 135, 266*t*
NADPH (nicotinamide adenine dinucleotide phosphate), 135, 267*t*
naphthodianthrone, 225, 285*t*
narcotic, 285*t*
nasal short posterior ciliary, 201
NATHAN I (Neurological Assessment of Thioctic Acid in Neuropathy) trial, 161–162
NATHAN II (Neurological Assessment of Thioctic Acid in Neuropathy) trial, 161
National Academy of Medicine, 230
National Cancer Institute, 7
National Health Interview Survey (NHIS), 1–3
National Institutes of Health (NIH), 8, 238
National Institutes of Health National

Center for Complementary and Integrative Health (NCCIH), 1, 6
National Library of Medicine, 4
National Osteoporosis Foundation, 233
National Toxicology Program (NTP), 7
Native American population, 2
Natural Medicines, 2, 12, 223, 237, 239, 243, 245
natural product, 1
Natural Products Association, 223
nausea, 261*t*, 263*t*, 272*t*–273*t*, 277*t*, 286*t*
nefazodone, 221, 284*t*
neolinustatin, 68
neomirtilline, 34, 249*t*
nephrolithiasis, 231
nephropathy
    α-lipoic acid, 160, 273*t*–274*t*
    benfotiamine, 166, 275*t*
    berberine, 28, 248*t*
    fish oil (ω-3 fatty acid), 277*t*
    milk thistle, 106, 262*t*
    turmeric, 141, 268*t*–269*t*
nephrotoxicity, 7
nephrotoxin, 219
nerve conduction velocity (NCV), 162
nervousness, 76, 256*t*
Neuropathy Impairment Score-Lower Limbs (NIS-LL), 161–162
neural tube defect, 138
neuroinflammatory lipid peroxidation, 141, 269*t*
neurologic disorder, 170
neuropathic pain, 6
neuropathy, 100, 141, 166–167, 268*t*–269*t*, 273*t*–276*t*
Neuropathy Impairment Score (NIS), 161–162
Neuropathy Symptom Score, 167
neuroprotective properties, 198
New England Journal of Medicine, 4
New York Heart Association (NYHA), 172–173
niacin, 221, 284*t*
night contrast sensitivity, 35
NIH-funded Drug-Induced Liver Injury Network (DILIN) study, 4
nitric oxide, 193, 214, 279*t*, 283*t*
non-alcoholic fatty liver disease (NAFLD)
    berberine, 28, 248*t*

coenzyme Q10 (CoQ10), 276t
fish oil (ω-3 fatty acid), 277t
flaxseed, 68, 255t
milk thistle, 262t
tea, 134, 266t
turmeric, 141, 268t
nonalcoholic steatohepatitis (NASH), 106,
262t
nonbotanical product, 1, 12. *See also under
specific supplement*
nonmainstream practice, 1
non-nucleoside reverse transcriptase
inhibitor, 194
non-steroidal anti-inflammatory (NSAID),
24, 252t
nonsulfonylurea secretagogue, 82
nopal (*Opuntia streptacantha Lemaire*), 2,
117–121, 263t
norepinephrine, 135, 227, 285t
Nrf2 (nuclear factor erythroid 2–related
factor 2), 160, 273t
NSF® International, 10, 239
N-terminal pro-Btype natriuretic peptide
(NT-proBNP), 172
nuclear factor-k B (NF-kB), 141, 160, 166,
180, 229, 268t–269t, 274t–275t, 277t, 286t
nutrition, 1
Nutrition Facts Label, 239

O

oat bran, 46
obesity
aloe, 20, 246t
α-lipoic acid, 160, 273t–274t
berberine, 248t
chia, 45–46, 251t
chromium, 252t
cinnamon, 253t
coenzyme Q10 (CoQ10), 175
diabetes comorbidities, 4
fenugreek, 62, 254t
fish oil (ω-3 fatty acid), 277t
flaxseed, 69, 255t
garcinia, 278t
ginseng, 77
glucomannan, 204–205, 281t
gymnema, 85
hibiscus, 282t

holy basil, 87, 258t
honey, 259t
magnesium, 103
microbiome dysfunction, 122
nopal, 117
probiotics, 122–124, 264t
psyllium, 129, 265t
tea, 134–135, 137–138, 266t–267t
turmeric, 141, 268t–269t
vinegar, 270t–271t
zinc, 155
ocular blood flow, 34, 198, 201, 249t, 280t
ocular disorder, 201
odds ratio (OR), 162
Office of Dietary Supplements (ODS), 8
oligosaccharide, 91, 259t
omega-3-carboxylic acid, 184
omega-3 fatty acid, 6, 232–233, 243, 255t,
276t. *See also* fish oil
omeprazole, 50
Omtryg® (Trygg Pharma, Inc.), 185
1,25-dihydroxyvitamin D (1,25[OH]2D),
229
1-deoxynojirimycin, 112, 263t
oolong tea, 134–137, 266t
ophthalmic disorder, 34
ophthalmoscopy parameter, 35
opioid withdrawal, 237
Opuntia streptacantha lemaire (nopal). *See*
nopal
oral anticoagulant, 42
oral contraceptive, 5, 166, 181, 225, 275t,
285t
oral diabetes agent, 30, 42, 57, 63, 88, 112
oral glucose tolerance test (OGTT)
bilberry, 35–36
bitter melon, 41
fenugreek, 63
ginkgo, 200
ginseng, 77
honey, 93
ivy gourd, 97–98
magnesium, 102
nopal, 119
zinc, 154
oral hypoglycemic drug, 3, 30–31, 84
oral medication, 21, 24
organic acid, 147, 208, 270t, 282t
organic anion-transporting polypeptide

(OATP), 24, 107, 142, 247t, 268t

ORIGIN (Outcome Reduction with Initial Glargine Intervention) trial, 182

orlistat, 230, 286t

oropharyngeal inflammation, 148, 270t

osteoarthritis, 141, 242

osteopathic manipulation, 1

osteoporosis, 229–230, 286t

O tenuiflorum L.; Formerly Known as *Ocimum sanctum L.* (holy basil). *See* holy basil

ovarian cancer, 107, 230

over-the-counter (OTC) supplement, 220

overweight, 77, 84, 123–124, 137, 156, 175

oxidative neural tissue damage, 141

oxidative stress, 68, 106, 109, 152, 160, 193, 201, 279t

oxide, 261t

oxygen consumption, 271t

oxygen transport, 200

oxylipin, 68, 255t

oxyntomodulin, 147, 271t

P

P2Y12 inhibitor, 34, 63

Pacific Islander population, 2

pain, 6, 273t

palatinose (isomaltulose), 91

palpitation, 247t

Panax ginseng C.A. Meyer (ginseng [Asian or Korean]). *See* ginseng

panaxoside, 75

Panax quinquefolius L. (ginseng [American]). *See* ginseng

pancreatic
    antioxidant effect, 259t
    β-cell, 34, 62, 82, 87, 193, 229, 238, 258t, 286t
    cancer, 230
    insulin production, 20
    insulin secretion, 91, 199
    islet cell, 152, 272t

pancreatitis, 123, 189, 277t–278t

parenteral nutrition, 49, 104

Parkinson's disease, 160, 170

paroxetine (Paxil®), 226

pathogenic microbe, 264t

PCBs (polychlorinated biphenyls), 181

p-coumaric acid compound, 87, 258t

pectin, 96, 260t, 263t

pentobarbital, 135

pentobarbitone-induced duration of sleep, 88

pentosane, 129, 265t

pentose phosphate pathway, 166

peptide Y-Y (PYY), 147, 259t, 271t

peripheral arterial disease (PAD), 70, 198, 200, 280t

peripheral
    circulation, 214
    circulatory problems, 198
    neuropathy, 160–161, 242–243, 275t
    resistance, 276t
    tissue glucose utilization, 147, 270t
    vascular disease, 5
    vasodilation, 253t

peroneal MNCV, 162

peroneal nerve conduction velocity, 167

peroneal SNCV, 162

peroxisome proliferator-activated receptor (PPARs), 56, 253t

peroxisome proliferator-activated receptor α (PPAR-α), 147, 180–181, 271t, 277t

peroxisome proliferator-activated receptor-g (PPARg), 28, 39, 238, 248t, 250t, 268t

peroxisome proliferator-activated receptor-g (PPARg) agonist, 106, 141, 262t

peroxynitrite, 160

persons with diabetes (PWD), 1–5, 9, 11, 238–240

Peter, EL, 42

p-glycoprotein, 39, 42, 107, 225, 250t

pharmacotherapy, 1

phenobarbital, 258t, 286t

phenol, 6

phenolic acid, 91, 214, 259t, 283t

phenolic acid derivative, 62

phenolic compound, 117, 214, 246t, 263t

phenolic constituent, 20

phenylketonuria, 129, 265t

phenytoin (Dilantin®), 92, 153, 199, 259t, 272t, 286t

phloroglucinol, 225

phosphatidylcholine, 107, 262t–263t

phosphatidylinositol- 3-kinase/protein

kinase B, 112, 263*t*

phosphodiesterase-5-inhibitor, 7

phosphoenolpyruvate, 50

phosphoenolpyruvate carboxykinase, 134, 266*t*

phosphofructokinase, 87, 258*t*

phosphofructose, 272*t*

phospholipid-protein interaction, 170

phosphorous, 45, 229, 251*t*, 286*t*

phosphorylation reaction, 152, 261*t*, 272*t*

photosensitivity, 225

phototoxicity, 225, 285*t*

physical activity, 1

physiologic effect, 180

Physiotherapy Evidence Database (PEDro) scale, 123–124

phytochemical, 6, 117, 263*t*

phytoestrogen, 68

phytosterol, 219, 284*t*

pine bark extract (*Pinus pinaster Ait*), 36, 214–218, 243, 283*t*

Pinus pinaster ait (pine bark extract). *See* pine bark extract

pioglitazone, 142, 268*t*

piperidine, 268*t*

piperine, 144

Plantago ovata (psyllium). *See* psyllium

plant alkaloid, 6

plaque stabilization, 180

plasma creatine kinase, 176

plasma glucose, 101, 136, 216. *See also* blood glucose; glucose

plasma sialic acid (PSA), 41

Plasma Thiobarbituric Acid Reactive Substances (TBARS), 152

platelet activating factor, 68, 280*t*

platelet aggregation, 20, 34, 181, 189, 198, 278*t*, 280*t*

platelet inhibition, 75

pleiotropic effect, 141

poison ivy, 147

polyisoprenoid tail, 170, 276*t*

polyketide, 219, 284*t*

polyneuropathy symptom, 167

polypeptide, 82

polypeptide P, 39–40, 250*t*

polyphenol

  banaba, 24

  bilberry, 34, 249*t*

  hibiscus, 208, 282*t*

  holy basil, 87, 258*t*

  tea, 134, 266*t*

  vinegar, 147, 270*t*

polyphenolic polymer, 56

polysaccharide, 129, 204, 265*t*, 281*t*

polysaccharide-D-glucose, 281*t*

polysaccharide-D-mannose, 281*t*

polyunsaturated fatty acid, 68

"Possibly Effective" rating, 245

"Possibly Ineffective" rating, 245

postprandial endothelial dysfunction, 167

postprandial glucose. *See also* glucose

  berberine, 29–31

  bitter melon, 42

  chia, 251*t*

  cinnamon, 56, 253*t*

  fenugreek, 62–64

  flaxseed, 68, 255*t*

  garlic, 195–196

  ginseng, 75–78

  glucomannan, 204, 281*t*

  gymnema, 83

  holy basil, 88

  honey, 92

  ivy gourd, 97–98

  mulberry, 113

  nopal, 118–119

  psyllium, 129–131, 265*t*

  vinegar, 148–149

  zinc, 155

potassium, 148

potassium depleter, 270*t*

potassium-sparing diuretic, 100, 261*t*

pravastatin, 210

prebiotic, 91, 204, 259*t*, 281*t*

prediabetes

  aloe, 21–22, 246*t*

  α-lipoic acid, 163

  banaba, 24–25, 247*t*

  bilberry, 34, 249*t*

  bitter melon, 39, 42, 250*t*

  chromium, 252*t*

  cinnamon, 56, 253*t*

  fenugreek, 254*t*

  fish oil (ω-3 fatty acid), 277*t*

  flaxseed, 68, 255*t*

  ginseng, 75, 256*t*

  magnesium, 100–101, 103

mulberry, 114
nopal, 119
probiotic, 124
tea, 137
turmeric, 142–143
vitamin D, 231
zinc, 152–154
prednisone, 153
preeclampsia, 100
Preferred Reporting Items for Systematic
  Reviews and Meta-Analyses (PRISMA),
  53
pregnancy
  aloe, 20
  berberine, 28
  chromium, 49
  coenzyme Q10 (CoQ10), 176
  fenugreek, 62
  flaxseed, 68, 255t
  garlic, 194
  ginseng, 76
  hibiscus, 208
  honey, 92
  magnesium, 104
  probiotic, 123
  red yeast rice, 219
  supplement use, 240
  tea, 135
  zinc, 155
pregnancy-related leg cramp, 100
pregnane x receptor, 225
prickly pear cactus, 2
probiotics (Lactobacillus species and
  Others), 1, 20, 122–128, 264t
procyanidin, 283t
product integrity, 11
product rating, 245
proinflammatory cytokine, 141, 269t
proinflammatory molecule, 152, 272t
proprotein convertase subtilisin/kesin type
  2 (PCSK9), 28, 248t
prostacyclin synthesis, 180, 278t
prostate cancer, 45, 68, 153, 230, 251t, 255t
prostate function, 272t
protease inhibitor, 40, 194, 221, 226, 279t,
  284t–285t
protein, 45, 62, 91, 96, 251t, 259t–260t
protein carbonyl activity, 141, 268t
protein kinase A (PKA), 24

protein kinase B (PKB/Akt), 166, 275t
protein synthesis, 152
proteinuria, 109
prothrombotic mediator production, 180,
  278t
proton pump inhibitor (PPI), 50, 100, 153,
  252t, 261t, 272t
protopanaxadiol, 256t
protopanaxatriol, 256t
pruritus, 220, 268t
psoriasis, 39
psychiatric disorder, 180, 225
psychiatric medication, 257t, 265t
psychomotor performance, 75
psyllium (Plantago ovata), 129–133, 265t
Pycnogenol®, 214–217
pyrophosphatase, 160, 273t
pyruvate dehydrogenase, 160, 273t
pyruvate kinase, 272t
pyruvic acid, 160, 273t

Q

Qigong, 1
QSYMBIO study, 172
quercetin, 34, 45, 198, 251t, 280t

R

radiation treatment, 122, 264t
raloxifine, 107, 262t
ramipril, 216
randomized controlled trials (RCTs)
  aloe, 21–22
  α-lipoic acid, 161–163
  banaba, 25
  benfotiamine, 167
  berberine, 29–31
  bilberry, 35–36
  bitter melon, 40–42
  chia, 45–47
  chromium, 50–53
  cinnamon, 57–59
  coenzyme Q10 (CoQ10), 171–176
  "Effective" rating, 245
  fenugreek, 63–65
  fish oil (ω-3 fatty acid), 181–184
  flaxseed, 69–72
  garcinia, 189–191
  garlic, 194–196

ginkgo, 199–201
ginseng, 77–78
glucomannan, 205
gymnema, 82–86
hibiscus, 209–210
holy basil, 88–89
honey, 92–94
ivy gourd, 97–98
magnesium, 101–103
milk thistle, 107–109
mulberry, 112–114
nopal, 118–119
pine bark extract, 215–217
probiotic, 123–125
psyllium, 130–132
red yeast rice, 221–222
St. John's wort, 226–227
tea, 135–138
turmeric, 142–144
vinegar, 148–149
vitamin D, 230–233
zinc, 153–156
rash, 220, 275t, 283t
rate ratios (RR), 182
reactive nitrogen species, 273t
reactive oxygen species, 267t, 273t, 276t
record keeping, 240
REDUCE-IT (Reduction of Cardiovascular
    Events with Icosapent Ethyl-Intervention
    Trial), 183–184
red yeast rice (*Monascus Purpureus Went*),
    25, 32, 171, 219–224, 276t, 284t
reginin A, 24, 247t
relaxation technique, 1
renal
    failure, 50
    function, 41, 45, 100, 232, 261t
    inflammation, 141, 269t
    toxicity, 50, 252t, 284t
R enantiomer, 160, 273t
renin angiotensin system (RAS) inhibitor,
    109
repaglinide, 142, 268t
respiratory infection, 5, 89
restlessness, 76, 135, 256t
resveratrol, 34
retina, 214
retinal capillary blood flow, 200–201
retinal edema, 144, 215

retinopathy
    α-lipoic acid, 160, 273t–274t
    benfotiamine, 168, 275t
    bilberry, 34–35, 249t
    case study, 242–243
    fish oil (ω-3 fatty acid), 277t
    ginkgo, 198, 200, 280t
    magnesium, 100
    pine bark extract, 214–215, 283t
    turmeric, 141, 268t–269t
retrobulbar blood vessel, 201
retrobulbar hemorrhage, 194, 199
revascularization event, 182
rhabdomyolysis, 219, 221, 284t
rheumatoid arthritis, 58
rhinorrhea, 62
rhododendron plant, 92
riboflavin, 129
rifampin, 286t
ringworm, 87
rivaroxaban, 40
RNA (ribonucleic acid), 152
rosiglitazone, 29
rubropunctamine, 284t

S

Saccharomyces boulardii, 122, 264t
Salba, 45
S-allyl-L-cysteine, 193, 279t
S-allyllmercaptocysteine, 193, 279t
Salvia hispanica L. (chia). *See* chia
saponin constituent, 20, 62, 246t, 254t
satiety, 147, 204, 271t, 281t
scorpion bite, 87
secoisolariciresinol diglucoside (SDG), 68,
    255t
"second meal effect", 265t
secretagogue, 200, 268t, 270t
sedation, 28, 285t
seizure, 39, 198–199, 237, 280t
seizure medication, 166
selective serotonin reuptake inhibitor
    (SSRI) antidepressant, 191
selective serotonin reuptake inhibitors
    (SSRIs), 4–5, 226–227, 278t, 285t
selenium, 175
self-care approach, 2
S enantiomer, 160, 273t

sensory nerve conduction velocity
(SNCV), 162
serotonergic antidepressant, 189, 285*t*
serotonin
reuptake, 189, 278*t*
reuptake inhibition, 225
syndrome, 4–5, 189, 226, 243, 278*t*, 285*t*
toxicity, 4–5, 242
sertraline (Zoloft®), 4–5, 226
serum advanced glycation end product, 41
serum creatinine, 112–113, 232, 263*t*
serum drug concentration, 284*t*
7 α–hydroxylase, 68, 255*t*
severe hypoglycemia, 39
severe interstitial nephritis, 50
sevoflurane, 20, 246*t*
sexual dysfunction, 75
sexual enhancement supplement, 7
short-chain fatty acid, 122, 147, 204, 246*t*
sibutramine, 7
sildenafil (Viagra®), 7
silidianin, 262*t*
Silybum marianum (milk thistle). *See* milk
thistle
silychristine, 262*t*
silymarin, 106–109, 262*t*
simvastatin, 208, 222
sirolimus, 107
skin eruption, 96
skin rash, 275*t*
sleep difficulties, 225, 285*t*
smoking, 170
smoking cessation, 237
snake bite, 87
Snellen test, 215
solar radiation protection, 134
sorbitol dehydrogenase, 141
sotolon, 62
soybean, 190
spasmolytic activity, 214
sperm, 87, 258*t*
spina bifida, 62
spinal epidural hematoma, 193–194
spironolactone, 100, 261*t*
sports performance enhancer, 75
SPRING trial, 123
stacking, 9
standardization, 8
standardized mean difference (SMD), 102,

162–163, 226
Standards of Medical Care, 238
star anise, 5–6
statin
banaba, 24, 247*t*
case study, 243
coenzyme Q10 (CoQ10), 170–171, 276*t*
fish oil (ω-3 fatty acid), 181, 183–184,
277*t*
garlic, 194, 279*t*
ginkgo, 199, 280*t*
hibiscus, 208, 210
psyllium, 129
red yeast rice, 219–221
St. John's wort, 5, 225, 285*t*
turmeric, 142, 268*t*
statin associated muscle symptoms
(SAMS), 176, 229, 276*t*
statin-associated myopathy symptoms
(SAMS), 170
statin-induced myalgia, 276*t*
statin-induced myopathy, 276*t*
statin-related myopathy, 171
Stephania tetranda, 7
steroid, 50, 100, 153, 230, 252*t*, 261*t*, 272*t*,
283*t*, 286*t*
steroidal saponin, 62
steroid use, 49
sterol regulatory element binding protein
(SREBP-1), 49, 147, 252*t*, 270*t*, 277*t*
sterol regulatory element binding protein
(SREBP-1c), 181
stigmasterol, 82, 257*t*
St. John's wort (*Hypericum perforatum L.*),
5, 8, 199, 225–228, 243, 284*t*–285*t*
stomach upset, 147, 247*t*
stool volume, 263*t*
STRENGTH trial (Statin Residual Risk
Reduction with Epanova in High
Cardiovascular Risk Patients with
Hypertriglyceridemia), 184
Streptococcus thermophilus, 122, 264*t*
stress, 75, 87
stroke, 163, 181–184, 194, 232
"structure and function" statement, 9
subarachnoid hemorrhage, 199
subdural hematoma, 199
"sugar destroyer", 82
"sugar-free" product, 265*t*

Suksomboon, N, 51
sulfate, 261*t*, 272*t*
sulfonylurea
    aloe, 20–21, 246*t*
    α-lipoic acid, 273*t*
    banaba, 24, 247*t*
    berberine, 248*t*
    bilberry, 249*t*
    bitter melon, 39, 41, 250*t*
    chromium, 252*t*
    cinnamon, 56, 58, 253*t*
    coenzyme Q10 (CoQ10), 174
    fenugreek, 63, 254*t*
    flaxseed, 255*t*
    garcinia, 278*t*
    garlic, 279*t*
    ginkgo, 199, 280*t*
    ginseng, 76, 256*t*
    glucomannan, 281*t*
    gymnema, 82–83, 257*t*
    holy basil, 258*t*
    ivy gourd, 97, 260*t*
    magnesium, 102, 261*t*
    milk thistle, 107, 262*t*
    mulberry, 263*t*
    nopal, 118, 263*t*
    pine bark extract, 283*t*
    psyllium, 265*t*
    St. John's wort, 5
    tea, 266*t*
    turmeric, 142
superoxide anion, 160
super-oxide dismutase (SOD), 152, 156, 272*t*
supplement, 4–8, 10–12. *See also under specific type*
surgery, 5, 10, 20, 238, 246*t*
swallowing disorder, 129, 265*t*
sweating, 262*t*
"sweet" taste, 257*t*
sympathetic nervous system (SNS), 135, 267*t*
sympathomimetic, 135, 266*t*
Symptomatic Diabetic Neuropathy (SYDNEY) Study, 161
systolic blood pressure (SBP)
    chia, 46–47
    cinnamon, 57
    coenzyme Q10 (CoQ10), 173, 175
    flaxseed, 70–71
    garlic, 194
    glucomannan, 205
    gymnema, 83
    hibiscus, 209–210
    magnesium, 103
    nopal, 119
    pine bark extract, 216–217
    tea, 137–138
    zinc, 154, 156

T

tachycardia, 135, 266*t*
tacrolimus, 100, 123, 215, 261*t*
tamoxifen, 107, 262*t*
tannin, 134, 266*t*
tartaric acid, 270*t*
taxifolin, 214, 262*t*, 283*t*
tea (*Camellia sinensis*), 134–140, 266*t*–267*t*
teratogenicity, 62, 219, 254*t*, 256*t*, 284*t*
terpenoid, 198, 280*t*
tetracyclic antidepressant, 226
tetracycline, 101, 153, 272*t*
tetrahydrocannabinol (THC), 238
Thai medicine, 96
theaflavin, 134, 266*t*
thearubigin, 134, 266*t*
theophylline concentration, 63, 254*t*
thermogenesis, 135, 267*t*
thiamine, 275*t*
thiamine deficiency, 166
thiobarbiturate acid reactive substance (TBARS), 141, 268*t*, 272*t*
thioctic acid. *See* α-lipoic acid
three3-hydroxy-3-methyl-glutaryl-CoA reductase (HMG-Co-A-reductase), 49–50, 219, 252*t*
throat obstruction, 204
thrombocytopenia, 50
thromboembolic event, 171
thromboembolism, 176
thromboxane A3, 180, 278*t*
thromboxane synthesis, 193
thyroid dysfunction, 20, 246*t*, 273*t*
thyroid function, 161, 221, 284*t*
thyroid supplement, 284*t*
thyroxine, 87, 161, 258*t*, 273*t*
tinnitus, 198

"Tips for Older Dietary Supplement Users", 10
"Tips for the Savvy Supplement User", 10
total symptom score (TSS), 162–163, 167
toxic hepatitis, 82, 257*t*
toxicity, 6–7, 226, 284*t*, 286*t*
tramadol, 191
transcription factor, 180
transforming growth factor β (TGF-β), 109
transforming growth factor β (TGF-β1), 141, 269*t*
transient receptor potential of vanilloid type 1 (TRPV1) and 2 (TRPV2) channels, 238
transketolase activity, 166, 275*t*
transporter gene activation, 225
trazodone, 199
treatment, 3
Treatment Trialists' Collaboration, 182
tremor, 247*t*
tricyclic antidepressant, 171, 226
triglyceride
    aloe, 21–22
    α-lipoic acid, 162–163
    berberine, 29, 31
    chia, 45, 251*t*
    chromium, 49–50, 52
    cinnamon, 59, 253*t*
    coenzyme Q10 (CoQ10), 174–175
    fenugreek, 63–65
    fish oil (ω-3 fatty acid), 181, 183–184, 277*t*
    flaxseed, 69, 71–72
    garcinia, 190
    garlic, 195
    glucomannan, 205
    gut microbiota, 122
    honey, 91
    magnesium, 103
    milk thistle, 108
    mulberry, 113
    nopal, 119
    production, 181
    red yeast rice, 221
    tea, 137–138
    turmeric, 142–144
    vinegar, 150
    zinc, 156
Trigonella foenum-graecum Linn.
    (fenugreek). *See* fenugreek
trigonelline, 62
triterpene, 96, 260*t*
triterpene saponin, 75, 82
trivalent chromium, 117, 252*t*
TSH (thyroid stimulating hormone), 225
tumor necrosis factor α (TNFα), 106, 141, 160, 180, 262*t*, 268*t*–269*t*, 274*t*, 277*t*
tumor necrosis factor β (TNFβ), 106, 262*t*
turmeric (*Curcuma longa Linn*), 26, 141–144, 242, 268*t*–269*t*
(20S)-protopanaxadiol (PPD), 75
(20S)-protopanaxatriol (PPT), 75
25-hydroxyvitamin D (25[OH] D), 229–231, 286*t*
"2018 Farm Bill", 237
type 1 diabetes (T1D)
    benfotiamine, 166–167
    bitter melon, 40
    chromium, 51
    cinnamon, 56, 58
    complementary health approaches (CHA), 2
    fenugreek, 63
    gymnema, 82–83
    honey, 92
    magnesium, 102–103
    vinegar, 148
    vitamin D, 230
    zinc, 154
type 2 diabetes (T2D)
    aloe, 20–21
    banaba, 25
    benfotiamine, 166–167
    berberine, 29–31
    bilberry, 35
    bitter melon, 40–41
    cannabidiol (CBD) supplement, 238
    chia, 46
    chromium, 51–53
    cinnamon, 56–58
    coenzyme Q10 (CoQ10), 174–175
    fenugreek, 63
    fish oil (ω-3 fatty acid), 182
    flaxseed, 69
    ginkgo, 200
    ginseng, 76, 78
    gymnema, 82–84
    hibiscus, 209–210

holy basil, 88
honey, 92–93
ivy gourd, 97
magnesium, 100–102, 261*t*
milk thistle, 107–108
mulberry, 112–113
nopal, 118
pine bark extract, 215–216
probiotics, 123–124
psyllium, 130–131
tea, 136–137
turmeric, 142–143
vinegar, 148–149
vitamin D, 230–232
zinc, 154, 156
tyrosine, 170
tyrosine kinase, 24, 49, 252*t*, 261*t*
tyrosine kinase activity, 100
tyrosine phosphatase, 24
tyrosine phosphorylation, 134, 160, 247*t*,
266*t*, 273*t*

U

ubiquinol, 276*t*
ubiquinone, 276*t*
ulcer, 91, 147
ultraviolet radiation-induced oxidative
stress, 214
unsaturated fatty acid, 219, 284*t*
urinary albumin excretion (UAE), 168, 216
urinary albumin to creatinine ratio
(UACR), 109
urinary incontinence, 112
urinary tract infection (UTI), 220
urinary tumor necrosis factor-α (TNF-α),
109
urine, 161, 273*t*
urine calcium:creatinine ratio, 231
ursolic acid, 87, 258*t*
U.S. Food & Drug Administration (FDA),
7–10, 91, 132, 186, 220, 237, 239, 245
U.S. Pharmacopeia (USP), 10, 239
US Preventive Services Task Force
Recommendation Statement, 233
"USP-verified mark", 10
uterine cancer, 107, 262*t*
uterine contraction, 62, 248*t*, 254*t*

V

Vaccinium myrtillus L. (bilberry). *See*
bilberry
varicose vein, 34
vascular cell adhesion molecule-1 (VCAM-
1), 180, 277*t*
vascular endothelial growth factor (VEGF),
141, 269*t*
vascular endothelial growth factor receptor
2 (VEGFR 2), 166
vascular event, 182, 184
vascular resistance, 201
vasculature dysfunction, 201
vasoconstrictive mediator production, 180,
278*t*
vasodilatation, 170
vasodilation, 180, 214, 276*t*, 283*t*
vasorelaxation, 34, 208, 249*t*, 282*t*
veisalgia, 117
venoarterial response, 144
venous insufficiency, 34, 214, 249*t*, 283*t*
verapamil, 40
Veronese, N, 102–103
vertigo, 161, 198, 273*t*
very low density lipoprotein (VLDL)
cholesterol, 84
very low density lipoprotein (VLDL)
secretion, 181, 277*t*
vibration perception threshold, 167
vicine, 39, 250*t*
vinblastine, 40
vincristine, 40
vinegar (*Acetic acid*), 147–151, 270*t*–271*t*
visceral fat, 147, 271*t*
viscosity, 281*t*
visual acuity, 34–35, 144, 215
VITAL (Vitamin D and w-3 Trial) study,
182–183
Vital-HF trial, 233
vitamin, 1–2, 91, 259*t*
vitamin A, 96, 204, 281*t*
vitamin B1 (thiamine). *See* benfotiamine
vitamin B6, 167
vitamin B12, 167
vitamin C, 50, 155–156, 160, 252*t*, 273*t*
vitamin D, 204, 229–235, 281*t*, 286*t*
Vitamin D and Omega-3 Trial to Prevent
and Treat DKD (VITAL-DKD), 232

vitamin E, 50, 155, 160, 181, 204, 252*t*, 273*t*, 281*t*
vitamin K, 135, 171, 204, 266*t*, 281*t*
vomit, 250*t*, 261*t*, 263*t*, 272*t*–273*t*, 286*t*
von Willebrand factor, 46

W

warfarin
  bilberry, 34
  case study, 242–243
  coenzyme Q10 (CoQ10), 276*t*
  fenugreek, 63
  fish oil (ω-3 fatty acid), 277*t*
  garlic, 194
  ginkgo, 5, 199
  ginseng, 76, 256*t*
  gymnema, 82, 257*t*
  holy basil, 88
  honey, 92
  St. John's wort, 225, 285*t*
  tea, 135, 266*t*
  turmeric, 142, 268*t*
weakness, 247*t*, 262*t*, 286*t*
website
  ConsumerLab.com, 10
  evaluation, 11
  "FDA 101: Health Fraud Awareness", 11
  LiverTox, 4
  Natural Medicines, 12
  "Tips for Older Dietary Supplement Users", 10
  "Tips for the Savvy Supplement User", 10
  U.S. Food & Drug Administration (FDA), 10–11

weight loss, 28–29, 93, 156, 164, 238, 257*t*, 263*t*, 286*t*
weight loss supplement
  banaba, 24
  chromium, 49
  garcinia, 4, 189–190
  glucomannan, 204
  gymnema, 82
  hibiscus, 208, 210
  ingredient, 7
  tea, 138
  vinegar, 147
wellness, 3
wheezing, 62
WHO (World Health Organization), 1
whole grain, 36
whortleberry (*Vaccinium arctostaphylos*), 34
withdrawal-like symptom, 225, 285*t*
wound, 91–93

X

Xuezhikang (XZK), 219, 221

Y

yoga, 1

Z

zinc, 50, 87, 152–158, 252*t*, 258*t*, 268*t*, 272*t*
Zinc Influx Transporters (ZIPs), 152

CPSIA information can be obtained
at www.ICGtesting.com
Printed in the USA
JSHW050526190221
11898JS00001B/1

9 781580 407687